Sampling of Populations

Sampling of Populations

Methods and Applications

Third Edition

PAUL S. LEVY

School of Public Health
University of Illinois at Chicago

STANLEY LEMESHOW

School of Public Health
University of Massachusetts

A Wiley-Interscience Publication
JOHN WILEY & SONS, INC.
New York • Chichester • Weinheim • Brisbane • Singapore • Toronto

Copyright © 1999 by John Wiley & Sons, Inc. All rights reserved

Published simultaneously in Canada.

For ordering and customer information call 1-800-CALL-WILEY

Library of Congress Cataloging-in-Publication Data:
Levy, Paul S.
   Sampling of populations : methods and applications / Paul S. Levy
Stanley Lemeshow. —3rd ed.
      p.   cm. —(Wiley series in probability and statistics.
Survey methodology section)
   "Wiley-Interscience publication."
   Includes bibliographical references and index.
   ISBN 0-471-15575-6 (cloth : alk. paper)
   1. Population—Statistical methods. 2. Sampling (Statistics)
I. Lemeshow, Stanley. II. Title. III. Series
HB849.49.L48   1999
304.6'01'51952—dc21   98-20498
                                                              CIP

Printed in the United States of America
10 9 8 7

To our wives, Virginia and Elaine,
and our sons and daughters

Contents

Tables

Table

Table

Table

Table

Boxes

Box

Getting Files from the Wiley ftp and Internet Sites

To download the files listed in this book and other material associated with it use an ftp program or a Web browser.

FTP ACCESS

If you are using an ftp program, type the following at your ftp prompt or URL prompt:

ftp:// ftp.wiley.com

Some programs may provide the first Up for you in which case you can type:

ftp.wiley.com

If log in parameters are required, log in as anonymous (e.g., User ID: anonymous). Leave password blank. After you have connected to the Wiley ftp site, navigate through the directory path of:

/public/sci_tech_med/populations

FILE ORGANIZATION

Under the populations directory are subdirectories that include MATLAB files for PC, Macintosh, and UNIX systems and Microsoft® Excel files. Important information is included in README files.

If you need further information about downloading the files, you can call Wiley's technical support at 212-850-6753.

LIST OF DATA SETS PROVIDED ON WEB SITE

Data Set

momsag.dta	tab9_1a.dta
workers.dta	tab9_lc.ssd
wloss2.ssd	i110pt1.ssd
jacktwin.ssd	i110pt2.dta
jacktwin2.dta	i110pt2.ssd
dogscats.ssd	hospslct.ssd
tab7pt1.ssd	exmp12_2.ssd
tab7pt1.dta	exmp12_2.dta
bhratio.dat	amblnce2.ssd
hospsamp.dta	

Preface To The Third Edition

The original edition of *Sampling of Populations: Methods and Applications* was published in 1980 by Lifetime Learning Publications (a Division of Wadsworth, Inc.) under the title *Sampling for Health Professionals*. Like other Lifetime Learning Books, its primary intended audience was the working professional; in this instance, the practicing statistician. With this as the target audience, the authors felt that such a book on sampling should have the following features:

- Presentation of the basic concepts and procedures of sample design and estimation methods in a user-friendly way with a minimum of mathematical formality and jargon.
- Compilation of important formulas in boxes that can be easily located by the user.
- Presentation of the various procedures for drawing a sample (e.g., systematic sampling, probability proportional to size sampling) in a step-by-step manner that the reader could easily follow (almost like a manual).
- Use of heuristic demonstrations and numerous illustrative examples rather than rigorous mathematical proofs for the purpose of giving the reader a clearer understanding of the rationale for certain procedures used in sampling.

Sampling for Health Professionals was well received both by reviewers and readers, and had a steady following throughout its existence (1980–91). In addition to having a strong following among practicing statisticians (its intended primary audience), it had been adopted as a primary text or recommended as additional reading by an unexpectedly large number of instructors of sampling courses in various academic units.

Based on the success of this first version of the book, we developed a greatly revised and expanded version that was published by John Wiley & Sons in 1991 under the title *Sampling of Populations: Methods and Applications.* Our purpose in that revision was to improve the suitability of the book for use as a text in applied sampling courses without compromising its readability or its suitability for the continuation and self-learning markets. The resulting first Wiley edition was a considerably updated and expanded version of the original work, but in much the same style and tone.

Although less than a decade has elapsed since the appearance of the first Wiley edition, there have been major developments both in the planning and conduct of sample surveys and in the analysis of data from sample surveys. In particular, refinements in telephone sampling and interviewing methodology have now made it generally more feasible and less expensive than face-to-face household interviewing. While the first edition contained some material on random digit dialing (RDD), it did not cover the various refinements of RDD or the use of list-assisted sampling methods and other innovations that are now widely used.

Also, "user friendly" computer software is much more readily available not only for obtaining standard errors of survey estimates, but also for performing statistical procedures such as contingency table analysis and multiple linear or logistic regression that take into consideration complexities in the sample design. In fact, at the writing of this new edition, modules for the analysis of complex survey data have begun to appear in major general statistical software packages (e.g., STATA). Such software is now widely used and has removed the necessity for many of the complicated formulas that appeared in Chapter 11 as well as elsewhere in the first Wiley edition. Likewise, the analysis methods that appear in Chapter 16 of that edition are a reflection of methods used historically when design-based analysis methodology was not in its present state of development and software was not readily available. We felt that the discussion in that chapter did not reflect adequately the present state of the art with respect to analysis strategies for survey data and we have totally revised it to reflect more closely current practice.

Both of us feel strongly that knowledge of telephone-sampling methodology and familiarity with computer-driven methods now widely used in the analysis of complex survey data should be part of any introduction to sampling methods, and, with this in mind, we have greatly enhanced and revised the material on survey data analysis, and attempted to introduce the use of appropriate software throughout the book in our discussion of the major sample designs and estimation procedures. In this new edition, there is an entire chapter on telephone sampling written specifically for this book by Robert Casady, formerly of the Bureau of Labor Statistics, and Jim Lepkowski of the University of Michigan Institute for Social Research. Both of these individuals have made considerable contributions in the area of telephone sampling and have developed very successful short courses on that topic.

In addition to adding material on the topics just mentioned, we have made other revisions based on our own experience with the book in sampling courses and on suggestions from students and colleagues. Some of these are listed below.

1. Exercises that seem to be ineffective have been modified or replaced. Some new exercises have been added.

2. The material on two-stage cluster sampling has been expanded and reorganized, with designs in which clusters are sampled with equal probability presented in Chapter 10 and designs in which clusters are sampled with unequal probability given in Chapter 11. The important class of probability proportional to size (PPS) sampling designs is now presented in Chapter 11 as a particular case of designs in which clusters are sampled with unequal probability. This appears to us a more natural way to present cluster sampling designs and has worked out very well in our classes.

3. In our presentation of many of the numerical illustrative examples, we include discussion of how the analysis would appear in one of the software packages that specializes in or includes analysis of survey data.

4. Chapters that deal with specific sampling designs now have a similar structure, with the following subsections:

   - How to take the sample
   - Estimation of population parameters
   - More theoretical discussion of sampling distributions of these estimates (if worthwhile)
   - Estimation of standard errors
   - Sample size determination
   - Optimization issues (if appropriate)
   - Summary, exercises, bibliography

5. We have greatly expanded the number of articles cited in the annotated reference list to include more recent articles of importance. In particular, one of us (PSL) was the Section Editor for Design of Experiments and Sample Surveys of the recently published *Encyclopedia of Biostatistics* and, as such, was responsible for the material on sample-survey methods. In that capacity, he solicited over 50 expository or review articles covering important topics in sampling methodology and written by experts on the particular topics. These are useful references for readers learning sampling for the first time as well as for more advanced readers, and we have cited many of them.

6. In the prior edition, we did not include in electronic form data sets used in the illustrative examples and exercises. In this edition, we make such data available on the Internet.

It is our feeling that one of the strengths of the earlier edition is its focus on the basic principles and methods of sampling. To maintain this focus, we omit or treat very briefly several very interesting topics that have seen considerable development in the last decade. We feel that they are best covered in more specialized texts on sampling. As a result, we do not cover to any extent topics such as *distance sampling, adaptive sampling*, and *superpopulation models* that are of considerable importance, but have been treated very well in other volumes. We did, however, include several topics that were not in the previous edition and that we feel are important for a general understanding of sampling methodology. Examples of such topics included in this edition are *construction of stratum boundaries and desired number of strata* (Chapter 6); *estimation of ratios for subdomains* (Chapter 7); *poststratified ratio estimates* (Chapter 7); *the Hansen-Hurwitz estimator and the Horvitz-Thompson estimator* (Chapter 11). From our experience with the first edition of *Sampling of Populations: Methods and Applications*, we feel that this book will be used by practicing statisticians as well as by students taking formal courses in sampling methodology. Both of us teach in schools of public health, and have used this book as the basic text for a one-semester course in sample-survey methodology. Our classes have included a mix of students concentrating in biostatistics, epidemiology, and other areas in the biomedical and social and behavioral sciences. In our experience, this book has been very suitable to this mix of students, and we feel that at least 80% of this material could be covered without difficulty in a single-semester course.

Several instructors have indicated that, in their courses on sampling theory, this book works well as a primary text in conjunction with a more theoretical text (e.g., W.G. Cochran, *Sampling Techniques*, 3rd ed., New York: Wiley, 1977), with the latter text used for purposes of providing additional theoretical background. Conversely, selected readings from our book have been used to provide sampling background to students in broader courses on survey research methodology (often taught in sociology departments).

The number of our students and colleagues who gave us helpful comments and suggestions on our earlier text and on the present volume are too numerous to mention and we are grateful to all of them. We would like to thank, in particular, Janelle Klar and Elizabeth Donohoe-Cook for carefully reading this manuscript and making valuable editorial and substantive suggestions. In addition, we would like to thank the two anonymous individuals who reviewed an earlier draft of this manuscript for the publisher. Although we did not agree with all of their suggestions, we did take into consideration in our subsequent revision many of their thoughtful and insightful comments. Most of all, however, we wish to recognize the pioneers of sampling methodology who have written the early textbooks in this field. In particular, the books by William Cochran, Morris Hansen, William Hurwitz and William Madow, Leslie Kish, and P.V. Sukhatme are statistical classics that are still widely studied by students, academics, and practitioners. Those of us who cut our teeth on these books and have made our careers in survey sampling owe them a great debt.

PAUL S. LEVY
STANLEY LEMESHOW

Chicago, Illinois
Amherst, Massachusetts
December, 1998

Sampling of Populations

PART 1

Basic Concepts

CHAPTER 1

Uses of Sample Surveys

1.1 WHY SAMPLE SURVEYS ARE USED

Information on characteristics of populations is constantly needed by politicians, marketing departments of companies, public officials responsible for planning health and social services, and others. For reasons relating to timeliness and cost, this information is often obtained by use of sample surveys. Such surveys are the subject of this book.

The following is an example of a sample survey conducted to obtain information about a health characteristic in a particular population. A health department in a large state is interested in determining the proportion of the state's children of elementary school age who have been immunized against the childhood infectious diseases (e.g., polio, diphtheria, tetanus, pertussis, etc.). For administrative reasons, this task must be completed in only one month.

At first glance this task would seem to be most formidable, involving the careful coordination of a large staff attempting to collect information, either from parents or from school immunization records on each and every child of elementary school age residing in that state. Clearly, the budget necessary for such an undertaking would be enormous because of the time, travel expenses, and number of children involved. Even with a sizable staff, it would be difficult to complete such an undertaking in the specified time frame.

To handle problems such as the one outlined above, this text will present a variety of methods for selecting a subset (a *sample*) from the original set of all measurements (the *population*) of interest to the researchers. It is the members of the sample who will be interviewed, studied, or measured. For example, in the problem stated above, the net effect of such methods will be that valid and reliable estimates of the proportion of children who have been immunized for these diseases could be obtained in the time frame specified and at a fraction of the cost that would have resulted if attempts were made to obtain the information concerning every child of elementary school age in the state.

More formally, a *sample survey* may be defined as a study involving a subset (or sample) of individuals selected from a larger population. Variables or characteristics of interest are observed or measured on each of the sampled individuals. These measurements are then aggregated over all individuals in the sample to obtain *summary statistics* (e.g., means, proportions, totals) for the sample. It is from these summary statistics that extrapolations can be made concerning the entire population. The validity and reliability of these extrapolations depend on how well the sample was chosen and how well the measurements were made. These issues constitute the subject matter of this text.

When all the individuals in the population are selected for measurement, the study is called a *census*. The summary statistics obtained from a census are not extrapolations, since every member of the population is measured. The validity of the resulting statistics, however, depends on how well the measurements are made. The main advantages of sample surveys over censuses lie in the reduced costs and greater speed made possible by taking measurements on a subset rather than on an entire population. In addition, studies involving complex issues requiring elaborate measurement procedures are often feasible only if a sample of the population is selected for measurement since limited resources can be allocated to getting detailed measurements if the number of individuals to be measured is not too great.

In the United States, as in many other countries, government agencies are mandated to develop and maintain programs whereby sample surveys are used to collect data on the economic, social, and health status of the people, and these data are used for research purposes as well as for policy decisions. For example, the National Center for Health Statistics (NCHS), a center within the United States Department of Health and Human Services, is mandated by law to conduct a program of periodic and ongoing sample surveys designed to obtain information about illness, disability, and the utilization of health care services in the United States [12]. Similar agencies, centers, or bureaus exist within other departments (e.g., the Bureau of Labor Statistics within the Department of Labor, the National Center for Educational Statistics within the Department of Education), which collect data relevant to the mission of their departments through a program of sample surveys. Field work for these surveys is often done by the U.S. Bureau of the Census, which also has its own program of surveys.

The surveys developed by such government agencies often have very complex designs and require very large and highly skilled staff (and hence, large budgets) for their execution. While the nature of the missions of these government agencies — provision of valid and reliable statistics on a wide variety of parameters for the United States as a whole and various subgroups of it — would justify these large budgets, such costs are rarely justified or at all feasible for most institutions that make use of sample surveys. The information needs of most potential users of sample surveys are far more limited in scope and much more focused around a relatively small set of particular questions. Thus, the types of surveys conducted outside of the federal government are generally simpler in design and "one-shot" rather than ongoing. These are the types of surveys on which we will focus in this text. We will, however, devote some discussion to more complex sample surveys, especially in Chapter 12, which discusses variance estimation methods that have been developed primarily to meet the needs of the very complex government surveys.

Sample surveys belong to a larger class of nonexperimental studies generally given the name "observational studies" in the health or social sciences literature. Most sample surveys can be put in the class of observational studies known as "cross-sectional studies." Other types of observational studies include cohort studies and case-control studies.

Cross-sectional studies are "snapshots" of a population at a single point in time, having as objectives either the estimation of the prevalence or mean level of some characteristics of the population or measurement of the relationship between two or more variables measured at the same point in time.

Cohort and case-control studies are used for analytic rather than descriptive purposes. For example, they are used in epidemiology to test hypotheses about the association between exposure to suspected risk factors and the incidence of specific diseases.

These study designs are widely used to gain insight into relationships. In the business world, for example, a sample of delinquent accounts might be taken (e.g., the "cases") along with a sample of accounts that are not delinquent (e.g., the "controls"), and the characteristics of each group compared for purposes of determining those factors that are associated with delinquency. Numerous examples of these study designs could be given in other fields.

As mentioned above, cohort and case-control studies are designed with the objective in mind of testing some statement (or *hypothesis*) concerning a set of independent variables (e.g., suspected risk factors) and a dependent variable (e.g., disease incidence). While such studies are very important, they do not make up the subject matter of this text. The type of study of concern here is often known as a *descriptive survey*. Its main objective is that of *estimating* the level of a set of variables in a defined population. For example, in the hypothetical example presented at the beginning of this chapter, the major objective is to estimate, through use of a sample, the proportion of all children of elementary school age who have been immunized for childhood diseases. In descriptive surveys, much attention is given to the selection of the sample since extrapolation is made from the sample to the population. Although hypotheses can be tested based on data collected from such descriptive surveys, this is generally a secondary objective in such surveys. Estimation is almost always the primary objective.

1.2   DESIGNING SAMPLE SURVEYS

In this section, we will discuss the four major components involved in designing sample surveys. These are sample design, survey measurements, survey operations, and statistical analysis and report generation.

1.2.1   Sample Design

In a sample survey, the major statistical components are referred to as the *sample design* and include both the sampling plan and the estimation procedures. The *sampling plan* is the methodology used for selecting the sample from the population. The *estimation procedures* are the algorithms or formulas used for obtaining estimates of population values from the sample data and for estimating the reliability of these population estimates.

The choice of a particular sample design should be a collaborative effort involving input from the statistician who will design the survey, the persons involved in executing the survey, and those who will use the data from the survey. The data users should specify what variables should be measured, what estimates are required, what levels of reliability and validity are needed for the estimates, and what restrictions are placed on the survey with respect to timeliness and costs. Those individuals involved in executing the survey should furnish input about costs for personnel, time, and materials as well as input about the feasibility of alternative sampling and measurement procedures. Having received such input, the statistician can then propose a sample design that will meet the required specifications of the users at the lowest possible cost.

1.2.2   Survey Measurements

Just as sampling and estimation are the statistician's responsibility in the design of a sample survey, the choice of measurements to be taken and the procedures for taking these measurements are the responsibility of those individuals who are experts in the subject matter of the survey and also of those individuals having expertise in the measurement sciences. The former (often called "subject matter persons") give the primary input into specifying the measurements that are needed in order to meet the objectives of the survey. Once these measurements are specified, the measurement experts — often psychologists or sociologists with special training and skills in survey research — begin designing the questionnaires or forms to be used in eliciting the data from the sample individuals. The design of a questionnaire or other survey instrument which is suitable for collecting valid and reliable data is often a very complex task; it requires considerable care and sometimes a preliminary study, especially if some of the variables to be measured have never been measured before by the survey process.

Once the survey instruments have been drafted, the statistician provides input with respect to procedures to be used to evaluate and assure the quality of the data. In addition, the statistician ensures that the data can be easily coded and processed for statistical analysis, and provides input into the estimation methods.

1.2.3 Survey Operations

Once the sample has been chosen and the measurement instruments or questionnaires drafted, pretested, and modified, the field work of the survey — including data collection — can begin. But before the data collection starts, there should be a dry run or *pilot survey* on a small sample, with the objective of testing the measurement instruments and eliminating any discernible imperfections in the survey procedures.

In order for the estimates from the survey to be valid and reliable, it is important that the data be collected in accordance with the survey design, and it is the task of those individuals responsible for survey operations to oversee and supervise the data collection procedures. The nature of the survey operations staff depends on the size and scope of the sample survey, the complexity of the measurements, and the nature of the survey (e.g., a one-shot survey vs. an ongoing survey). For example, the National Health and Nutrition Examination Survey (NHANES), a series of complex nationwide sample surveys conducted through NCHS by means of physical examinations and interviews, has a large operations staff and a very large operations budget [11,12]. On the other hand, a sample survey having only a limited set of objectives can be executed with a small operations staff.

1.2.4 Statistical Analysis and Report Writing

After the data have been collected, coded, edited, and processed, the data can be analyzed statistically and the findings incorporated into a final report. As in all components of a sample survey, considerable care should be taken in the interpretation of the findings of the survey. These findings are in the form of estimated characteristics of the population from which the sample was taken. These estimates, however, are subject to both sampling and measurement errors, and any interpretation of the findings should take these errors into consideration. In many projects involving sample surveys, ample time and resources are allocated to the design of the sample, the development of the measuring instruments or questionnaire, and the survey operations, but very little time and resources are allocated to the final statistical analysis and report writing. This situation is unfortunate, because the impact of the findings is often lost through lack of effort at this last stage. In this text, Chapter 16 is devoted to the analysis of data arising from sample surveys.

1.3   PRELIMINARY PLANNING OF A SAMPLE SURVEY

In the previous section we discussed the major components involved in a sample survey. From that discussion it should be evident that a sample survey can be a considerable undertaking, requiring much in the way of time and resources, both material and human. It should also be evident that serious consideration should be given to deciding whether or not to conduct a sample survey, and once the decision is made to go ahead, serious thought should be given to formulating the survey objectives and specifications before work on the survey design begins.

In the preliminary planning stage, those individuals contemplating a sample survey should formulate the objectives of the proposed survey. The objectives should include specification of the information to be gathered and of the population to which the findings of the survey will be extrapolated. Alternatives to a survey should be discussed, such as secondary analysis of data already collected. Careful consideration should be given to the use of the data collected from the proposed survey, especially to the decisions that will be made on the basis of the findings of the survey. This step will determine whether it is worthwhile to conduct the survey at all and, if so, how accurate the resulting estimates should be.

In the preliminary planning stage, thought should be given to the various subdomains of the population (e.g., age groups, sex groups, race groups) for which estimates are required, and to the level of accuracy required for these estimates. Additional thought should be given to the resources that are available in terms of budget and personnel and the time frame in which the data are needed. The resolution of these issues helps to determine whether it is feasible to plan and conduct a sample survey and, if so, to determine the required configuration of the survey in terms of its components.

EXERCISES

1.1   Means, proportions, and totals are examples of:
   a. Summary statistics
   b. Sample persons
   c. Survey reports
   d. Database elements

1.2   Sample surveys are *least* concerned with
   a. Production of summary statistics
   b. Production of valid and reliable estimates
   c. Describing characteristics of the population
   d. Testing hypotheses

1.3 Which of the following is most correct concerning what is included in the sample design?
   a. The sampling plan and statistical reports
   b. The sampling plan and estimation procedures
   c. The sampling plan and cost estimates
   d. The estimation procedures and quality control measures

1.4 Sample surveys belong to a larger class of studies called:
   a. Cohort studies
   b. Observational studies
   c. Case-control studies
   d. Quasi experiments

1.5 Which of the following best describes estimates obtained from a census?
   a. Both sampling and measurement errors present
   b. Sampling errors but not measurement errors present
   c. Measurement errors but not sampling errors present
   d. Neither sampling nor measurement errors present

1.6 Feedback from a pilot study will generally yield which of the following benefits?
   a. Lowering of measurement errors
   b. Lowering of sampling errors
   c. Decrease in costs
   d. All of the above

1.7 You are the chief executive officer of a hospital and wish to know within a very short time the proportion covered by third-party carriers other than Medicare or Medicaid of all inpatient admissions within 1998. How would you go about determining this proportion?

1.8 As the same CEO as in Exercise 1.7, you wish to estimate the mean out-of-pocket costs per inpatient admission. How could you go about determining this?

BIBLIOGRAPHY

The following general texts in sampling theory have been used for many years and can give the reader additional perspectives on sampling. The first two have been reissued in the Wiley "Classics" Series.

1. Cochran, W. G., *Sampling Techniques*, 3rd ed., Wiley, New York, 1977.

2. Hansen, M. H., Hurwitz, W. N., and Madow, W. G., *Sample Survey Methods and Theory*, Vols. 1 and 2, Wiley, New York, 1953.

3. Kish, L., *Survey Sampling*, Wiley, New York, 1965.

4. Mendenhall, W., Ott, L., and Scheaffer, R. L., *Elementary Survey Sampling*, Duxbury Press, Belmont, Calif., 1971.

The text by Cochran [1] emphasizes the theoretical development of sampling methodology, but at the same time gives the reader a sense of how the methods are used. The text by Hansen et al. [2] uses the notation and approaches taken historically by the major government agencies involved in sample surveys (e.g., Bureau of the Census, Bureau of Labor Statistics, etc.). The book by Kish [3] is comprehensive and contains a wide variety of advanced sampling techniques. Mendenhall et al. [4] give a very readable presentation of basic sampling techniques.

The following more recent texts are much more specialized. The text by Sudman [5] addresses a wide variety of issues that are often encountered in the planning of sample surveys. Hedayat and Sinha [6] have written a book that emphasizes theoretical issues. The recent books by Thompson [7] and by Thompson and Seber [8] discuss in detail methods of sampling that are used in the estimation of wildlife populations and in other areas of ecology. The book by Kalton [9] gives a highly readable introduction to sampling that can be valuable to nonstatisticians as well as statisticians. It reflects the author's wide experiences as a sampling statistician. The very recent text by Lehtonen and Pahkinen [10] places a high emphasis on methods for analysis of data from complex sample surveys.

5. Sudman, S., *Applied Sampling*, Academic Press, New York, 1976.

6. Hedayat, A. S., and Sinha, B. K., *Design and Inference in Finite Population Sampling*, Wiley, New York, 1991.

7. Thompson, S. K., *Sampling*, Wiley, New York, 1992.

8. Thompson, S. K., and Seber, G., *Adaptive Sampling*, Wiley, New York, 1996.

9. Kalton, G., *Introduction to Survey Sampling*, Sage University Paper 35: Quantitative Applications in the Social Sciences, 07-035. Sage Publications, Newbury Park, Calif., 1989.

10. Lehtonen, R., and Pahkinen, E. J. *Practical Methods for Design and Analysis of Complex Surveys*, Rev. Ed., Wiley, Chichester, U.K., 1994.

The following relate to the major surveys conducted by the National Center for Health Statistics (NCHS).

11. National Center for Health Statistics, *Catalog of Publications 1980–1987*, U.S. Department of Health and Human Services, Hyattsville, Md., 1988.

12. National Center for Health Statistics, *Plan and Operation of the Health and Nutrition Examination Survey. United States, 1971–1973*, Vital and Health Statistics, Series 1, No. 10a. DHEW Publication No. (HRA) 76-1310, U.S. Government Printing Office, Washington, D.C., 1973.

Both the Encyclopedia of Statistical Sciences *[13] and the more recent* Encyclopedia of Biostatistics *[14] contain expository articles on many topics in survey sampling. Volume 6 in the* Handbook of Statistics *series [15] deals exclusively with sampling methodology and contains 24 chapters authored by experts on various aspects of sampling. Chapter 1, written by D. R. Bellhouse [16], gives an excellent historical overview of sampling methodology.*

13. Kotz, S., and Johnson, N. L., *Encyclopedia of Statistical Sciences*, Vol. 76, Wiley, New York, 1986.

14. Armitage, P., and Colton, T., Eds., *The Encyclopedia of Biostatistics*, Wiley, Chichester, U.K., 1998.

15. Krishnaiah, P. R., and Rao, C. R., Eds. *Handbook of Statistics*, Vol. 6, *Sampling*, Elsevier, Amsterdam and New York, 1988.

16. Bellhouse, D. R., A brief history of random sampling methods. In *Handbook of Statistics*, Vol. 6, *Sampling*, Krishnaiah, P. R., and Rao, C. R., Eds., Elsevier, Amsterdam and New York, pp. 1–14, 1988.

CHAPTER 2

The Population and the Sample

In the previous chapter we discussed sample surveys as studies that estimate the distribution and levels of characteristics of a population by means of measurements on a subset of individuals selected from that population. In this chapter we develop the foundations of sampling methodology by first defining the components of a population in terms that are meaningful with respect to taking a sample from it. Once these properties of the population have been defined and discussed, we then begin the development of sampling methodology.

2.1 THE POPULATION

The *population* (or *universe* or *target population*) is the entire set of individuals to which findings of the survey are to be extrapolated. In this text we use the terms universe, target population, and population interchangeably.

The individual members of the population whose characteristics are to be measured are called *elementary units* or *elements* of the population. For example, if we are conducting a sample survey for purposes of estimating the number of persons living in Illinois who have never visited a dentist, the universe consists of all persons living in Illinois, and each person living in Illinois is an elementary unit or element. If we are conducting a sample survey of hospital medical records for purposes of estimating the number of hospital discharges in a given year having specified diagnoses, each hospital discharge occurring during the year is an element, and the totality of such discharges constitutes the universe or population.

In the conduct of sample surveys, it is often not feasible to sample the elementary units directly. This is because lists of elementary units from which the sample can be taken are often not readily available, and can be constructed only at considerable cost. Often, however, elementary units can be associated with other types of units for which lists are either available or can be readily constructed for purposes of sampling. These types of units are known as *enumeration units* or *listing units*. An enumeration unit or listing unit may contain one or more elementary units and can be identified prior to the drawing of the sample. For example, suppose that a sample survey is being planned in western Massachusetts for purposes of determining the number of persons in Hampshire County who are immunized for measles. The population in this instance consists of all persons living in this county, and the elementary units are all persons living in the county. It is very unlikely that an accurate and up-to-date list of all persons living in this county will be available or easily obtainable. If it were, a sample could then be drawn from this list. However, it is conceivable that a list of all households in the county is available or at least can be constructed without great difficulty or expense. If such a list is available, a sample of households can be drawn, and those persons residing in the households are taken as the sample elementary units. The households are the enumeration units.

If a sample is to be drawn from a list of enumeration units, it is necessary to specify by some algorithm the elementary units that are to be associated with each enumeration unit. Such an algorithm is called an *enumeration rule* or *counting rule*. In the household survey mentioned above for estimating the number of persons in Hampshire County who are immunized for measles, the elementary units are the persons living in the county, and the enumeration units are the households. The counting rule in this example might specify that all individuals living in a particular household are associated with the household.

In the Hampshire County example, the counting rule is obvious and straightforward. Sometimes, however, the counting rule that associates elementary units with enumeration units is not so obvious. For example, suppose that we wish to estimate the number of persons in California who have a relatively rare and severe disease such as systemic lupus erythematosis (SLE). It would make sense in this instance to take a sample survey of health care providers (e.g., physicians and hospitals), and to obtain from them information about the individuals under their care for the particular disease. Since an individual with the disease may be receiving or may have received care from several sources, there is more than one reasonable way of linking cases (elementary units) with sources (enumeration units). For example, one counting rule may allow a case to be linked to the health care provider (source) that is responsible for primary care for that person at the time of the survey. A second counting rule might allow a case to be linked to all sources that have ever treated that person. A third might link the case to the source that first diagnosed the disease in that individual. Over the past two decades there has been a rapidly growing body of work based on the realization that the choice of an appropriate counting rule can improve considerably the reliability of estimates in a sample survey [3].

The primary purpose of almost every sample survey is to estimate certain values relating to the distributions of specified characteristics of a population (universe). These values are most often in the form of means, totals or aggregates, and proportions or ratios. They may also be percentiles, standard deviations, or other features of a distribution. For example, in a household survey in which a sample of Chicago residents is taken, we may wish to estimate the average number of acute illness episodes per person (a population mean), the total days of work or school lost among all members of the population because of acute illness (a population total or aggregate), and the proportion of persons having two or more acute illnesses within the past year (a population proportion). We might also wish to estimate the median annual household expenditure for health care and the standard deviation of the distribution of days lost from work due to acute illness. In the ensuing discussion, we develop formal notation for discussing the concepts mentioned above.

2.1.1   Elementary Units

The *number of elementary units* in the population is denoted by N, and each elementary unit will be identified by a label in the form of a number from 1 to N. A *characteristic* (or *variable*) will be denoted by a letter such as $\mathscr{X}$ or $\mathscr{Y}$. The *value* of a *characteristic* $\mathscr{X}$ in the ith elementary unit will be denoted by X_i. For example, in a survey of hospital discharges occurring in a hospital over a particular year, the population might be the set of all hospital discharges occurring during the time period, and each discharge would be an elementary unit. If 2000 discharges occurred during the year, then N would be equal to 2000, and each discharge would be given (for the purposes of the survey) an identifying label in the form of a number from 1 to 2000. Let us suppose that we are interested in the distribution of number of days hospitalized (length of stay) among the discharges. Then X_1 would represent the length of stay with respect to the hospital discharge labeled "1"; X_2, the length of stay with respect to the hospital discharge labeled "2", and so on.

2.1.2   Population Parameters

We mentioned above that the objectives of a survey include estimation of certain *values* of the distribution of a specified variable or characteristic in a population. These values for a population are called *parameters*, and for a given population a parameter is constant. Definitions of those parameters most often of interest in terms of estimation are given in the ensuing discussion.

POPULATION TOTAL. The *population total* of a characteristic $\mathscr{X}$ is generally denoted by X and is the sum of the values of the characteristic over all elements in the population. The population total is given by

$$X = \sum_{i=1}^{N} X_i$$

POPULATION MEAN.　The *population mean* with respect to a characteristic $\mathscr{X}$ is given by

$$\bar{X} = \frac{\sum_{i=1}^{N} X_i}{N}$$

POPULATION PROPORTION.　When the characteristic being measured represents the presence or absence of some *dichotomous* attribute, it is often desired to estimate the proportion of elementary units in the population having the attribute. If the attribute is denoted by $\mathscr{X}$, and if X is the total number of elementary units in the population having the attribute, then P_x denotes the *population proportion* of elements having the attribute and is given by

$$P_x = \frac{X}{N}$$

It should be noted that a population proportion is a population mean for the special situation in which the variable $\mathscr{X}$ is given by

$$X_i = \begin{cases} 1 & \text{if attribute } \mathscr{X} \text{ is present in element } i \\ 0 & \text{if attribute } \mathscr{X} \text{ is not present in element } i \end{cases}$$

Thus $X = \sum_{i=1}^{N} X_i$ would represent the total number or elements having the attribute.

POPULATION VARIANCE AND STANDARD DEVIATION.　The variance and the standard deviation of the distribution of a characteristic in a population are of interest because they measure the *spread* of the distribution. The *population variance* of a characteristic $\mathscr{X}$ is denoted by σ_x^2 and is given by

$$\sigma_x^2 = \frac{\sum_{i=1}^{N} (X_i - \bar{X})^2}{N}$$

The *population standard deviation*, denoted σ_x is simply the square root of the variance and is given by

$$\sigma_x = \left(\frac{\sum_{i=1}^{N} (X_i - \bar{X})^2}{N} \right)^{1/2}$$

When the characteristic being considered is a dichotomous attribute, it can be shown that the population variance as defined above reduces to the expression

$$\sigma_x^2 = P_x(1 - P_x)$$

For convenience in later reference, the formulas given above are summarized in Box 2.1.

Now let us see how these formulas may be used in practice.

Illustrative Example. Suppose we are interested in the distribution of household visits made by physicians in a community over a specified year. The 25 physicians in the community are labeled from 1 to 25 and the number of visits made by each physician is shown in Table 2.1.

In this instance the elementary units are physicians and there are 25 of them. In other words, $N = 25$. If we let X_i = the number of physician visits made by physician i, the population mean, total, variance, and standard deviation are given below (see formulas in Box 2.1):

$$\bar{X} = 5.08 \text{ visits} \qquad \sigma_x^2 = 67.91 \text{ (visits)}^2$$
$$X = 127 \text{ visits} \qquad \sigma_x = 8.24 \text{ visits}$$

If we let $\mathcal{Y}$ represent the attribute of having performed one or more household visits during the specified time period, we have

$$P_y = \frac{14}{25} = .56$$

where P_y is the proportion of physicians in the population who performed one or more household visits during the period. We also have

$$\sigma_y^2 = (.56) \times (1 - .56) = .246 \qquad \text{and} \qquad \sigma_y = \sqrt{.246} = .496$$

Another population parameter which is of importance in sampling theory is the *coefficient of variation*, denoted by V_x. The coefficient of variation of a distribution is the ratio of the standard deviation of the distribution to the mean of the distribution:

$$V_x = \frac{\sigma_x}{\bar{X}} \qquad (2.7)$$

The coefficient of variation represents the spread of the distribution relative to the mean of the distribution. For the distribution of household visits in the illustrative example above, the coefficient of variation is given by

$$V_x = \frac{8.24}{5.08} = 1.62$$

BOX 2.1   POPULATION PARAMETERS

Total

$$X = \sum_{i=1}^{N} X_i \qquad (2.1)$$

Mean

$$\bar{X} = \frac{\sum_{i=1}^{N} X_i}{N} \qquad (2.2)$$

Proportion

$$P_x = \frac{X}{N} \qquad (2.3)$$

Variance

$$\sigma_x^2 = \frac{\sum_{i=1}^{N}(X_i - \bar{X})^2}{N} \qquad (2.4)$$

Standard Deviation

$$\sigma_x = \left(\frac{\sum_{i=1}^{N}(X_i - \bar{X})^2}{N} \right)^{1/2} \qquad (2.5)$$

Variance, Dichotomous Attribute

$$\sigma_x^2 = P_x(1 - P_x) \qquad (2.6)$$

In these definitions N is the number of elementary units in the population and X_i is the value of the ith elementary unit.

Table 2.1 Number of Household Visits Made During a Specified Year

Physician	No. of Visits	Physician	No. of visits
1	5	14	4
2	0	15	8
3	1	16	0
4	4	17	7
5	7	18	0
6	0	19	37
7	12	20	0
8	0	21	8
9	0	22	0
10	22	23	0
11	0	24	1
12	5	25	0
13	6		

For a dichotomous attribute $\mathscr{Y}$, it can be shown that the coefficient of variation V_y is given by

$$V_y = \left(\frac{1 - P_y}{P_y}\right)^{1/2} \tag{2.8}$$

For the distribution of physicians with respect to the attribute of having performed one or more household visits during the specified time period (see the illustrative example), the coefficient of variation is given by

$$V_y = \left(\frac{.44}{.56}\right)^{1/2} = .886$$

The square of the coefficient of variation, V_x^2 is known as the *relative variance* or *rel–variance* and is a parameter that is widely used in sampling methodology □

Illustrative Example. As an illustration of the use of the coefficient of variation as a descriptive statistic, let us suppose that we wish to obtain some insight into whether cholesterol levels in a population are more variable than systolic blood pressure variables in the same population. Let us suppose that the mean systolic blood pressure level in the population is 130 mmHg (millimeters of mercury) and the standard deviation is 15 mmHg. Let us suppose further that the mean cholesterol level is 200 mg/100 ml (milligrams per 100 milliliters) and that the standard deviation is 40 mg/100 ml. Examination of the respective standard deviations does not tell us in any meaningful way which characteristic has more variability in the population because they are measured in different units (millimeters of mercury vs. milligrams per 100 milliliters in this instance). Comparison of the two variables can be made, however, by examination of the respective coefficients of variation; 15/130 or .115, for systolic blood pressure vs. 40/200 or .200 for cholesterol. The coefficients of variation can be compared because they are dimensionless numbers. Thus, since the coefficient of variation for cholesterol level is greater than that for systolic blood pressure, we would conclude that cholesterol has more variability than systolic blood pressure in this population. □

In the example given above, the standard deviation could not be used to compare the variability of two variables because the variables were not measured in the same units of measurement. Let us now consider two variables that are measured in the same measurement units, for example, systolic blood pressure and diastolic blood pressure. Suppose that the mean diastolic blood pressure in the population is 60 mmHg, with a standard deviation equal to 8 mmHg, and that systolic blood pressure has a mean and a standard deviation as given in the previous example (i.e., $\bar{X} = 130$ mmHg and $\sigma_x = 15$ mmHg). Then in absolute terms, systolic blood pressure is more variable than diastolic blood pressure ($\sigma_x = 15$ mmHg for systolic vs. 8 mmHg for diastolic). In relative terms, however, as measured by the coefficient of variation, diastolic blood pressure has the greater variability. The coefficients of variation are 8/60 or .133 for diastolic and 15/130 or .115 for systolic. In the design of sample surveys, relative variation is often of more concern than absolute variation — hence the importance of the coefficient of variation.

2.2 THE SAMPLE

In Section 2.1 we introduced concepts relating to the universe or target population. We emphasize that the parameters of the population discussed in Section 2.1—such as the mean level of a characteristic, the total amount of a characteristic in a population, or the proportion of elements in the population having some specified attribute—are almost always unknown. Thus, the primary objectives of a sample survey are to take a sample from the population and to estimate population parameters from that sample. In this section, we introduce certain concepts relating to samples and we discuss how estimates of population parameters are made from the sample.

2.2.1 Probability and Nonprobability Sampling

Sample surveys can be categorized into two very broad classes on the basis of how the sample was selected, namely probability samples and nonprobability samples. A probability sample has the characteristic that every element in the population has a known, nonzero probability of being included in the sample. A nonprobability sample is one based on a sampling plan that does not have this feature. In probability sampling, because every element has a known chance of being selected, unbiased estimates of population parameters that are linear functions of the observations (e.g., population means, totals, proportions) can be constructed from the sample data. Also, the standard errors of these estimates can be estimated under the condition that the second-order inclusion probabilities (i.e., joint probability of including any two enumeration units) are known. This gives the users of the survey estimates insight into how much value can be placed on the estimates. Nonprobability sampling, on the other hand, does not have this feature, and the user has no firm method of evaluating either the reliability or the validity of the resulting estimates. These issues and concepts will be addressed later in this chapter.

Nonprobability samples are used quite frequently, especially in market research and public opinion surveys. They are used because probability sampling is often a time-consuming and expensive procedure and, in fact, may not be feasible in many situations. An example of nonprobability sampling is the so-called quota survey in which interviewers are told to contact and interview a certain number of individuals from certain demographic subgroups. For example, an interviewer might be told to interview five black males, five black females, ten white males, and ten white females, with the selection of the specific individuals within each of these categories left in the hands of the interviewer. It is highly likely that such a method of selecting a sample can lead to estimates that are very biased. For example, as a matter of convenience, the interviewer might choose the five black males and five black females from only upper socioeconomic neighborhoods, which may not be representative of the black community as a whole.

Another type of nonprobability sampling that is sometimes used is called *purposive* or *judgmental* sampling. In this type of sampling, individuals are selected who are considered to be most representative of the population as a whole. For example, we may attempt to estimate the total number of blood samples drawn during a given year in an outpatient clinic by choosing a few "typical" days and reviewing the clinic records for those sampled days. If we had the resources to sample only a few days, this approach might lead to more valid and reliable estimates than the approach of using a random sample of days, because the judgmental approach would be likely to avoid the possibility of including unusual days (e.g., days in which the patient load was atypically high, low, or unusual in some other way). The disadvantage of judgmental sampling is that no insight can be obtained mathematically concerning the reliability of the resulting estimates.

In this text we will consider only probability samples, since we feel very strongly that sample surveys should yield estimates that can be evaluated statistically with respect to their expected values and standard errors.

2.2.2 Sampling Frames, Sampling Units, and Enumeration Units

In probability sampling, the probability of any element appearing in the sample must be known. For this to be accompolished, some "list" should be available from which the sample can be selected. Such a list is called a *sampling frame* and should have the property that every element in the population has some chance of being selected in the sample by whatever method is used to select elements from the sampling frame. A sampling frame does not have to list all elements in the population. For example, if a city directory is used as a sampling frame for a sample survey in which the elements are residents of the city, then clearly the elements would not be listed at all in the sampling frame, which is, in this instance, a listing of (presumably) all households in the city. Since this is a probability survey, however, every element has some chance of being selected in the sample if this sampling frame contains, in reality, all households in the city.

Often a particular sampling design specifies that the sampling be performed in two or three stages; this design is called a *multistage sampling design*. For example, a household survey conducted in a large state might have a sampling design specifying that a sample of counties be drawn within the state; that within each county selected in the sample, a sample of minor civil divisions (townships) be drawn; and that within each minor civil division a sample of households be drawn. In multistage sampling, a different sampling frame is used at each stage of the sampling. The units listed in the frame are generally called *sampling units*. In the example mentioned above, the sampling frame for the first stage is the list of counties within the state, and each county is a sampling unit for this stage. The list of townships within each of the counties selected in the sample at the first stage is the sampling frame for the second stage, and each township is a sampling unit for this stage. Finally, the list of households within each township sampled at the second stage is the sampling frame for the third and final stage, and each household is a sampling unit for this stage. The sampling units for the first stage are generally called *primary sampling units* (PSUs). The sampling units for the final stage of a multistage sampling design are called *enumeration units* or *listing units*; these have been discussed earlier.

2.2.3 Sampling Measurements and Summary Statistics

Let us suppose that in some way we have taken a sample of n elements from a population of N elements and that we measure each sample element with respect to some variable $\mathcal{X}$. For convenience we label the sample elements from 1 to n (no matter what their original labels were in the population); we let x_1 denote the value of $\mathcal{X}$ for the element labeled "1"; we let x_2 denote the value of $\mathcal{X}$ for the element labeled "2"; and so on. Having taken the sample, we can then compute for the sample such quantities as totals, means, proportions, and standard deviations, just as we did for the population. However, when these quantities are calculated for a sample, they are not parameters in the true sense of the word, since they are subject to sampling variability (a true parameter is a constant). Instead, these sample values are generally referred to as *statistics*, as *summary statistics*, or as *descriptive statistics*. Definitions of some statistics that are used in many sample designs, either for descriptive purposes or in formulas for population estimates, are given in the following discussion; others will be introduced as needed.

SAMPLE TOTAL. The *sample total* of a characteristic is generally denoted by x and is the sum of the values of the characteristic over all elements in the sample:

$$x = \sum_{i=1}^{n} x_i$$

SAMPLE MEAN. The *sample mean* with respect to a characteristic $\mathscr{X}$ is generally denoted by $\bar{x}$ and is given by

$$\bar{x} = \frac{\sum_{i=1}^{n} x_i}{n}$$

SAMPLE PROPORTION. When the characteristic $\mathscr{X}$ being measured represents presence or absence of some dichotomous attribute, the *sample proportion* is generally denoted by p_x and is given by

$$p_x = \frac{x}{n}$$

where x is the number of sample elements having the attribute.

SAMPLE VARIANCE AND STANDARD DEVIATION. For any characteristic $\mathscr{X}$ the *sample variance* s_x^2 is given by

$$s_x^2 = \frac{\sum_{i=1}^{n}(x_i - \bar{x})^2}{n - 1}$$

When the characteristic $\mathscr{X}$ is a dichotomous attribute, the sample variance s_x^2 as defined above reduces to

$$s_x^2 = \frac{np_x(1 - p_x)}{n - 1}$$

If the sample size n is large (say greater than 20), we can use the following approximation:

$$s_x^2 \approx p_x(1 - p_x)$$

The *sample standard deviation* is simply the square root of the sample variance:

$$s_x = \left(\frac{\sum_{i=1}^{n}(x_i - \bar{x})^2}{n - 1} \right)^{1/2}$$

For convenience in later reference, these formulas are summarized in Box 2.2.

2.2.4   Estimation of Population Characteristics

An estimate of the population total X can be obtained from the sample total x as given by

$$x' = \left[\frac{N}{n} \right](x) \tag{2.15}$$

In other words, if we multiply the sample total x by the ratio of the number of elements in the population to the number in the sample, we can use the resulting statistic x' as an estimate of the population total X.

An estimate $\hat{\sigma}_x^2$ of the population variance σ_x^2 is given by

$$\hat{\sigma}_x^2 = \left(\frac{N-1}{N} \right)(s_x^2) \tag{2.16}$$

If the number of elements N in the population is moderately large, then the expression $(N - 1)/N$ in equation (2.16) will be numerically close to unity and we can use the approximation

$$\hat{\sigma}_x^2 \approx s_x^2$$

We emphasize here that the sample statistics and estimates of population characteristics presented above would not be used for every sample design. As we discuss specific sample designs in later chapters, we will present the methods of estimating population characteristics that are specific to the particular design being discussed.

   Illustrative Example.   Let us illustrate these concepts by using the data on physician household visits given in Table 2.1. Suppose that in some way we take a sample of nine physicians in the population and suppose that our sample includes the nine physicians listed in Table 2.2.

   The sample mean, total, and variance for these data are (see the formulas in Box 2.2)

BOX 2.2 SAMPLE STATISTICS

Total

$$x = \sum_{i=1}^{n} x_i \qquad (2.9)$$

Mean

$$\bar{x} = \frac{\sum_{i=1}^{n} x_i}{n} = \frac{x}{n} \qquad (2.10)$$

Proportion

$$p_x = \frac{x}{n} \qquad (2.11)$$

where in Equation (2.11) x is the number of sample elements having the dichotomous attribute.

Variance

$$s_x^2 = \frac{\sum_{i=1}^{n}(x_i - \bar{x})^2}{n - 1} \qquad (2.12)$$

Variance, Dichotomous Attribute

$$s_x^2 = \frac{np_x(1 - p_x)}{n - 1} \qquad (2.13)$$

Standard Deviation

$$s_x = \left(\frac{\sum_{i=1}^{n}(x_1 - \bar{x})^2}{n - 1} \right)^{1/2} \qquad (2.14)$$

In these definitions n is the number of elements in the sample and x_1 is the value of the ith element.

Table 2.2   Sample Data for Number of Household Visits

Physician	No. of Visits	Physician	No. of Visits
1	5	17	7
6	0	19	37
7	12	21	8
12	5	25	0
13	6		

$$x = 80 \qquad \bar{x} = 8.89 \qquad s_x^2 = 125.11$$

The sample proportion with one or more household visits is

$$p_y = .78$$

The sample variance with respect to having made one or more household visits is

$$s_y^2 = .1944$$

If we wish to estimate from this sample, the total, X, of all household visits made by physicians in the population during the specified time period, we first obtain the sample total, x, of household visits among the nine sample physicians. Then we obtain x' by multiplying x by N/n, where in this case $N = 25$ and $n = 9$. A summary of population parameters and sample estimates (based on the formulas above and in Boxes 2.1 and 2.2) follows.

Population Parameter	**Estimate from Sample**
$X = 127$	$x' = \frac{25}{9}(80) = 222.22$
$\bar{X} = 5.08$	$\bar{x} = 8.89$
$\sigma_x^2 = 67.91$	$\hat{\sigma}_x^2 = \left(\frac{24}{25}\right)(125.11) = 120.11$
$P_y = .56$	$p_y = \frac{7}{9} = .78$
$\sigma_y^2 = .246$	$\hat{\sigma}_y^2 = \left(\frac{24}{25}\right)(.1944) = .1866$ $\qquad \square$

We see from the summary of calculations in the example above that the estimates of population parameters from the particular sample taken are neither equal to the population parameters being estimated nor even very close to the true values of these parameters. If we had taken a different sample, we would have obtained different estimates of these parameters, which may have been either closer or further away from the true parameter values. Since we never really know the true values of the population parameters that we are estimating from a sample, we never know how good or how bad our population estimates really are. If, however, our sampling plan uses probability sampling, then we can get some mathematical insight into how far away our estimates are likely to be from the unknown true values. In order to do this, we must know something about the distribution of our population estimates over all possible samples that can arise from the particular sampling plan being used. In the next section we develop methodology for obtaining such information from probability samples.

2.3 SAMPLING DISTRIBUTIONS

In the previous section we discussed estimation of population parameters from a sample. In this section we consider the distribution of these estimates of population parameters over all possible samples that can be generated by using a particular sampling plan.

Let us suppose that a particular sampling plan and estimation procedure could result in T possible samples from a given population and that a particular sample results in an estimate $\hat{d}$ of a population parameter d. The relative frequency distribution of $\hat{d}$ over the T possible samples is called the *sampling distribution* of $\hat{d}$ with respect to the specified sampling plan and estimation procedure.

To illustrate a sampling distribution, let us examine the following example.

Illustrative Example. Suppose that a hypothetical community has six schools. This population of six schools is given in Table 2.3. Now suppose that we wish to take a sample of two of these schools for estimating the total number of students not immunized for measles among the six schools in the community.

Table 2.3   Data for Number of Students Not Immunized for Measles Among Six Schools in a Community

School	No. of Students	Students Not Immunized for Measles	
		Total	Proportion
1	59	4	.068
2	28	5	.179
3	90	3	.033
4	44	3	.068
5	36	7	.194
6	57	8	.140
Total	314	30	.096

Let us specify a sampling plan in which six identical sealed envelopes, each containing a card numbered from 1 to 6, are placed in a hat and are thoroughly shuffled. Two envelopes are then drawn from the hat and the two schools corresponding to the two numbers on the cards in the selected envelopes are included in the sample. Suppose that information concerning immunization status for measles is elicited from each child in the sample schools. The total number of students not immunized for measles is obtained by inflating the sample totals over the two sample schools by the ratio N/n, where $N = 6$ and $n = 2$. This procedure yields 15 possible samples, each having the same chance of being selected. In terms of the notation described in the definition of a sampling distribution, we have $T = 15$, $d = X = 30$, and each $\hat{d} = x'$, where X and x' are the population total and estimated population total, respectively. The 15 possible samples obtained from this sampling plan, along with values of x' are listed in Table 2.4.

Since each of the 15 samples listed in Table 2.4 has the same chance (1/15) of being selected, we can obtain the frequency distribution of x'. Table 2.5 represents the sampling distribution of the estimated total x'.

The relative frequencies in the last column of Table 2.5 show the fraction of all samples that take on the corresponding values of x'. Using these relative frequencies, we can draw a picture of the sampling distribution of x' as shown in Figure 2.1.

Sampling distributions can be described by certain characteristics. For our purposes, the two most important are the mean and the variance (or its square root, the standard deviation). These are defined next.

Table 2.4   Possible Samples and Values of x'

Sample	Sample Schools	x'
1	1,2	27
2	1,3	21
3	1,4	21
4	1,5	33
5	1,6	36
6	2,3	24
7	2,4	24
8	2,5	36
9	2,6	39
10	3,4	18
11	3,5	30
12	3,6	33
13	4,5	30
14	4,6	33
15	5,6	45

Table 2.5 Sampling Distributions for Data of Table 2.4

x'	Frequency	Relative Frequency
18	1	1/15
21	2	2/15
24	2	2/15
27	1	1/15
30	2	2/15
33	3	3/15
36	2	2/15
39	1	1/15
45	1	1/15

The *mean of the sampling distribution* of an estimated parameter $\hat{d}$ with respect to a particular sampling plan that yields T possible samples resulting in C possible values of $\hat{d}$ is also known as the *expected value* of $\hat{d}$, denoted by $E(\hat{d})$, and is defined as

$$E(\hat{d}) = \sum_{i=1}^{C} \hat{d}_i \pi_i \qquad (2.17)$$

where $\hat{d}_i$ is a particular value of $\hat{d}$ and π_i, is the probability of obtaining that particular value of $\hat{d}$. (Note that if each sample is equally likely, then $\pi_i = f_i/T$, where f_i is the number of times that a particular value, d_i, of $\hat{d}$ occurs).

The *variance* $\mathrm{Var}(\hat{d})$ *of the sampling distribution* of an estimated parameter $\hat{d}$ with respect to a particular sampling plan is given by

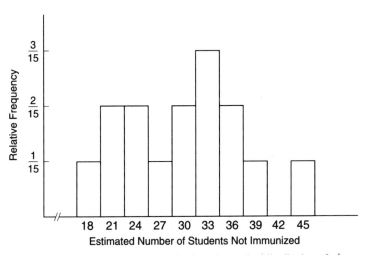

Figure 2.1 Relative frequency distribution of sampling distribution of x'.

$$\text{Var}(\hat{d}) = \sum_{i=1}^{C} [\hat{d}_i - E(\hat{d})]^2 \pi_i \tag{2.18}$$

The algebraic equivalent of this equation which can be used for computations is

$$\text{Var}(\hat{d}) = \sum_{i=1}^{C} \hat{d}_i^2 \pi_i - E^2(\hat{d}) \tag{2.19}$$

The *standard deviation* $\text{SE}(\hat{d})$ *of the sampling distribution* of an estimated parameter $\hat{d}$ is more commonly known as the *standard error* of $\hat{d}$ and is simply the square root of the variance $\text{Var}(\hat{d})$ of the sampling distribution of $\hat{d}$:

$$\text{SE}(\hat{d}) = [\text{Var}(\hat{d})]^{1/2} \tag{2.20}$$

Using these general equations, we can derive expressions for the mean and variance (and hence the standard error) of the sampling distribution for means, totals, and proportions. For convenience in later reference, these expressions are summarized in the next two boxes. □

When each sample does not have the same probability of selection, or if we wish to compute means and variances of sampling distributions directly from a sampling distribution such as the one given in Table 2.5, then we must use the expressions given in Box 2.4.

Now let us see how some of these formulas can be used in practice. We will use the data given in the previous example

Illustrative Example. For the previous example we have $\hat{d} = x'$, $T = 15$, $C = 9$, and the π_i are the relative frequencies associated with any particular value of x'. The mean $E(x')$ of the sampling distribution of x' for the example is (using the expressions in Box 2.4)

$$\begin{aligned}
E(x') &= \sum_{i=1}^{9} x_i'(f_i/15) \\
&= 18(1/15) + 21(2/15) + 24(2/15) + 27(1/15) \\
&\quad + 30(2/15) + 33(3/15) + 36(2/15) + 39(1/15) \\
&\quad + 45(1/15) \\
&= 30
\end{aligned}$$

BOX 2.3 MEAN AND VARIANCE OF SAMPLING DISTRIBUTION WHEN EACH SAMPLE HAS SAME PROBABILITY (1/T) OF SELECTION

For Totals

$$E(x') = \frac{\sum_{i=1}^{T} x_i'}{T} \qquad \mathrm{Var}(x') = \frac{\sum_{i=1}^{T} [x_i' - E(x')]^2}{T} \qquad (2.21)$$

where x_i' is the sample total computed from the ith possible sample selected from the population. Note that some of the values of x_i' may be the same from sample to sample, but each realization appears in the sum even if there is duplication.

For Means

$$E(\bar{x}) = \frac{\sum_{i=1}^{T} \bar{x}_i}{T} \qquad \mathrm{Var}(\bar{x}) = \frac{\sum_{i=1}^{T} [\bar{x}_i - E(\bar{x})]^2}{T} \qquad (2.22)$$

For Proportions

$$E(p_y) = \frac{\sum_{i=1}^{T} p_{y_i}}{T} \qquad \mathrm{Var}(p_y) = \frac{\sum_{i=1}^{T} [p_{y_i} - E(p_y)]^2}{T} \qquad (2.23)$$

In these expressions, T is the number of possible samples.

The variance $\mathrm{Var}(x')$ of the sampling distribution of x' is

$$\begin{aligned}
\mathrm{Var}(x') = &\; (18 - 30)^2(1/15) + (21 - 30)^2(2/15) + (24 - 30)^2(2/15) \\
&+ (27 - 30)^2(1/15) + (30 - 30)^2(2/15) + (33 - 30)^2(3/15) \\
&+ (36 - 30)^2(2/15) + (39 - 30)^2(1/15) + (45 - 30)^2(1/15) \\
= &\; 52.8
\end{aligned}$$

The standard error of x' is

$$\mathrm{SE}(x') = \sqrt{52.8} = 7.27 \qquad \square$$

BOX 2.4   MEAN AND VARIANCE OF SAMPLING DISTRIBUTION WHEN EACH SAMPLE DOES NOT HAVE SAME PROBABILITY OF SELECTION*

For Totals

$$E(x') = \sum_{i=1}^{C} x'_i \pi_i \qquad \text{Var}(x') = \sum_{i=1}^{C} [x'_i - E(x')]^2 \pi_i \qquad (2.24)$$

For Means

$$E(\bar{x}) = \sum_{i=1}^{C} \bar{x}_i \pi_i \qquad \text{Var}(\bar{x}) = \sum_{i=1}^{C} [\bar{x}_i - E(\bar{x})]^2 \pi_i \qquad (2.25)$$

For Proportions

$$E(p_y) = \sum_{i=1}^{C} p_{y_i} \pi_i \qquad \text{Var}(p_y) = \sum_{i=1}^{C} [p_{y_i} - E(p_y)]^2 \pi_i \qquad (2.26)$$

In these expressions C is the number of possible unique values of a statistic, and $\pi_i = f_i/T$ is the proportion of the same yielding the ith unique value, where f_i is the frequency of occurrences in the sampling distribution of the ith realization and T is the number of possible samples.

*Or when possible values of the totals, means or proportions do not occur with the same relative frequency over all possible samples.

2.4   CHARACTERISTICS OF ESTIMATES OF POPULATION PARAMETERS

In the previous section we introduced the concept of the sampling distribution of an estimate of a population parameter with respect to a particular sampling plan. Also, we introduced the concepts of the mean of the sampling distribution of a population estimate and the standard error of the estimate. We can now discuss certain properties of population estimates in terms of these concepts. It would seem intuitively clear that a desirable property of a sampling plan and estimation procedure is that it should yield estimates of population parameters of which the mean of the sampling distribution is equal to, or at least close to, the true unknown parameter, and for which the standard error is very small. In fact, the accuracy of an estimated population parameter is evaluated in terms of these two characteristics. In this section we introduce the concepts that are used in the evaluation of sample designs.

2.4.1 Bias

The *bias* $B(\hat{d})$ of an estimate $\hat{d}$ of a population parameter d is defined as the difference between the mean $E(\hat{d})$ of the sampling distribution of $\hat{d}$ and the true value of the unknown parameter d. In other words,

$$B(\hat{d}) = E(\hat{d}) - d \qquad (2.27)$$

An estimator $\hat{d}$ is said to be *unbiased* if $B(\hat{d}) = 0$. In other words, $\hat{d}$ is an unbiased estimator if the mean of the sampling distribution of $\hat{d}$ is equal to d.

In the example considered in the previous section, the estimate x' of the total number of children not immunized for measles is an unbiased estimator of the true population total X, since it was demonstrated that $E(x') = 30 = X$.

We emphasize that the same estimation procedure that is unbiased for one sampling plan can be biased for another sampling plan. The next example illustrates this idea.

Illustrative Example.   Let us consider the same population of six schools used in the previous example, but now let us use the following sampling plan. Place cards with numbers from 1 to 10 in ten sealed envelopes, and place the sealed envelopes in a hat. Take one envelope from the hat and choose schools in the sample according to the procedure shown in Table 2.6. This procedure is a probability sample since each school has a known, nonzero probability of being selected in the sample. The distribution of estimated totals if this procedure were used is shown in Table 2.7.

Since each of the 10 possible samples is equally likely, we have the distribution of x' that is shown in Table 2.8. From the distribution in Table 2.8 we see that the mean $E(x')$ of the sampling distribution of x' under this sampling plan is given by

$$\begin{aligned} E(x') &= 18(1/10) + 21(2/10) + 24(2/10) + 27(1/10) \\ &\quad + 33(1/10) + 36(2/10) + 39(1/10) \\ &= 27.9 \end{aligned}$$

Thus, since the population total X is equal to 30, the estimated population total x' is not an unbiased estimate of the true population total X under this sampling plan.

Table 2.6   Sampling Procedure for Population of Six Schools

Number Picked	Schools Chosen in Sample	Number Picked	Schools Chosen in Sample
1	1 and 2	6	2 and 3
2	1 and 3	7	2 and 4
3	1 and 4	8	2 and 5
4	1 and 5	9	2 and 6
5	1 and 6	10	3 and 4

Table 2.7   Possible Samples and Values of x'

Sample	Sample schools	x'
1	1,2	27
2	1,3	21
3	1,4	21
4	1,5	33
5	1,6	36
6	2,3	24
7	2,4	24
8	2,5	36
9	2,6	39
10	3,4	18

Table 2.8   Sampling Distribution of x'

x'	π
18	1/10
21	2/10
24	2/10
27	1/10
33	1/10
36	2/10
39	1/10
Total	1

2.4.2   Mean Square Error

The mean square error of population estimate $\hat{d}$, denoted by $\text{MSE}(\hat{d})$, is defined as the mean of the squared differences over all possible samples between the values of the estimate and the true value d of the unknown parameter. In terms of the notation developed in the last section, the mean square error of $\hat{d}$ is defined by the relation

$$\text{MSE}(\hat{d}) = \sum_{i=1}^{C}(\hat{d}_i - d)^2 \pi_i \tag{2.28}$$

Notice the difference between the mean square error of an estimate and the variance of an estimate. The mean square error of an estimate is the mean value of squared deviations about the true value of the parameter being estimated; the variance of an estimate is the mean value of the squared deviations about the mean value of the sampling distribution of the estimate. If the estimate is unbiased — or, in other words, if the mean of the sampling distribution of the estimate is equal to the true value of the parameter — then the mean square error of the estimate is equal to the variance of the estimate, since the deviations are taken about the same entity. In general, the mean square error of the estimate is related to its bias and variance by the following relation:

$$\text{MSE}(\hat{d}) = \text{Var}(\hat{d}) + B^2(\hat{d}) \tag{2.29}$$

In other words, the mean square error of a population estimate is equal to the variance of the estimate plus the square of its bias. □

Illustrative Example. In the example involving the six schools, the first sampling plan discussed yielded an unbiased estimate of the population total. The mean square error of this estimate is given by

$$\text{MSE}(x') = 52.8 + 0^2 = 52.8$$

In other words, the MSE is equal to the variance of the estimate.

In the example involving the same six schools and the sampling plan that yielded a biased estimate x' of X, the variance of x' is (from Equation (2.24))

$$\begin{aligned}
\text{Var}(x') = {}& (18 - 27.9)^2(1/10) + (21 - 27.9)^2(2/10) + (24 - 27.9)^2(2/10) \\
& + (27 - 27.9)^2(1/10) + (33 - 27.9)^2(1/10) + (36 - 27.9)^2(2/10) \\
& + (39 - 27.9)^2(1/10) \\
= {}& 50.49
\end{aligned}$$

Thus, the MSE for x' is

$$\text{MSE}(x') = 50.49 + (30 - 27.9)^2 = 54.9$$

Note that the second sampling plan yields an estimator x' that has smaller variance but larger overall mean square error than the equivalent estimate yielded by the first sampling plan. □

Illustrative Example. Let us look at another example of the use of the mean square error. Suppose a survey is being planned to evaluate the seriousness of burn injuries that occur in the United States. In connection with the survey, three students are being trained at survey headquarters in the assessment of a patient's body suffering third-degree burns (this is called *full-thickness burn area*).

To assess the students' progress, a senior burn surgeon uses sets of photographs taken of ten patients, each of whom suffered full-thickness burn areas of 37%. These ten patients, whose total burn injuries were equal in total percentage of the body involved rather than in specific body parts involved, were selected from among many seen by the surgeon.

Let us call the three students Dave, Don, and Virginia. Table 2.29 shows the means and variances of the ten burn area estimates made by each student. Now let us evaluate each of these estimates.

The average burn assessment made by Dave happens to equal the true average of the photographs under consideration (i.e., bias $= 37 - 37 = 0$). However, the variability in his measurements is large and, as a result, his mean square error is large (i.e., MSE $= 0^2 + 64 = 64$).

Don tended to overestimate the actual full-thickness burn area (i.e., bias $= 42 - 37 = 5$), but he did so consistently. As a result, the mean square error for his readings (MSE $= 5^2 + 9 = 34$) is smaller than Dave's. Stated differently, the mean of the squared deviations of each of Don's assessments of burn area about the true burn area is smaller than Dave's.

Virginia's assessment of burn area overestimated the true values (i.e., bias $= 50 - 37 = 13$), but there is little variability in these assessments. The resulting mean square error (MSE $= 13^2 + 9 = 178$) is the largest of the three students.

Pictorially, the relationship among bias, variability, and mean square error is seen in Figure 2.2 where it is assumed that the measurements are normally distributed with the stated means and variances. Notice that while the mean of Dave's distribution is equal to the true value, it would not be unusual for any one of his assessments to miss the true value by a wide margin (as indicated by the wide spread of his distribution). For instance, suppose we let $\Pr(\mathcal{X} > C)$ represent the probability that a particular realization of the random variable $\mathcal{X}$ exceeds the value C. Then the probability that Dave misses the true burn area by more than 10 percentage points is given by

Table 2.9 Data for the Burn Area Estimates

Student	Mean (%)	Variance $(\%)^2$
Dave	37	64
Don	42	9
Virginia	50	9

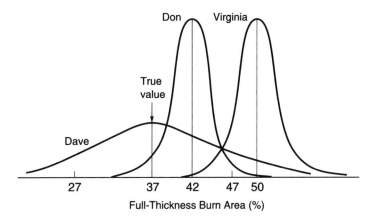

Figure 2.2 Relationship among bias, variability, and MSE for data of Table 2.9.

$$\Pr(\mathcal{X} > 47) + \Pr(\mathcal{X} < 27) = \Pr\left(z > \frac{47 - 37}{\sqrt{64}} = 1.25\right)$$
$$+ \Pr(z < -1.25) = .21$$

where z is the standard normal deviate.

Don's burn measurements are usually high, but it is not often that he would be more than 10 percentage points away from the true value. For Don

$$\Pr(\mathcal{X} > 47) + \Pr(\mathcal{X} < 27) = \Pr\left(z > \frac{47 - 42}{\sqrt{9}} = 1.67\right)$$
$$+ \Pr(z < -5.00) = .05$$

Finally, as reflected by her large MSE, the probability that Virginia misses the target burn area by more than 10 percentage points is quite high:

$$\Pr(\mathcal{X} > 47 + \Pr(\mathcal{X} < 27) = \Pr\left(z > \frac{47 - 50}{\sqrt{9}} = -1\right)$$
$$+ \Pr(z < -7.67) = .84$$

We have seen in this example that, when evaluating particular estimates, it is important to examine both bias and variance. Both these entities play important roles in determining the size of the mean square error. □

2.4.3 Validity, Reliability, and Accuracy

In earlier sections we spoke of the desirability of using sample designs that yield reliable and valid estimates. However, we have never defined just what the terms "reliable" and "valid" mean in terms of characteristics of estimates.

We now have developed enough concepts and notation concerning estimates to be able to define these two terms as well as a third term, the "accuracy" of an estimate, which we will see is derived from the validity and reliability.

The *reliability* of an estimated population characteristic refers to how reproducible the estimator is over repetitions of the process yielding the estimator. If we assume that there is no measurement error in the survey, then the reliability of an estimator can be stated in terms of its sampling variance or, equivalently, its standard error. The smaller the standard error of an estimator, the greater is its reliability.

The *validity* of an estimated population characteristic refers to how the mean of the estimator over repetitions of the process yielding the estimate, differs from the true value of the parameter being estimated. Again, if we assume that there is no measurement error, the validity of an estimator can be evaluated by examining the bias of the estimator. The smaller the bias, the greater is the validity.

The *accuracy* of an estimator refers to how far away a particular value of the estimate is, on average, from the true value of the parameter being measured. The accuracy of an estimator is generally evaluated on the basis of its MSE or, equivalently, on the basis of the square root of its MSE (denoted by RMSE and called "root mean square error"). The smaller the MSE of an estimate, the greater is its accuracy.

2.5   CRITERIA FOR A GOOD SAMPLE DESIGN

Throughout the remainder of this book we will be discussing various sample designs and showing how manipulation of the sampling plan, estimation procedure, or counting rule can affect the reliability and validity of the resulting estimates. We will limit our discussion to probability samples, because these are the only sampling plans that allow the reliability of the estimates to be evaluated from the data collected in the survey. Since the accuracy of an estimate involves both its reliability and its validity, and since accuracy is measured by the mean square error, one of our criteria for choosing a sample design will be the size of the mean square errors anticipated for the resulting estimates.

In addition to the mean square error criterion, the cost involved in conducting a survey according to a specified sample design will be used as a criterion for evaluating the particular sample design. The criteria of cost and accuracy can be combined into a composite criterion by first deciding on the total cost to be allocated to the survey, and then choosing the sample design that will yield estimates having the lowest MSE at that particular cost. Conversely, we might make specifications on the MSEs of the estimates and choose the sample design that yields estimates meeting these specified MSEs at the lowest possible cost.

Finally, in addition to accuracy and cost, a third criterion we will use is *feasibility* in executing a particular sample design. No matter how cost-efficient a particular design is, it is of no use if it is not feasible to execute the design.

2.6 SUMMARY

In this chapter we discussed and developed concepts concerning populations, samples, and estimates.

We defined what we mean by a population and we discussed how the elements of a population are often grouped for purposes of sampling into enumeration units or listing units. We showed how the elementary units and enumeration units are often linked by a counting rule. We defined certain parameters that characterize the distribution of variables in the population. The parameters discussed include the population mean, total or aggregate, proportion, variance, standard deviation, coefficient of variation, and relative variance or rel–variance.

We discussed the concept of taking a sample from a population, and we distinguished between probability samples and nonprobability samples. We discussed the use of sampling frames in selecting samples from a population and the use of a multistage selection of a sample. Summary statistics for samples such as the sample mean, sample total, sample proportion, and sample variance were introduced, and their use in obtaining estimates of population characteristics or variables was discussed.

Concepts relating to the sampling distribution of estimates were developed, including the mean of the sampling distribution of an estimate, its variance and standard error, its bias, and its mean square error. The concepts of reliability, validity, and accuracy of an estimated population characteristic were then defined in relation to the concepts of variance, bias, and mean square error.

EXERCISES

2.1 The accompanying table presents a population of five hospitals denoted by A, B, C, D, and E. The total number of beds is given for each hospital.

Hospital	Number of Beds
A	160
B	220
C	850
D	510
E	110

    a. Compute the mean number $\bar{X}$ of beds and the standard deviation σ_x of the distribution of number of beds in the population of five hospitals.

    b. How many samples of two hospitals can be drawn from this population of five hospitals?

    c. List each of the possible samples of two hospitals and compute the mean number of beds per hospital for each sample.

    d. Assuming each of the samples listed in part (c) is equally likely, compute the mean, $E(\bar{x})$, and variance, $\text{Var}(\bar{x})$ of the distribution of sample means, $\bar{x}$. How does $E(\bar{x})$ compare with the population mean $\bar{X}$?

    e. Calculate the standard error of $\bar{x}$. How does $\text{SE}(\bar{x})$ compare with the population standard deviation σ_x?

    f. How many different samples of four hospitals can be drawn from this population? List each of these samples plus the sample mean $\bar{x}$ for each sample.

    g. Calculate $E(\bar{x})$ and $\text{Var}(\bar{x})$ for the sample means listed in part (f). How do these compare with the values of $E(\bar{x})$ and $\text{Var}(\bar{x})$ obtained in part (d)?

2.2 For each of the following problems indicate how you would carry out a sample and specify these entities:

    a. The population

    b. The variable(s)

    c. The elementary unit

    d. The frame

    e. The enumeration unit

        1. Suppose we wish to estimate the average cost of an appendectomy in a certain state. There are 27 hospitals in this state.

        2. Suppose we wish to do a nutritional survey in order to estimate the average amount of fiber consumed by individuals in a certain city. Suppose there is no list of families available for the city but there is a map of the city showing each block in detail.

        3. Suppose we are interested in the proportion of calves who die prior to the first year of life at all dairy farms in a particular state.

2.3 Suppose that a survey is being planned for purposes of estimating the average number of hours spent exercising daily by adults (18 years of age or older) living in a certain community. A list of all individuals living in the town is not available; however, a list of all households is available at the office of the town clerk. For simplicity, suppose this list consists of nine households and that the information you would collect, were you to visit each household is, as shown in the accompanying table.

    a. Define these:

        1. Population

        2. Elementary unit

        3. Enumeration unit

     4. Frame

     5. Variable

b. Devise a sampling plan to estimate the average daily time expenditure on exercising by adults living in the community.

c. Select all samples of two households from this frame and compute the average exercising time per person for each sample.

d. Compute the expected value of your estimate and compare this to the actual population parameter.

e. Calculate the standard error of your estimate.

Household	No. of Adults	Aggregate Number of Hours Spent Exercising by All Adults
1	2	1
2	3	3
3	2	7
4	5	8
5	3	4
6	1	0
7	2	1
8	3	2
9	2	0

2.4 As part of an AIDS education program, 120 intravenous drug users seronegative for HIV (Human Immunodeficiency Virus) at a first screening were given instructions on sterilizing their needles with bleach and practicing "safe sex." One year after the program's inception, a sample of 30 of these subjects was taken by numbering the participants from 1 to 120 and taking all subjects whose numbers are divisible by 4 (e.g., 4, 8, 12, etc.).

    a. What is the chance of each individual being chosen in the sample?

    b. If subjects 1, 3, 4, 8, 29, and 65 are seropositive for HIV, what is the proportion of seroconverted subjects for this population?

    c. What is the proportion of seroconverted subjects in the sample? Is this an unbiased estimate of the population proportion?

2.5 As part of a marketing program, a city block containing 4 households was selected and a sample of 3 households was sampled as follows: Jeremiah, the research assistant, identified the households and numbered each household from 1 to 4. He then was to list all combinations of the 4 households 2 at a time. These are:

| 1 and 2 | 1 and 3 | 1 and 4 |
| 2 and 3 | 2 and 4 | 3 and 4 |

Unfortunately, Jeremiah got this job because he was related to the Department Chairman, and he was very careless. He forgot the combination 3 and 4. He chose a random number between 1 and 5 (it turned out to be 4) which corresponded to the combination 2 and 3. Thus households 2 and 3 were sampled. The variable of interest was out-of-pocket medical expenses incurred by the household. These were as follows for the 4 households

Household	Expenses ($)
1	345.00
2	126.00
3	492.00
4	962.00

a. Based on Jeremiah's sampling procedure, what is the mean, standard error, and MSE of the estimated mean out-of-pocket medical expenses?

b. Is the estimate derived from this sampling procedure unbiased?

c. Does every household have the same chance of appearing in the sample? Why or why not?

2.6 It is desired to perform a quality control audit of laboratory data from a large clinical trial for purposes of estimating the proportion of laboratory values in the database that are invalid. There are 394 patients in the clinical trial, and each person has had from 60 to 200 laboratory determinations during the course of the trial. The sampling plan chosen was to select a random sample of 10 patients and for each sample person take a random sample of 10 laboratory determinations, which would then be checked against the patient medical record for accuracy.

a. What are the elementary units in this sample design?

b. What are the sampling units in this sample design?

c. Does each person in the population have an equal chance of being selected in the sample?

d. Does each laboratory determination in the population have an equal chance of being selected in the sample?

2.7 Data from the sample described in Exercise 2.6 are shown below:

Subject	Total Invalid Laboratory Values in 10 Sampled
1	1
2	0
3	2
4	0
5	1
6	0
7	0
8	0
9	0
10	1

Based on these data, what is the estimated proportion of laboratory results that are invalid?

2.8 The following table shows the total number of laboratory determinations for the 10 sample patients described in Exercise 2.6 as well as the number of invalid determinations among the 10 determinations sampled:

Subject	Total Laboratory Values	Total Invalid Laboratory Values in 10 Sampled
1	103	1
2	123	0
3	93	2
4	200	0
5	128	1
6	165	0
7	132	0
8	189	0
9	176	0
10	180	1

Based on these data, estimate the proportion of laboratory values that are invalid using *all* of the data in the above table.

2.9 Match the term in column 1 with the most appropriate term in column 2.

Column 1	Column 2
1. MSE	A. $\sum_{i=1}^{n} x_i$
2. Reliability	B. Population
3. Bias	C. Accuracy
4. Universe	D. $\sum_{i=1}^{N} X_i$
5. Sample Total	E. Validity
6. Population Total	F. Variance

BIBLIOGRAPHY

The sampling texts cited in Chapter 1 [1–16] all develop the concepts discussed in this chapter, each in its own way. The following sampling text by Hajek [1] presents in Chapter 1 an especially good discussion of the concepts developed in this chapter.

1. Hajek, J. H., *Sampling from a Finite Population*, Marcel Dekker, New York and Basel, 1981.

The concept of counting rule will be developed further in a later chapter when we discuss the topic of network sampling. The following articles give examples of the use of counting rules in sample surveys.

2. Sirken, M. G., Household surveys with multiplicity. *Journal of the American Statistical Association*, 65: 257, 1970.

3. Sirken, M. G., and Levy, P. S., Multiplicity estimation of proportions based on ratios of random variables. *Journal of the American Statistical Association*, 69: 68, 1974.

4. Czaja, R., and Blair, J., Using network sampling in victimization surveys. *Journal of Quantitative Criminology*, 6: 186, 1990.

5. Sirken, M. G., Network sampling. In *The Encyclopedia of Biostatistics*, Armitage, P. A., and Colton, T., Eds. Wiley, Chichester, U.K., 1998.

The following expository articles appearing in The Encyclopedia of Biostatistics *provide a more complete discussion of some of the topics discussed in this chapter.*

6. King, B., Quota, representative, and other methods of purposive sampling. In *The Encyclopedia of Biostatistics*, Armitage, P. A., and Colton, T., Eds. Wiley, Chichester, U.K., 1998.

7. Warnecke, R. B., Sampling frames. In *The Encyclopedia of Biostatistics*, Armitage, P. A., and Colton, T., Eds. Wiley, Chichester, U.K., 1998.

8. Xia, Z., Probability sampling. In *The Encyclopedia of Biostatistics*. Armitage, P. A., and Colton, T., Eds. Wiley, Chichester, U.K., 1998.

PART 2

Major Sampling Designs and Estimation Procedures

CHAPTER 3

Simple Random Sampling

In Chapter 2 we laid a foundation for our discussion of sampling by setting forth general concepts concerning the universe or target population, the sample, sampling distributions, and desirable properties of population estimates. Beginning in this chapter, we build upon that foundation by relating these concepts to specific sampling plans and estimation procedures that are widely used in sample surveys. We begin this process by discussing those sampling plans in which the elementary units themselves serve as the sampling units. Such sampling procedures are sometimes referred to as *element sampling*. In this chapter we discuss a method of element sampling—namely, simple random sampling—that is important not because it is widely used in actual sample surveys but because it provides the foundation upon which the statistical theory of sampling is constructed. Thus, while in practice you may never decide to select a design based on simple random sampling (we discuss why this is so in Section 3.8), we devote this chapter to its discussion because of its contribution to sampling theory.

3.1 WHAT IS A SIMPLE RANDOM SAMPLE?

Let us suppose we have a population of N elements and we wish to take a sample of n of these elements. It can be shown from the mathematical theory of permutations and combinations that the number T of possible samples of n elements from a population of N elements is denoted by $\binom{N}{n}$ and is given by

$$T = \binom{N}{n} = \frac{N!}{n!(N-n)!} \tag{3.1}$$

where $n! = n(n-1)(n-2)\cdots(1)$ and $0! = 1$. For example, if a population contains 25 elements and we wish to take a sample of 5 elements, then from Relation (3.1) with $N = 25$ and $n = 5$, we have the following:

$$T = \frac{25!}{(5!)(25 - 5)!} = 53,130$$

Thus, there are 53,130 possible samples of 5 elements from a population of 25 elements.

With this relation in mind, we have the following definition of simple random sampling.

A *simple random sample* of n elements from a population of N elements is one in which each of the $\binom{N}{n}$ possible samples of n elements has the same probability of selection, namely $1/\binom{N}{n}$.

It should be mentioned that the type of sampling discussed above, and throughout this volume, is known as *sampling without replacement*. In sampling without replacement, a particular element can appear only once in a given sample, whereas if sampling is done with replacement, a given element can appear more than once in a particular sample. In practice, almost all sampling is done without replacement. Sampling with replacement is of interest primarily for theoretical reasons, since the mathematical theory of this type of sampling is less unwieldy than the theory of sampling without replacement. Under certain conditions, results derived under assumptions of sampling with replacement are approximately true even if the sampling is done without replacement. For discussions of sampling with replacement, you may wish to consult a more mathematical sampling text such as Cochran [1], Hansen et al. [2], or Kish [3].

3.1.1   How to Take a Simple Random Sample

The first step in taking a simple random sample is to assign a number from 1 to N to each element in the population. The next step is to pick a sample of n of these numbers by use of some random process such as a table of random numbers, a computer, or a calculator with a random number generator. Whatever procedure is used must ensure that the numbers selected are all different and that none are greater than N. Once the numbers are chosen, the population elements corresponding to these numbers are taken as the sample.

For example if we want to take a random sample of six physicians from the list of 25 physicians in Table 2.1, we could use the random number table in the Appendix (Table A.l). Using two-digit numbers, and beginning at some arbitrary point (e.g., row 7, first two digits in column 1, we proceed down the column until six different numbers between 01 and 25 are chosen. All numbers equal to 00 or greater than 25 are discarded. For this example the numbers we get are 09, 10, 07, 02, 01, and 05. These random numbers identify those individuals who will be studied in the sample. (If you work through this example by referring to Table A.1, you will note that we encounter the numbers 07 and 02 twice. Since we are sampling without replacement, they are discarded the second time we encounter them. Also note that when we come to the bottom of a particular column, we proceed to the top line of the very next column on that same page. We do not proceed to the next page of random numbers until we run out of columns on the current page.)

3.1.2 Probability of an Element Being Selected

In simple random sampling there are $\binom{N}{n}$ possible samples of n elements from a population of N elements and each sample has a probability of $1/\binom{N}{n}$ of being selected. Also in simple random sampling, the probability of any element being selected is equal to n/N, the ratio of the sample size to the population size. This can be demonstrated very simply by the following argument. The number of samples of n elements not containing a particular element is equal to $\binom{N-1}{n}$, the number of ways in which the $N - 1$ other elements can combine in groups of size n. The probability of any element not being included is therefore equal to $\binom{N-1}{n}/\binom{N}{n}$, which is equal to $(N - n)/N$. The probability of a particular element being included is therefore equal to $1 - [(N - n)/N]$, or n/N.

In virtually all of the standard statistical software packages, procedures based on random number generators are available for selecting simple random samples with or without replacement. Where feasible, the use of the computer for generating samples can take much of the drudgery out of the sampling process. The user, however, should be careful to ensure that the methodology used to take the computer-generated sample conforms to the specified sampling design.

One of the most useful sampling programs is the module, SAMPLE [7] written for Version 5 of SYSTAT, which is a widely used general-purpose statistical package. At this time, it appears to be the only sampling module that is integrated with a general-purpose PC-based statistical program and that has the capability of taking samples from a wide variety of sampling plans commonly used in sample surveys (e.g., simple random sampling, systematic sampling, stratified random sampling, and probability proportional to size sampling).

3.2 ESTIMATION OF POPULATION CHARACTERISTICS UNDER SIMPLE RANDOM SAMPLING

3.2.1 Estimation Formulas

Under simple random sampling, the following estimates x', $\bar{x}$, p_y, and s_x^2 are the estimates of population totals, means, proportions and variances that are invariably used in simple random sampling designs:

$$x' = \frac{N \sum\limits_{i=1}^{n} x_i}{n}$$

$$\bar{x} = \frac{\sum\limits_{i=1}^{n} x_i}{n}$$

$$p_y = \frac{\sum\limits_{i=1}^{n} y_i}{n}$$

(where y_i is a dichotomous variable with values 0 or 1)

$$\hat{\sigma}_x^2 = \left(\frac{N-1}{N}\right) s_x^2$$

where

$$s_x^2 = \frac{\sum\limits_{i=1}^{n} (x_i - \bar{x})^2}{n-1}$$

These estimates are used because, as will be discussed in the next section, they are unbiased estimates of the corresponding population parameters. The estimated variances of x', $\bar{x}$, and p_y, are shown in Box 3.1.

3.2.2 Numerical Computation of Estimates and Their Standard Errors

Historically, production of estimates and their standard errors from sample survey data has required use of special-purpose programs or macros, and could not be done routinely by direct use of modules in the standard general-purpose statistical packages (e.g. SAS, SPSS, BMDP). Even for simple random sampling, the estimated standard error of a sample mean or proportion obtained from most general statistical software packages will overestimate the true standard error by the factor, $\sqrt{N/(N-n)}$. In general, computation of appropriate estimates and their standard errors from sample survey data has required use of programs such as SUDAAN, WESVAR and PC-CARP, which are not general-purpose statistical packages, but were written for the primary purpose of performing analysis of data from sample surveys.

More recently, however, the manufacturers of general-purpose statistical packages have shown interest in developing such modules. One such widely used general statistical package, STATA, has incorporated into Version 5.0 a set of commands that can compute estimates and their standard errors for a wide variety of sample designs, and it is likely that the other major packages will have similar capability in the near future. Because we anticipate a great

---

BOX 3.1   ESTIMATED TOTALS, MEANS, PROPORTIONS, AND VARIANCES UNDER SIMPLE RANDOM SAMPLING, AND ESTIMATED VARIANCES AND STANDARD ERRORS OF THESE ESTIMATES

Estimate	**Estimated Variance and Standard Error of Estimate**

Total

$$x' = \frac{N}{n} \sum_{i=1}^{n} x_i$$

$$\widehat{\mathrm{Var}}(x') = N^2 \left(\frac{N-n}{N}\right)\left(\frac{s_x^2}{n}\right)$$

$$\widehat{\mathrm{SE}}(x') = N \sqrt{\frac{N-n}{N}} \left(\frac{s_x}{\sqrt{n}}\right)$$

Mean

$$\bar{x} = \frac{\sum_{i=1}^{n} x_i}{n}$$

$$\widehat{\mathrm{Var}}(\bar{x}) = \left(\frac{N-n}{N}\right)\left(\frac{s_x^2}{n}\right)$$

$$\widehat{\mathrm{SE}}(\bar{x}) = \sqrt{\frac{N-n}{N}} \frac{s_x}{\sqrt{n}}$$

Proportion

$$p_y = \frac{\sum_{i=1}^{n} y_i}{n}$$

$$\widehat{\mathrm{Var}}(p_y) = \left(\frac{N-n}{N}\right)\frac{p_y(1-p_y)}{n-1}$$

$$\widehat{\mathrm{SE}}(p_y) = \sqrt{\frac{N-n}{N}} \sqrt{\frac{p_y(1-p_y)}{n-1}}$$

where y is a dichotomous variable having values 0 or 1.

---

increase in the availability of such software, we will include in many of our numerical illustrative examples discussion of how computation of estimates and their standard errors would be accomplished by the use of STATA and/ or SUDAAN. The former is a general-purpose statistical package that has recently added modules for analysis of survey data, while the latter has been developed specifically for analysis of sample survey data and has been very widely used. Our choice of these two packages should not imply our endorsement of them over other software products. We have chosen them because of our current familiarity with them.

Illustrative Example.   A sample of hospitals was taken in Illinois for purposes of examining compliance with respect to screening of newborns and their mothers for hepatitis B surface antigen (HBsAG), a marker for infection with the hepatitis B virus. This was a relatively large survey having a complex sampling design, and will be used throughout this book to illustrate major concepts and procedures. For this particular example, we will illustrate the use of STATA for computation of estimates and standard errors, and will assume that we have a simple random sample of 25 birth records taken from a total of 773 births that occurred in one of the sample hospitals during the year.

The relevant data are organized into a file containing 25 records, each having the following variables:

hospno: The identification number of the hospital (hospno = 13 in this instance)

birth: The total number, N, of births that occurred in the hospital during the year ($N = 773$)

weight1: The reciprocal of the sampling fraction ($N/n = 773/25 = 30.92$)

momsag: Whether or not the mother's antigenic status with respect to HBsAg appears on the newborn's record (momsag = 1 if yes; 0 if no).

The file containing 25 records with variables in the order (hospno birth weight1 momsag) is shown opposite.

In order for STATA to process data for a particular sampling design, every record must have certain information on it that is required for that design. For a simple random sample, the following two variables are required:

1. The sampling weight, N/n. In this file, it is located in the variable *weight1*, and is equal to 773/25 or 30.92 for each record.
2. The number of enumeration units, N, in the population. This is necessary for computation of the expression $(N - n)/N$, which is a factor in the formula for a standard error of an estimate. In this file, it is located in the variable, *birth*, and is equal to 773 for each record.

The data must then be put into a STATA data file, which has the extension, *dta*. There are various ways in which this can be done, and the reader is referred to the STATA manual [9] for further information. We will name the resulting file *momsag.dta*.

hospno	birth	weight1	momsag
13	773	30.92	0
13	773	30.92	1
13	773	30.92	1
13	773	30.92	1
13	773	30.92	1
13	773	30.92	1
13	773	30.92	1
13	773	30.92	1
13	773	30.92	1
13	773	30.92	1
13	773	30.92	1
13	773	30.92	1
13	773	30.92	1
13	773	30.92	1
13	773	30.92	1
13	773	30.92	1
13	773	30.92	0
13	773	30.92	1
13	773	30.92	1
13	773	30.92	1
13	773	30.92	1
13	773	30.92	1
13	773	30.92	1
13	773	30.92	1

The data can then be processed from the following set of commands:

```
use a:\momsag
.svyset pweight weight1
.svyset fpc birth
.svymean momsag
.svytotal momsag
```

The first command indicates that the data set *momsag.dta*, located on a floppy diskette in the A drive, is to be used. The next two commands set the two parameters necessary for a simple random sample to be processed: The command *svyset pweight weight1* indicates that the sampling weight, N/n, which STATA refers to by the term *pweight*, is located in the variable named *weight1*. The command *svyset fpc birth* sets the parameter, N, used in computing the factor $(N - n)/N$ used in the formulas for the standard errors of estimates. In this instance, it indicates that this factor is located in the variable named *birth*.

Finally, the last two commands instruct the program to estimate the mean and total of the variable, *momsag*. STATA generates the following output:

```
.svymean momsag

Survey mean estimation

pweight:    weight1                        Number of obs     =    25
Strata:     < one >                        Number of strata  =     1
PSU:        < observations >               Number of PSUs    =    25
FPC:        birth                          Population size   =   773
```

Mean	Estimate	Std. Err.	[95% Conf. Interval]		Deff
momsag	.92	.0544746	.8075699	1.03243	1

Finite population correction (FPC) assumes simple random sampling without replacement of PSUs within each stratum with no subsampling within PSUs.

```
.svytotal momsag

Survey total estimation

pweight:    weight1                        Number of obs     =    25
Strata:     < one >                        Number of strata  =     1
PSU:        < observations >               Number of PSUs    =    25
FPC:        birth                          Population size   =   773
```

Mean	Estimate	Std. Err.	[95% Conf. Interval]		Deff
momsag	711.16	42.10889	624.2515	798.0685	1

Finite population correction (FPC) assumes simple random sampling without replacement of PSUs within each stratum with no subsampling within PSUs.

□

The estimated total shown above and its estimated standard error are exactly what would be obtained from the appropriate formulas given in Box 3.1. The estimated mean in the printout is the mean of a dichotomous variable having value 0 or 1 and would be interpreted as a proportion. Likewise, it and its standard error are exactly what would be obtained from the appropriate formulas shown in Box 3.1.

The term *PSU* shown in the output stands for *Primary Sampling Unit*, and in the case of simple random sampling is the enumeration unit (which is the hospital record in this example). In other sampling designs, the primary sampling unit and enumeration unit may not be the same. The term *Deff* shown in the output is a term known as the *design effect*, and is the ratio of the variance of an estimate from a particular sampling design to that of an estimate from a simple random sample of the same number of enumeration units. It will be discussed in subsequent sections of this text.

The reasons why we use the estimates shown in Box 3.1 and their estimated variances and standard errors are discussed in Section 3.3.

3.3 SAMPLING DISTRIBUTIONS OF ESTIMATED POPULATION CHARACTERISTICS

The estimates resulting from a simple random sample are unbiased estimates of the corresponding population parameters. Let us illustrate this idea through an example.

Illustrative Example.   As a simple example, let us consider the population of six schools shown in Table 2.3, and let us suppose that we wish to estimate, from a simple random sample of three schools, the total number of children in the six schools not immunized for measles. Using the estimated total $x' = (N/n)x = (6/3)x$, we have the estimates shown in Table 3.1 for the $\binom{6}{3}$ or 20 samples of 3 schools from a population of 6 schools.

Note that each school appears in 10 of the 20 possible samples. Thus, the probability of any particular school appearing in the sample is 10/20, which is also equal to n/N or 3/6.

The sampling distribution of the estimated total x' (with $n = 3$) for the data in Table 3.1 is shown in Table 3.2. From Table 3.2 we see that the 20 equally likely samples yield 11 different values of x'.

The mean, the variance, and the standard deviation of the sampling distribution of x' are as follows:

Table 3.1   Possible Samples of Three Schools and Values of x'

Schools in Sample	x'	Schools in Sample	x'
1,2,3	24	2,3,4	22
1,2,4	24	2,3,5	30
1,2,5	32	2,3,6	32
1,2,6	34	2,4,5	30
1,3,4	20	2,4,6	32
1,3,5	28	2,5,6	40
1,3,6	30	3,4,5	26
1,4,5	28	3,4,6	28
1,4,6	30	3,5,6	36
1,5,6	38	4,5,6	36

Table 3.2 Sampling Distribution of the x' in Table 3.1

x'	f	$\pi = f/T$
20	1	.05
22	1	.05
24	2	.10
26	1	.05
28	3	.15
30	4	.20
32	3	.15
34	1	.05
36	2	.10
38	1	.05
40	1	.05
Total	20	1.00

$$E(x') = \sum_{i=1}^{11} x_i'\pi_i = 20(.05) + 22(.05) + \cdots + 40(.05) = 30$$

$$\text{Var}(x') = \sum_{i=1}^{11} [x_i' - E(x')]^2\pi_i = (20 - 30)^2(.05) + (22 - 30)^2(.05)$$

$$+ \cdots + (40 - 30)^2(.05) = 26.4$$

$$\text{SE}(x') = \sqrt{\text{Var}(x')} = \sqrt{26.4} = 5.138$$

We note that for the six schools given in Table 2.3, the population parameters X, σ_x^2, and σ_x are

$$X = 30 \qquad \sigma_x^2 = 3.67 \qquad \sigma_x = 1.915$$

We further note that, for the sampling distribution of x' shown in Table 3.2,

$$E(x') = X = 30$$

That is, the estimated total in simple random sampling appears to be an unbiased estimate of the true population total. □

It can be demonstrated that the variance, $\text{Var}(x')$, and standard deviation, $\text{SE}(x')$, of the sampling distribution of x' are given by

$$\text{Var}(x') = \left(\frac{N^2}{n}\right)(\sigma_x^2)\left(\frac{N - n}{N - 1}\right)$$

and

$$SE(x') = \left(\frac{N}{\sqrt{n}}\right)(\sigma_x)\left(\frac{N-n}{N-1}\right)^{1/2}$$

For the example shown above

$$\text{Var}(x') = \left(\frac{6^2}{3}\right)(3.67)\left(\frac{6-3}{6-1}\right) = 26.4$$

which is the same result that we got through direct computation.

Thus, we see that for simple random sampling, the estimated population total, x', is an unbiased estimate of the population total X. The standard error of x' given by the equation above is directly proportional to σ_x, the standard deviation of the distribution of $\mathcal{X}$ in the population, and inversely proportional to the square root of the sample size, n. The standard error also depends on the square root of the factor $(N-n)/(N-1)$, which is known as the *finite population correction*, and is often denoted fpc.

We can obtain some insight into the role played by the fpc by examining its value for a hypothetical population containing $N = 10{,}000$ elements and for sample sizes as given in Table 3.3. From this table we see that if the sample size, n, is very much less than the population size, N, then the fpc is very close to unity and thus will have very little influence on the numerical value of the standard error $SE(x')$ of the estimated total, x'. On the other hand, as n gets closer to N, the fpc decreases in magnitude and thus will cause a reduction in the value of $SE(x')$.

If we write the fpc in the form $\sqrt{\text{fpc}}$, we have

$$\sqrt{\text{fpc}} = \sqrt{\frac{N-n}{N-1}} = \sqrt{\frac{N}{N-1}} \times \sqrt{1-\frac{n}{N}}$$

Table 3.3   Values of the fpc ($N=10{,}000$)

Sample Size, n	$\text{fpc} = \sqrt{\dfrac{N-n}{N-1}}$
1	1.0000
10	.9995
100	.9950
500	.9747
1000	.9487
5000	.7071
9000	.3162

In this form we see that its value depends primarily on the ratio of n to N rather than on their absolute magnitudes. It makes sense intuitively that the fpc is a factor in the value of $SE(x')$, since n being close to N implies that most of the elements in the population are in the sample. This further implies that the relatively few elements not sampled would have very little effect on the distribution of x'.

A presentation similar to the one given above for the properties of a sample total under simple random sampling could be given for the properties of the sampling distribution of sample means $\bar{x}$ and sample proportions p_y having an attribute $\mathcal{Y}$. We will not discuss each sampling distribution separately, but we summarize their properties in Box 3.2. We see from Box 3.2 that, under simple random sampling, sample totals, means, and proportions are unbiased estimates of the corresponding population parameters.

3.4 COEFFICIENTS OF VARIATION OF ESTIMATED POPULATION PARAMETERS

In the previous chapter we defined the coefficient of variation V_x of the distribution of a variable $\mathcal{X}$ in a population as the standard deviation of the distribution of $\mathcal{X}$ divided by the mean value of $\mathcal{X}$ in the population. Similarly, we define the *coefficient of variation* $V(\hat{d})$ of an estimate $\hat{d}$ of a population parameter d as its standard error $SE(\hat{d})$ divided by the true value d of the parameter being estimated. In other words,

$$V(\hat{d}) = \frac{SE(\hat{d})}{d} \tag{3.5}$$

The square $V^2(\hat{d})$ of the coefficient of variation of an estimated parameter is known as the *relative variance* (or rel–variance) *of the estimated parameter*.

The coefficient of variation of an estimated parameter measures the sampling variability of the estimate relative to the value of the parameter being estimated and is used in assessing the reliability of the estimate. As we will see later on, it appears as a factor in many important results in sampling theory.

Box 3.3 presents the coefficients of variation for estimated totals, means, and proportions for a simple random sample.

The results shown in Box 3.3 are obtained by substituting the values of the standard errors shown in Box 3.2 into the formula for the coefficient of variation of an estimate [Equation (3.5)]. For example, the coefficient of variation of an estimated total x' is, according to Box 3.2 and Equation (3.5)

$$V(x') = \frac{\left(\dfrac{N}{\sqrt{n}}\right)(\sigma_x)\sqrt{\dfrac{N-n}{N-1}}}{X}.$$

BOX 3.2 POPULATION ESTIMATES, AND MEANS AND STANDARD ERRORS OF POPULATION ESTIMATES UNDER SIMPLE RANDOM SAMPLING

Total, x'

$$x' = \frac{N \sum_{i=1}^{n} x_i}{n} = \left(\frac{N}{n}\right)(x) \qquad E(x') = X$$

$$SE(x') = \left(\frac{N}{\sqrt{n}}\right)(\sigma_x)\sqrt{\frac{N-n}{N-1}} \qquad (3.2)$$

Mean, $\bar{x}$

$$\bar{x} = \frac{\sum_{i=1}^{n} x_i}{n} = \frac{x}{n} \qquad E(\bar{x}) = \bar{X}$$

$$SE(\bar{x}) = \left(\frac{\sigma_x}{\sqrt{n}}\right)\sqrt{\frac{N-n}{N-1}} \qquad (3.3)$$

Proportion, p_y

$$p_y = \frac{\sum_{i=1}^{n} y_i}{n} = \frac{y}{n} \qquad E(p_y) = P_y$$

$$SE(p_y) = \sqrt{\frac{P_y(1-P_y)}{n}}\sqrt{\frac{N-n}{N-1}} \qquad (3.4)$$

The notation used in these formulas is defined in Boxes 2.1 and 2.2; n is the number of elements in the sample taken from a population of N elements.

BOX 3.3   COEFFICIENTS OF VARIATION OF POPULATION ESTIMATES UNDER SIMPLE RANDOM SAMPLING

Total, x'

$$V(x') = \left(\frac{V_x}{\sqrt{n}}\right)\sqrt{\frac{N-n}{N-1}} \qquad (3.6)$$

Mean, $\bar{x}$

$$V(\bar{x}) = \left(\frac{V_x}{\sqrt{n}}\right)\sqrt{\frac{N-n}{N-1}} \qquad (3.7)$$

Proportion, p_y

$$V(p_y) = \sqrt{\frac{1-P_y}{nP_y}}\sqrt{\frac{N-n}{N-1}} \qquad (3.8)$$

In these formulas V_x is the coefficient of variation for the variable $\mathcal{X}$, P_y is the population proportion, n is the number of elements in the sample, and N is the number of elements in the population.

But $X = N\bar{X}$, and so

$$V(x') = \left(\frac{1}{\sqrt{n}}\right)\left(\frac{\sigma_x}{\bar{X}}\right)\sqrt{\frac{N-n}{N-1}}$$

Since $\sigma_x/\bar{X}$ is by definition the coefficient of variation of the distribution of $\mathcal{X}$ in the population, we have

$$V(x') = \left(\frac{V_x}{\sqrt{n}}\right)\sqrt{\frac{N-n}{N-1}}$$

The other results displayed in Box 3.3 can be derived in a similar way. Note that under simple random sampling, the coefficient of variation of an estimated mean $\bar{x}$ is the same as that of an estimated total.

3.5   RELIABILITY OF ESTIMATES

The standard error of an estimate is a measure of the sampling variability of the estimate over all possible samples. Under the assumption that measurement error is nonexistent or negligible, the *reliability of an estimate* can be judged by the size of the standard error; the larger the standard error, the lower is the reliability of the estimate (see Section 2.4).

If we make the assumption that the estimates discussed in the previous section have, for reasonably large values of n (say, greater than 20), distributions that are close to the normal or Gaussian distribution, then we can use normal theory to obtain approximate confidence intervals for the unknown population parameters being estimated. For example, approximate $100(1 - \alpha)\%$ *confidence intervals* for the population total are given by

$$x' \pm z_{1-(\alpha/2)}\left(\frac{N}{\sqrt{n}}\right)(\sigma_x)\sqrt{\frac{N-n}{N-1}}$$

where $z_{1-(\alpha/2)}$ is the $100[1 - (\alpha/2)]$ percentile of the standard normal distribution. For example, for a 95% confidence interval, $\alpha = .05$ and $z_{1-(\alpha/2)} = z_{.975} = 1.96$.

Since σ_x is an unknown population parameter, it must be estimated from the sample. If we replace σ_x in the formula above by

$$\hat{\sigma}_x = \sqrt{\left(\frac{N-1}{N}\right)(s_x^2)}$$

we obtain the following approximate confidence interval for the population total X:

$$x' \pm z_{1-(\alpha/2)}(N)\sqrt{\frac{N-n}{N}}\left(\frac{s_x}{\sqrt{n}}\right)$$

Illustrative Example.   Suppose that a simple random sample of 9 of the 25 physicians listed in Table 2.1 is taken for the purpose of estimating the total X of household visits made by physicians in the population. Let us suppose that the physicians chosen are 13, 3, 17, 1, 14, 12, 7, 18, 4. The sample data are given in Table 3.4. The sample statistics are (from formulas in Boxes 2.2 and 3.2):

Table 3.4 Sample Data for Number of Household Visits

Physician	No. of Visits	Physician	No. of Visits
1	5	13	6
3	1	14	4
4	4	17	7
7	12	18	0
12	5		

$$x = 44 \qquad s_x = 3.48 \qquad x' = \left(\frac{25}{9}\right)(44) = 122.22$$

From the previous formula we obtain the upper limit of the 95% confidence interval for X with $z_{1-(\alpha/2)} = z_{.975} = 1.96$:

$$122.22 + 1.96(25)\sqrt{\frac{25-9}{25}}\left(\frac{3.48}{\sqrt{9}}\right) = 122.22 + 45.47 = 167.69$$

Likewise, the lower 95% confidence interval for X is

$$122.22 - 45.47 = 76.75$$

Note that the true population total, $X = 127$, is covered by this confidence interval.

These 95% confidence intervals have the following usual interpretation: if we were to repeatedly sample n elements from this population according to the same sampling plan, and if, for each sample, confidence intervals were calculated, 95% of such confidence intervals would include the true unknown population parameter. □

Box 3.4 summarizes the estimated variances of the sampling distribution for the total, mean, and proportion, and gives the form of the corresponding confidence interval.

It should be emphasized that the confidence intervals obtained by using the equations in Box 3.4 are based on the assumption that the estimate (e.g., x') is normally distributed. The extent to which this assumption is violated depends on such considerations as the nature of the distribution of the variable in the population and the size of the sample. If the variable has a nearly symmetric distribution and the sample size is not small, then the confidence coefficients expressed in the confidence intervals will be approximately correct. If the data are badly skewed, however, and the sample size is small, the confidence coefficients may be misleading (Exercise 3.1 illustrates the situation using the data in Table 2.1). For linear estimates such as those discussed in this chapter, the

BOX 3.4 ESTIMATED VARIANCES AND 100(1 − α)% CONFIDENCE INTERVALS UNDER SIMPLE RANDOM SAMPLING

Total, x'

$$\widehat{\text{Var}}(x') = N^2 \left(\frac{N-n}{N}\right)\left(\frac{s_x^2}{n}\right)$$

and

$$x' \pm z_{1-(\alpha/2)}(N)\sqrt{\frac{N-n}{N}}\left(\frac{s_x}{\sqrt{n}}\right) \qquad (3.9)$$

Mean, $\bar{x}$

$$\widehat{\text{Var}}(\bar{x}) = \left(\frac{N-n}{N}\right)\left(\frac{s_x^2}{n}\right)$$

and

$$\bar{x} \pm z_{1-(\alpha/2)}\sqrt{\frac{N-n}{N}}\left(\frac{s_x}{\sqrt{n}}\right) \qquad (3.10)$$

Proportion, p_y

$$\widehat{\text{Var}}(p_y) = \left(\frac{N-n}{N}\right)\left(\frac{p_y(1-p_y)}{n-1}\right)$$

and

$$p_y \pm z_{1-(\alpha/2)}\sqrt{\frac{N-n}{N}}\sqrt{\frac{p_y(1-p_y)}{n-1}} \qquad (3.11)$$

In these equations n is the number of elements in the sample, N is the number of elements in the population, s_x^2 is the sample variance, and $z_{1-(\alpha/2)}$ is the $100[1 − (\alpha/2)]$th percentile of the standard normal distribution.

Note that we may substitute the relation involving $\hat{\sigma}_x^2$ for s_x^2 [see Equation (2.16)] in the expressions for $\widehat{\text{Var}}(x')$ and $\widehat{\text{Var}}(\bar{x})$. Also note that, since $\widehat{\text{SE}}(\hat{d}) = \sqrt{\widehat{\text{Var}}(\hat{d})}$, the confidence interval may be written in terms of the estimated standard error. That is, we may write the confidence intervals as

$$x' \pm z_{1-(\alpha/2)}[\widehat{\text{SE}}(x')] \qquad \bar{x} \pm z_{1-(\alpha/2)}[\widehat{\text{SE}}(\bar{x})] \qquad p_y \pm z_{1-(\alpha/2)}[\widehat{\text{SE}}(p_y)]$$

central limit theorem of statistics gives a theoretical anchor to the assumption of normality. This theorem states, in effect, that if statistics such as means, totals, and proportions are based on large enough sample sizes, their sampling distributions tend to be normal, irrespective of the nature of the underlying distribution of the original observations.

Confidence intervals can be obtained for population means and proportions from the appropriate sample estimates in a manner analogous to that shown above for totals.

3.6 ESTIMATION OF PARAMETERS FOR SUBDOMAINS

Often the objectives of sample surveys include estimation of parameters not only for the population as a whole, but also for certain *subdomains* (subgroups or subsets) of the population. For example, a nationwide health survey of households might require estimates for the nation as a whole, but also for groups defined by age, sex, race, geographical area, or combinations of these. Often the subdomains are identified before the sample is taken, and the sample is drawn separately within each subdomain. This type of sampling plan will be considered in our discussion of stratified sampling in Chapters 5 and 6. Sometimes, however, a simple random sample is drawn from the population as a whole and estimates are expressed separately for each subdomain of interest. It is this type of sampling plan that is considered in this section. We will illustrate the procedure by use of an example.

Illustrative Example. Let us consider the population of six families living on one city block and shown in Table 3.5. Using these data, we find that the average (or mean) out-of-pocket medical expense per family is $296.67 for the total population, $316.67 for white families, and $276.67 for black families.

Table 3.5   Race and Out-of-Pocket Medical Expenses for Six Families (1987)

Family	Race	Out-of-Pocket Medical Expenses (dollars)
1	W	500
2	B	350
3	B	430
4	W	280
5	W	170
6	B	50

Let us suppose that we wish to take a simple random sample of four households from the population of six households for purposes of estimating the average per household medical expenditure for the population as a whole and for each race separately. The procedure for obtaining such an estimate for the population as a whole was discussed earlier, so, in this example, we will consider only estimates for the desired subdomains.

We can construct estimates for a particular subdomain (e.g., the black population) in the following way. Let

$$Y_i = \begin{cases} 1 & \text{if the } i\text{th family is black} \\ 0 & \text{if otherwise} \end{cases}$$

$X_i = $ the out-of-pocket expenses of the ith family

$Z_i = X_i Y_i$

For the six families in the population we have the value of X_i, Y_i, and Z_i shown in Table 3.6.

Letting Y and Z denote population totals and y and z denote sample totals in the usual way, we see that $Z = \$830$ and $Y = 3$ and that the average out-of-pocket medical expense per family for black families is equal to the ratio

$$\frac{Z}{Y} = \frac{\$830}{3} = \$276.67$$

Let us estimate Z/Y from the sample by the ratio, z/y, constructed from the sample elements. For samples of $n = 4$ elements, the distribution of z/y is given in Table 3.7.

If we calculate the mean $E(z/y)$ of the sampling distribution of z/y and the standard error $SE(z/y)$, we have

$$E(z/y) = \$276.67 = \frac{Z}{Y} \quad \text{and} \quad SE(z/y) = \$96.77$$

Table 3.6 Data for a Subdomain Based on the Families Listed in Table 3.5

Family	Race	X_i	Y_i	Z_i
1	W	500	0	0
2	B	350	1	350
3	B	430	1	430
4	W	280	0	0
5	W	170	0	0
6	B	50	1	50

Table 3.7 Sampling Distribution of z/y

Sample Elements	z	y	z/y
1,2,3,4	780	2	390
1,2,3,5	780	2	390
1,2,3,6	830	3	276.67
1,2,4,5	350	1	350
1,2,4,6	400	2	200
1,2,5,6	400	2	200
1,3,4,5	430	1	430
1,3,4,6	480	2	240
1,3,5,6	480	2	240
1,4,5,6	50	1	50
2,3,4,5	780	2	390
2,3,4,6	830	3	276.67
2,3,5,6	830	3	276.67
2,4,5,6	400	2	200
3,4,5,6	480	2	240

Thus, we see that, in this instance, the subdomain sample mean z/y is an unbiased estimate of the population mean Z/Y.   □

The ratio, z/y, is a special case of a ratio estimate, which will be described in detail in Chapter 7. In general, ratio estimates are not unbiased, although the magnitude of their bias is often small. However, as in the instance described above, when the denominator is a count of the elementary units and simple random sampling is used, this ratio is unbiased. In other words, what we have shown above empirically, is true in general for simple random sampling, namely that the sample mean of a variable among members of a subgroup is an unbiased estimator of the population mean for that subgroup (conditional on the sample size in the subgroup being nonzero).

A simple precise expression for the *standard error of an estimated mean for a subgroup* is not available. However, the following approximation is valid if the expected number, $E(y)$, of elements from the subdomain falling in the sample is greater than or equal to 20:

$$SE(z/y) = \left[\frac{\sigma_z}{\sqrt{E(y)}}\right] \times \sqrt{\frac{Y - E(y)}{Y - 1}} \qquad (3.12)$$

where z/y is the mean level of z among the y elements in the sample belonging to the subdomain and σ_z is the standard deviation of the distribution of the variable $\mathscr{Z}$ among members of the subgroup in the population as given by

$$\sigma_z = \left[\frac{\sum_{i=1}^{Y}(Z_i - \bar{Z})^2}{Y}\right]^{1/2}$$

Since Y, $E(y)$, and σ_z are not usually known, they are generally estimated by y' (which is equal to $(N/n)y$), y, and

$$\hat{\sigma}_z = \left(\frac{y'-1}{y'}\right)^{1/2} \times \sqrt{\sum_{i=1}^{y}(z_i - \bar{z})^2/(y-1)}$$

where z_i represents the value of the variable $\mathscr{Z}$ for the ith sample element and $\bar{z}$ is the sample mean of the z_i. Substituting the estimates y, y', and $\hat{\sigma}_z$ into Equation (3.12), we then have the *estimate of the standard error* $\widehat{SE}(z/y)$ of an estimated mean for a subgroup:

$$\widehat{SE}(z/y) = \left(\frac{\hat{\sigma}_z}{\sqrt{y}}\right)\sqrt{\frac{y'-y}{y'-1}} \qquad (3.13)$$

Note that the approximation given by Equation (3.12) cannot be used for the data in Table 3.5 since the average number of elements in the subgroup falling into the subgroup is equal to 2 [i.e., $E(y) = (n/N)Y$ over all possible samples], which is considerably less than 20.

Now let us illustrate how we would estimate a subgroup mean and its standard error by using the preceding equations.

Illustrative Example. Let us consider the data in Table 3.8 obtained from a random sample of 40 workers taken from a population of 1200 workers.

If we are interested in estimating the mean forced vital capacity (fvc) among workers having high exposure to pulmonary stressors, we have the following calculations:

$$y = 28 \qquad n = 40 \qquad N = 1200$$

$$y' = \left(\frac{N}{n}\right)(y) = \left(\frac{1200}{40}\right)(28) = 840$$

$$z = \sum_{i=1}^{n} z_i = 81 + 64 + \cdots + 84 = 2215$$

$$\frac{z}{y} = \frac{2215}{28} = 79.11$$

Table 3.8 Cumulative Exposure to Pulmonary Stressors and Forced Vital Capacity Among Workers in a Sample Taken at a Plant Employing 1200 Workers

worker	exposure[†]	fvc[*]	popsize	wt1
1	3	81	1200	30
2	3	64	1200	30
3	2	85	1200	30
4	2	91	1200	30
5	3	60	1200	30
6	1	97	1200	30
7	1	82	1200	30
8	1	99	1200	30
9	3	96	1200	30
10	3	91	1200	30
11	1	71	1200	30
12	3	88	1200	30
13	2	84	1200	30
14	3	85	1200	30
15	3	77	1200	30
16	3	76	1200	30
17	3	62	1200	30
18	3	67	1200	30
19	3	91	1200	30
20	2	99	1200	30
21	2	70	1200	30
22	1	64	1200	30
23	3	72	1200	30
24	2	72	1200	30
25	3	95	1200	30
26	3	96	1200	30
27	3	62	1200	30
28	3	67	1200	30
29	3	95	1200	30
30	1	87	1200	30
31	3	84	1200	30
32	3	89	1200	30
33	3	89	1200	30
34	3	65	1200	30
35	3	67	1200	30
36	3	69	1200	30
37	3	80	1200	30
38	3	98	1200	30
39	3	65	1200	30
40	3	84	1200	30

[*]Percentage of value expected on the basis of age, sex, and height.
[†]'1' = low; '2' = medium; '3' = high.

$$\hat{\sigma}_z = \sqrt{\frac{y'-1}{y'}\left(\frac{\sum_{i=1}^{y}(z_i - \bar{z})^2}{y-1}\right)^{1/2}}$$

$$= \sqrt{\frac{840-1}{840}}\sqrt{\frac{81 - 79.11)^2 + \cdots + (84 - 79.11)^2}{28 - 1}}$$

$$= 12.55$$

$$\widehat{SE}(z/y) = \left(\frac{\hat{\sigma}_z}{\sqrt{y}}\right)\sqrt{\frac{y'-y}{y'-1}} = \left(\frac{12.55}{\sqrt{28}}\right)\sqrt{\frac{840 - 28}{840 - 1}} = 2.33$$

Thus we would estimate from this sample that there are a total of 840 workers having high exposure to pulmonary stressors, that their average fvc is 79.11% and that a 95% confidence interval for the estimated mean is

$$z/y - (1.96)[\widehat{SE}(z/y)] \leqslant \frac{Z}{Y} \leqslant z/y + (1.96)[\widehat{SE}(z/y)]$$

$$79.11 - (1.96)(2.33) \leqslant \frac{Z}{Y} \leqslant 79.11 + (1.96)(2.33)$$

$$74.54 \leqslant \frac{Z}{Y} \leqslant 83.69 \qquad \square$$

The statements that would be used to estimate the average fvc for each of the groups classified by exposure level are shown below from the STATA data file, *workers.dta*, that contains the data shown in Table 3.8:

```
use "a:\workers.dta", clear
.svyset fpc popsize
.svyset pweight wtl
.svymean fvc, by (exposure)
```

Note that the only two parameters required by STATA for a simple random sample are the total number of enumeration units, N (present for each record on the variable named *popsize*), and the sampling weight, N/n (present for each record on the variable named *wtl*). The statement, *svymean fvc, by (exposure)*, indicates that the estimation of the mean level of the variable, *fvc*, is to be performed separately for each exposure level. Differences between the confidence intervals shown below and those shown earlier are due to the fact that we based our confidence interval on the normal distribution (as has been done traditionally in finite population sampling), whereas STATA bases their confidence intervals on the Student's t-distribution with $n - 1$ degrees of freedom (in this instance with 39 degrees of freedom, the 97.5 percentile is 2.02, as compared to 1.96 for the normal distribution).

The resulting STATA output is shown below:

Survey mean estimation							
pweight:	wt1			Number of obs		=	40
Strata:	< one >			Number of strata		=	1
PSU:	< observations >			Number of PSUs		=	40
FPC:	popsize			Population size		=	1200
Mean Subpop	Estimate	Std. Err.	[95% Conf. Interval]			Deff	
fvc							
exposure = = 1	83.33333	5.177446	72.86096	93.80571		1	
exposure = = 2	83.5	4.110476	75.18578	91.81422		1	
exposure = = 3	79.10714	2.321226	74.41202	83.80227		1	

Finite population correction (FPC) assumes simple random sampling without replacement of PSUs within each stratum with no subsampling within PSUs.

3.7   HOW LARGE A SAMPLE DO WE NEED?

One of the most important problems in sample design is that of determining how large a sample is needed for the estimates obtained in the sample survey to be reliable enough to meet the objectives of the survey. In this section, we will formulate this problem in very general terms and then show how it may be solved for a particular sample design, for example, for simple random sampling of elementary units.

In determining sample size, the first step is to specify the level of reliability needed for the resulting estimates (see Section 2.4). In general, the larger the sample, the greater will be the reliability of the resulting estimates. Validity, on the other hand, is a function of the measurement process rather than the sample size and will not, in general, be improved with an increase in sample size. An improvement in validity requires an improvement in the measuring process.

In determining the level of reliability needed for estimates, the statisticians and subject matter persons should examine the objectives of the survey. For example, suppose that from a hospital admitting 20,000 patients annually, a survey of hospital patients is to be taken for the purpose of determining the proportion of the 20,000 patients that received optimal care as defined by specified standards. The quality care review committee planning the survey may feel that some remedial action should be taken if fewer than 80% of the patients are receiving optimal care. In this instance, the committee would be concerned about overestimates of the true proportion, but would probably not be too concerned if the estimated proportion were 80% when the true proportion were 75%. The statistician might formulate this by saying that the user would like to be "virtually certain" that the estimated proportion differs from the true proportion by no more than 100[80–75)/75]% or 6.67% of the true proportion.

Now let us see what is meant here by "virtual certainty." In terms of reliability, if we assume that the sample estimates are normally distributed with a mean equal to the unknown population estimate, we know that for approximately 997 of every 1000 samples, the true population parameter will lie within three standard errors of the estimate (see Figure 3.1). In terms of the example mentioned above, if p_y is the estimated proportion, P_y, is the true unknown population proportion, and $SE(p_y)$ is the standard error of p_y, we can be virtually certain that P_y is greater than $p_y - 3 \times SE(p_y)$ and less than $p_y + 3 \times SE(p_y)$. The statistician's problem, then, is to choose a sample large enough so that $3 \times SE(p_y) \leqslant .0667 \times P_y$ when P_y is approximately equal to .80 (see the next example).

As it is used here, "virtual certainty" is but one of the many potential levels of confidence that may be employed in the construction of confidence intervals and the determination of necessary sample sizes. This particular level of confidence need not always be used. However, "virtual certainty" along with "95% confidence" are the levels most frequently specified in the determination of sample sizes for sample surveys.

Illustrative Example. Let us suppose that our design uses a simple random sample of records from a hospital admitting 20,000 patients annually. From Box 3.2 we see that $3 \times SE(p_y)$ is given by

$$3 \times SE(p_y) = 3 \times \sqrt{\frac{P_y(1 - P_y)}{n}} \sqrt{\frac{N - n}{N - 1}}$$

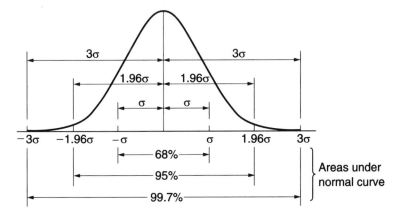

Figure 3.1 Areas under normal curve within ±1, ±1.96 and ±3 standard errors of the mean.

We want our sample large enough (see the discussion above) so that

$$3 \times \text{SE}(p_y) \leqslant .0667 P_y$$

or

$$3 \times \text{SE}(p_y) = 3 \times \sqrt{\frac{P_y(1 - P_y)}{n}} \sqrt{\frac{N - n}{N - 1}} \leqslant .0667 P_y$$

Solving this relation for n, we obtain

$$n \geqslant \frac{9 N P_y(1 - P_y)}{(N - 1)(.0667)^2 P_y^2 + 9 P_y(1 - P_y)}$$

Setting $P_y = .80$ and $N = 20,000$, we obtain $n \geqslant 494$. (It should be noted that in all sample size calculations the resulting value of n is rounded up to the nearest integer.) Thus, we need a sample of 494 patients or more to be virtually certain of obtaining estimates having the reliability required for meeting the objectives of the survey.   □

The example above can be generalized to any population proportion P_y under simple random sampling. If we wish to be virtually certain that the sample estimate p_y differs in absolute value from the true unknown proportion P_y by no more than εP_y, then the *sample size n* must satisfy the relation given by

$$n \geqslant \frac{9 N P_y(1 - P_y)}{(N - 1)\varepsilon^2 P_y^2 + 9 P_y(1 - P_y)}$$

The value of ε is set by the investigator to reflect the objectives of the survey.

If the population size N is very much greater than the required sample size n, the relation above can be approximated by the formula

$$n \geqslant \frac{9(1 - P_y)}{\varepsilon^2 P_y}$$

This relation shows that the required sample size depends on three factors: 9, ε^2, and $(1 - P_y)/P_y$. The factor 9 is the virtual certainty factor; the ε^2 factor represents the specifications set on our estimate in terms of the maximum relative difference allowed between it and the unknown true population proportion, P_y. The third factor $(1 - P_y)/P_y$ is the square of the coefficient of variation (or the relative variance) of the dichotomous variable (in this instance, receiving or not receiving optimal care) upon which the proportion,

P_y, is based. From the approximation formula for n we see that the more stringent (i.e., smaller) we make ε, the greater will be the sample size n.

The sample sizes required under simple random sampling for the estimation of population totals and means can be derived in a similar way and have similar forms to those shown above for proportions. The required sample sizes for totals, means, and proportions are summarized in Box 3.5. In this summary z is the *reliability coefficient*, which is based on the assumption that the sampling distribution of the particular estimate under consideration is normal. That is, for virtual certainty, $z = 3$. If 95% confidence is desired, z is 1.96.

With regard to the equations in Box 3.5, we note that parameters such as V_x^2, the rel–variance with respect to the distribution of a variable $\mathcal{X}$ in a population are generally *not known*. Thus, in order to calculate required sample sizes, statisticians must usually make educated guesses.

Illustrative Example. As another illustration of how sample size might be determined, let us suppose that a sample survey of retail pharmacies is to be conducted in a state that contains 2500 pharmacies. The purpose of the survey is to estimate the average retail price of 20 tablets of a commonly used vasodilator drug. An estimate is needed that is within 10% of the true value of the average retail price in the state. A list of all pharmacies is available and a simple random sample will be taken from that list. A phone survey of 20 of the $N = 1000$ pharmacies in another state showed an average price of $7.00 for the 20 tablets with a standard deviation of $1.40.

We can use information from the phone survey for purposes of estimating sample size for the proposed study. We estimate V_x^2 as*

$$\hat{V}_x^2 = \frac{\hat{\sigma}_x^2}{\bar{x}^2} = \frac{[(N-1)/N]s_x^2}{\bar{x}^2} = \frac{[999/1000](1.40)^2}{(7.00)^2} = .04$$

With $\varepsilon = .1$ and $N = 2500$, we obtain from the exact formula (3.15),

$$n = \frac{9(2500)(.04)}{9(.04) + 2499(.1)^2} = 35.5 \approx 36$$

Thus, a sample of 36 pharmacies is needed for purposes of this study. Note that the approximation $9V_x^2/\varepsilon^2$ would yield the same value of n. □

---

*The estimate of V_x^2 is derived as follows: $V_x^2 = \sigma_x^2/\bar{X}^2$ from Equation (2.7). Hence, $\hat{V}_x^2 = \hat{\sigma}_x^2/\hat{\bar{X}}^2$. But $\hat{\sigma}_x^2 = [(N-1)/N]s_x^2$ from Equation (2.16) and the estimate of $\bar{X}$ is $\bar{x}$. Thus, it follows that

$$\hat{V}_x^2 = \frac{\hat{\sigma}_x^2}{\hat{\bar{X}}^2} = \frac{[(N-1)/N]s_x^2}{\bar{x}^2}$$

BOX 3.5   EXACT AND APPROXIMATE SAMPLE SIZES REQUIRED UNDER SIMPLE RANDOM SAMPLING

	Exact	Approximate

Total, x'

$$n \geqslant \frac{z^2 N V_x^2}{z^2 V_x^2 + (N-1)\varepsilon^2} \qquad\qquad n \geqslant \frac{z^2 V_x^2}{\varepsilon^2} \qquad (3.14)$$

Mean, $\bar{x}$

$$n \geqslant \frac{z^2 N V_x^2}{z^2 V_x^2 + (N-1)\varepsilon^2} \qquad\qquad n \geqslant \frac{z^2 V_x^2}{\varepsilon^2} \qquad (3.15)$$

Proportion, p_y

$$n \geqslant \frac{z^2 N P_y(1-P_y)}{(N-1)\varepsilon^2 P_y^2 + z^2 P_y(1-P_y)} \qquad n \geqslant \frac{z^2(1-P_y)}{\varepsilon^2 P_y} \qquad (3.16)$$

In these equations z is the reliability coefficient (e.g., $z = 3$ for virtual certainty and $z = 1.96$ for a 95% confidence level), N is the population size, V_x^2 is the relative variance for the variable $\mathscr{X}$, ε is the value set by the investigator (i.e., the sample estimate $\hat{d}$ should not differ in absolute value from the true unknown population parameter d by more than εd), and P_y is the unknown population proportion.

In actual practice, one variable is rarely singled out as the basis for calculation of sample size. Usually several of the most important variables are chosen and sample sizes are calculated for each of these variables. The final sample size chosen might then be the largest of these calculated sample sizes. If funds are not available to take the largest of these calculated sample sizes, then, as a compromise measure, the median or mean of the calculated n's might be taken.

We also emphasize that the sample size selected to meet specifications for the reliability of an estimated characteristic in a population as a whole would not be large enough to estimate the characteristic in a subdomain of the population. For example, 500 individuals may be an adequate sample size to be virtually certain of estimating the prevalence of hypertension within 10% of the true prevalence in the population as a whole. But the estimated prevalence of hypertension in males based on the sample findings is not likely to be as reliable an estimate, since it is based on a sample size that is considerably smaller than 500. Thus, in calculating sample sizes, one should specify the particular subdomains or subgroups for which estimates are needed and the levels of reliability that are desired for the estimates in each subdomain.

3.8 WHY SIMPLE RANDOM SAMPLING IS RARELY USED

Simple random sampling is very important as a basis for development of the theory of sampling. Under simple random sampling any particular sample of n elements from a population of N elements can be chosen and, in addition, is as likely to be chosen as any other sample. In this sense, it is conceptually the simplest possible method, and hence it is one against which all other methods can be compared.

Although simple random sampling is conceptually simple, it can be expensive and often not feasible in practice since it requires that all elements be identified and labeled *prior* to the sampling. Often this prior identification is not possible, and hence a simple random sample of elements cannot be drawn.

Also, since a simple random sampling plan gives each possible sample of n units an equal chance of being selected, it may result in samples that are spread out over a large geographic area. Such a geographic distribution of the sample would be very costly to implement in situations where household interviews are required.

The fact that every element has an equal chance of being selected in the sample is likely to result in samples in which subdomains have representation in the sample in proportion to their distribution in the population. While this might be good for some types of surveys, it would not be good for those surveys in which interest is focused on subgroups that are composed of a small proportion of the population. For example, a simple random sample of households in Chicago is not likely to be an efficient design for estimating health behaviors among Chicago residents of Korean extraction.

In other words, even though it might be possible for a simple random sample of elements to be taken, there are other sampling methods which might be more appropriate for meeting the objectives of specific surveys. In the remainder of this book, we will discuss these other methods.

3.9 SUMMARY

In this chapter we introduced the concept of a simple random sample, and we noted its importance as the foundation of sampling theory. We presented general expressions for the mean, variance, standard error, coefficient of variation, and relative variance of estimated totals, means, and proportions under simple random sampling. We discussed the use of confidence intervals for purposes of evaluating the reliability of estimates for sample designs in general, and we illustrated their use for simple random sampling in particular. We showed how to estimate characteristics for subdomains when a simple random sample of the population as a whole has been drawn. We presented methodology for calculating the sample size required under simple random sampling for estimating population characteristics with specified reliability. Finally, we discussed the disadvantages of simple random sampling with respect to its often not being feasible, cost efficient, or appropriate when estimates of characteristics are required for subdomains that are composed of a relatively small proportion of the total population.

EXERCISES

3.1 From the data in Table 2.1, using simple random sampling, take ten different samples of six physicians. For each sample compute approximate 95% confidence intervals for the average number of household visits per physician. For how many of these calculated 95% confidence intervals is the true population mean $\bar{X}$ within the boundaries of the intervals? If this number is much higher or lower than expected, how do you explain it? (Start with the first random number in the upper left-hand corner of Table A.1 in the Appendix and read down the columns, going no further than row 35.)

3.2 How many simple random samples of 15 elements can be taken from a population containing 65 elements?

3.3 From the data in Table 3.8 estimate the proportion of all workers in the plant having a fvc less than 70% of that expected on the basis of age, sex, and height. Give a 95% confidence interval for this estimated proportion.

3.4 From the data in Table 3.8 on the workers having low or medium exposure to pulmonary stressors, estimate the proportion who have an fvc below 90% of that expected on the basis of age, sex and height. Give 95% confidence interval for this proportion.

3.5 From the data in Table 3.8 estimate the proportion of workers in the plant having low or medium exposure to pulmonary stressors. Give 95% confidence intervals for this estimated proportion.

3.6 A survey of workers is to be taken in a large plant that makes products similar to those made in the plant from which the data in Table 3.8 are obtained. The purposes of the survey are to estimate (a) the proportion of all workers having an fvc below 70% and (b) the mean fvc among all workers. Estimates are needed within 5% of the true value of the parameter being estimated. How large a sample of workers is required? The plant employs 5000 workers.

3.7 A community within a city contains 3000 households and 10,000 persons. For purposes of planning a community satellite to the local health department, it is desired to estimate the total number of physician visits made during a calendar year by members of the community. For this information to be useful, it should be accurate to within 10% of the true value. A small pilot survey of 10 households, conducted for purposes of gathering preliminary information, yielded the accompanying data on physician visits made during the previous calendar year. Using these data as preliminary information, determine the sample size needed to meet the specifications of the survey.

Household	No. of Persons in Household	No. of Physician Visits Per Person During Previous Year
1	3	4.0
2	6	4.5
3	2	8.0
4	5	3.4
5	2	0.5
6	3	7.0
7	4	8.5
8	2	6.0
9	6	4.0
10	4	7.5

3.8 A section of a random number table is reproduced here:

06	97	37	77
08	00	39	81
14	08	58	01
22	17	24	19
75	73	12	79
69	59	32	53
54	03	48	44

a. Starting with the first random number in the upper left-hand corner of this table and reading down the columns, select a sample of 6 of the 25 physicians listed in Table 2.1.

   b. Estimate the mean number $\bar{X}$ of houshold visits made by physicians in the population, and construct a 90% confidence interval for $\bar{X}$.

   c. Estimate the total number X of household visits made by the physicians in the population and construct a 95% confidence interval for X. How does this confidence interval compare to the one given in the Illustrative Example in Section 3.5?

   d. Estimate with virtual certainty, the proportion of physicians in the population making two or more household visits per year.

3.9 A community in the San Francisco Bay area consists of approximately 50,000 persons, of whom approximately 40% are Caucasians, 25% are African American, 20% are Hispanic, and 15% are Asian. It is desired to estimate in this community, the proportion of persons who are not covered by some form of health insurance. One would like to be 95% certain that this estimate is within 15% of the true proportion, which is believed to lie somewhere between 10% and 20% of the total population. Assuming simple random sampling, how large a sample is needed?

3.10 In the previous example, if a simple random sample of the entire population is to be taken, how large a sample is required in order to be 95% certain of estimating within 10% of the true value, the proportion of the Asian population not covered by some form of health insurance (again assuming that the true value lies between 10% and 20%).

3.11 A city contains 20 neighborhood health clinics and it is desired to take a sample of 5 of these clinics for purposes of estimating the total number of persons from all these clinics who had been given, during the past 12 month period, prescriptions for a recently approved antidepressant drug. If one assumes that the mean number of patients seen at these clinics is 1500 per year with the standard deviation of this distribution among clinics being equal to 300, and that approximately 5% of all patients regardless of clinic are given this drug, is a simple random sample of 5 of these clinics likely to yield an estimate that is within 20% of the true value?

3.12 A company containing 700 employees is planning to test employees for working under the influence of illicit drugs (e.g., cannabis, cocaine). During the course of a year, a sample of 3 days will be selected for testing, and on each of these days, a simple random sample of 50 employees will be selected to be tested. Employees will *not* be excluded from being tested on the second or third testing date even if they had been tested on previous occasions. If an employee is always working under the influence of cocaine, what is his/her chances of being detected in this testing program (assume that anyone under the influence of one of the illicit drugs who is sampled and tested will have a positive test for that drug)?

3.13 In the previous exercise, what is the employee's chance of being detected if he/she is "under the influence" on the job only 10% of the time?

BIBLIOGRAPHY

The "classic" sampling texts listed below all give very complete discussions of simple random sampling.

1. Cochran, W. G., *Sampling Techniques*, 3rd ed., Wiley, New York, 1977.

2. Hansen, M. H., Hurwitz, W. N., and Madow, W. G., *Sample Survey Methods and Theory*, Vols. 1 and 2, Wiley, New York, 1953.

3. Kish, L., *Survey Sampling*, Wiley, New York, 1965.

The other sampling texts referenced in the previous chapters all develop the concepts of simple random sampling, each in its own way. The following articles in the Encyclopedia of Biostatistics *also treat various aspects of simple random sampling.*

4. Xia, Z., Sampling with and without replacement. In *The Encyclopedia of Biostatistics*, P. A. Armitage and T. Colton, Eds., Wiley, Chichester, U.K., 1998.

5. Levy, P. S., Simple random sampling. In *The Encyclopedia of Biostatistics*, Armitage, P. A., and Colton, T., Eds., Wiley, Chichester, U.K., 1998.

6. Levy, P. S., Design effect. In *The Encyclopedia of Biostatistics*, Armitage, P. A., and Colton, T., Eds., Wiley, Chichester, U.K., 1998.

The software package, SAMPLE, originally developed as a module for Version 5.0 of the general-purpose statistical package, SYSTAT, is a very useful program for selecting samples from a wide variety of commonly used designs, including simple random sample. Later versions of SYSTAT, however, no longer support this module.

7. Frankel, M. R., and Spencer, B.D., *SAMPLE: A Supplementary Module for SYSTAT*, SYSTAT Inc., Evanston, Ill., 1990.

Within the SAS system, algorithms are proposed for taking simple random samples with and without replacement. These are discussed in Chapter 12 of the following reference.

8. SAS Institute Inc., *SAS^R Language and Procedures: Usage 2, Version 6*, 1st ed., SAS Institute Inc., Cary, N.C., 1991.

In our discussion of software for obtaining estimates and their standard errors from sample survey data, we mentioned the software packages: STATA, SUDAAN, WESVAR, and PC CARP. References to these are listed below:

9. STATA Corporation, *STATA Technical Bulletin STB-31*, STATA Corporation, College Station, Tex., 1996.

10. Shah, B. V., Barnwell, B. G., and Bieler, G.S., *SUDAAN User's Manual, Version 6.4*, 2nd Ed., Research Triangle Institute, Research Triangle Park, N.C., 1996.

11. Brick, J. M., Broene, P., James, P., and Severynse, J., *A User's Guide to WesVarPC*, Westat, Inc., Rockville, Md., 1996.

12. Fuller, W. A., Kennedy, W., Schell, D., Sullivan, G., and Park, H. J., *PC CARP*, Statistical Laboratory, Iowa State University, Ames, Iowa, 1989.

EPI INFO, a PC software package in the public domain, was written for applied epide-miologists and has word processing, database, and statistical analysis modules. It has a module, CSAMPLE, that has the capability of producing estimates and their standard errors from survey data having a variety of sample designs. At the time of this writing, it is in Version 6.

13. Dean, A. G., Dean, J. A., Coulombier, D., Brendel, K. A., Smith, D. C., Burton, A. H., Dicker, R. C., Sullivan, K., Fagan, R. F., and Arner, T G., *Epi Info, Version 6: A Word Processing, Database, and Statistics Program for Epidemiology on Microcomputers*, Centers for Disease Control and Prevention, Atlanta, Ga., 1994.

The article listed below reviews several software packages that can analyze data from sample surveys, including the programs listed above.

14. Carlson, B. L., Software for the statistical analysis of sample survey data. In *The Encyclopedia of Biostatistics*, Armitage, P. A., and Colton, T. Eds., Wiley, Chichester, U.K., 1998.

The books listed below treat sample-size requirements for a wide variety of estimation and hypothesis testing scenarios, including finite-population sampling.

15. Lemeshow, S., Hosmer, D. W., Klar, J., and Lwanga, S. K., *Adequacy of Sample Size in Health Studies*, Wiley, Chichester, U.K., 1990.

16. Lwanga, S. K., and Lemeshow, S., *Sample Size Determination in Health Studies*, World Health Organization, Geneva, Switzerland, 1991.

The software program listed below includes algorithms for estimation of sample size for simple random sampling from a finite population.

17. Elashoff, J. D., *nQuery Advisor[R] Version 2.0 User's Guide*, Statistical Solutions Ltd., Cork, Ireland, 1997.

CHAPTER 4

Systematic Sampling

In the previous chapter, we introduced the concept of simple random sampling of elements and discussed its importance as being "conceptually" the simplest kind of sampling since every possible combination of n elements from a population of N elements has the same chance of being selected. We also discussed some of the problems associated with simple random sampling, including difficulties that may preclude drawing a sample by that method. In this chapter we discuss a type of sampling known as systematic sampling. Systematic sampling is widely used in practice because it is easy to apply and can be easily taught to individuals who have little training in survey methodology. In fact, systematic sampling, either by itself or in combination with some other method, may be the most widely used method of sampling.

4.1 HOW TO TAKE A SYSTEMATIC SAMPLE

Perhaps the best way to describe the procedure of systematic sampling is through an example. The next illustration serves as an introduction to this important sampling method.

Illustrative Example. Let us suppose that as part of a cost-containment and quality-of-care review program, a sample of inpatient medical records is selected on an ongoing basis for a detailed audit. The total number of records in the population is not likely to be known in advance of the sampling since the records are to be sampled on an ongoing basis, and so, it would not be possible to use simple random sampling to choose the records. However, it may be possible to guess the approximate number of records that would be available for selection per time period and to select a sample of one in every k records as they become available, where k is an integer having a particular value chosen to meet the requirements of the study.

For example, suppose it is anticipated that there will be available ten new discharge records per day and that a total sample of 300 records per year is desired. Then the total number of records available per year is estimated to be $10 \times 365 = 3650$. To obtain something in the neighborhood of 300 records per year in the sample, k should be the largest integer in the quotient $3650/300$. Since the value of the quotient is 12.17, k would be equal to 12. This value of k is known as the *sampling interval*. Thus, we would take a sample of 1 from every 12 records.

One way to implement this procedure is to identify each record as it is created with a consecutive number beginning with 1. (There are stamping devices that can do this easily). At the beginning of the study, a random number between 1 and 12 is chosen as the starting point. Then, that record and every twelfth record beyond it would be chosen. For example, if the random number is 4, then the records chosen in the sample would be 4, 16, 28, 40, 52, and so on.   □

To generalize, a systematic sample is taken by first determining the desired sampling interval k, choosing a random number j between 1 and k, and selecting the elements labeled $j, j + k, j + 2k, j + 3k \ldots$. Note that the sampling fraction for such a survey is $1/k$.

A slight modification of this method based on the decimal system is especially useful if the elements to be sampled are already numbered consecutively and if the actual drawing of the sample is to be done by unskilled personnel. If a sample of 1 in k units is specified (where k is, for example, a two-digit number), we may select a random two-digit number between 01 and k. If the number selected is j, then the two-digit numbers $j, j + k, j + 2k$, and so on, are selected until a three-digit number is reached. All elements ending in the two-digit numbers selected are then included in the sample. For example, if $k = 12$, a random two-digit number between 01 and 12 is chosen (e.g., 07). The two-digit sample numbers are then determined (e.g., 07, 19, 31, 43, 55, 67, 79, and 91), and all records ending with these two digits would be included in the sample (e.g., 07, 19, 31, 43, 55, 67, 79, 91, 107, 119, 131, 143, 155, 167, 179, 191, 207, 219, 231, etc.). This procedure is sometimes easier to use than the first procedure mentioned, especially if the individuals drawing the sample are unskilled, since they could be instructed to pull only those records ending with the specified digits. Our discussion of the properties of estimates from systematic random samples, however, will be based on the first method described.

Systematic samples can be taken easily from data files that are on a computer. The module, *SAMPLE*, in the statistical package, *SYSTAT*, can take a systematic sample of either a fixed number, n, or a fixed proportion, r, of records using a sampling procedure that is a modification of that described above [1].

4.2 ESTIMATION OF POPULATION CHARACTERISTICS

If a systematic sample of 1 in k elements yields a sample of n elements, then the *sample total*, x', the *sample mean*, $\bar{x}$, and the *sample proportion*, p_y, are calculated from the sample in the same manner as they were calculated for simple random sampling (see Box 3.1). The *estimated population total* x' for systematic sampling is given by

$$x' = \left(\frac{N}{n}\right)x \qquad (4.1)$$

and when $k = N/n$ is an integer, we have

$$x' = kx$$

It is not necessary that N be known prior to the sampling (as is the case when every kth person entering an emergency room is selected), N can be determined by counting the number of elements remaining after the last one is chosen and adding that remainder to nk.

Let us illustrate these ideas with an example.

Illustrative Example. Let us take a systematic random sample of one in six physicians from the list given in Table 2.1. We first take a random number between 1 and 6: for example, we choose 5. The physicians selected in the sample then are 5, 11, 17, and 23. The corresponding values of $\mathscr{X}$, the number of household visits, are shown in Table 4.1.

The estimated mean number $\bar{x}$ of household visits per physician is

$$\bar{x} = \frac{x}{n} = \frac{14}{4} = 3.5$$

The estimated total number x' of visits made by all the physicians in the population is

Table 4.1 Systematic Sample of One in Six Physicians (from Table 2.1)

Sample Number (i)	Physician Number	No. of Visits (x_i)
1	5	7
2	11	0
3	17	7
4	23	0
Total		14

$$x' = \left(\frac{N}{n}\right)x = \left(\frac{25}{4}\right)14 = 87.5$$

The estimated proportion p_y of physicians making one or more household visits is

$$p_y = \frac{y}{n} = \frac{2}{4} = .50$$

$\square$

Estimates of totals, means, and proportions along with estimates of their variances and standard errors are given for systematic sampling in Box 4.1. If the population N is known, then these expressions do not differ from those given for simple random sampling (see Box 3.1). The properties of these estimates under systematic sampling will be discussed in the next two sections. We will see that these expressions are appropriate only if there is no relationship between the variable being estimated and the ordering of the sampling frame from which the systematic sample is taken.

4.3 SAMPLING DISTRIBUTION OF ESTIMATES

In a simple random sample of n elements from a population containing N elements, every one of the $\binom{N}{n}$ total samples not only has a chance of being selected but also has the *same* chance of being selected. In a systematic sample of 1 in k elements, there are only k possible samples, and the particular sample selected depends on the random number initially selected.

Let us compare these two sampling methods in a specific example.

Illustrative Example.   Suppose that, from the listing in Table 2.1, a sample of one in five physicians is desired. The five possible samples are listed in Table 4.2 along with estimates $\bar{x}$, x', and p_y of the population parameters $\bar{X}$, X, and P_y. Since each of the five possible samples listed in Table 4.2 has the same chance, namely, 1/5, of being selected, the mean, $E(\bar{x})$, of the sampling distribution of the estimated mean is (see Box 2.3)

$$E(\bar{x}) = \left(\frac{1}{5}\right)(2.6 + 4.8 + 1.4 + 9.2 + 7.4) = 5.08 = \bar{X}$$

In other words, $\bar{x}$ is an unbiased estimate of $\bar{X}$. Similarly,

---

BOX 4.1 ESTIMATED TOTALS, MEANS, AND VARIANCES UNDER SYSTEMATIC SAMPLING, AND ESTIMATED VARIANCES AND STANDARD ERRORS OF THESE ESTIMATES*

Estimate	Estimated Variance and Standard Error of Estimate

Total

x' $\dfrac{N}{n}\sum\limits_{i=1}^{n} x_i$

$$\hat{Var}(x') = N^2 \left(\frac{N-n}{N}\right)\left(\frac{s_x^2}{n}\right)$$

$$\hat{SE}(x') = N\sqrt{\frac{N-n}{N}}\left(\frac{s_x}{\sqrt{n}}\right)$$

Mean

$\bar{x}$ $\dfrac{\sum\limits_{i=1}^{n} x_i}{n}$

$$\hat{Var}(\bar{x}) = \left(\frac{N-n}{N}\right)\left(\frac{s_x^2}{n}\right)$$

$$\hat{SE}(\bar{x}) = \sqrt{\frac{N-n}{N}}\left(\frac{s_x}{\sqrt{n}}\right)$$

Proportion

p_y $\dfrac{\sum\limits_{i=1}^{n} y_i}{n}$

$$\hat{Var}(p_y) = \left(\frac{N-n}{N}\right)\frac{p_y(1-p_y)}{n-1}$$

$$\hat{SE}(p_y) = \sqrt{\frac{N-n}{N}}\sqrt{\frac{p_y(1\ p_y)}{n-1}}$$

where y is a dichotomous variable having values 0 or 1.

The sampling interval, k, can be substituted for N/n, and kn can be substituted for N in those situations where the number, N, of elements in the population cannot be determined.

*Note: Estimated variances and standard errors may be seriously biased under certain conditions noted above.

$$E(x') = \left(\frac{1}{5}\right)(65 + 120 + 35 + 230 + 185) = 127 = X.$$

$$E(p_y) = \left(\frac{1}{5}\right)(.4 + .6 + .4 + .8 + .6) = .56 = P_y$$

Table 4.2   Five Possible Samples of One in Five Physicians Chosen from Table 2.1

Random Number Chosen (Physician in Sample)	Estimated Mean (Total) [Proportion]
1 (1, 6, 11, 16, 21)	2.6 (65) [.4]
2 (2, 7, 12, 17, 22)	4.8 (120) [.6]
3 (3, 8, 13, 18, 23)	1.4 (35) [.4]
4 (4, 9, 14, 19, 24)	9.2 (230) [.8]
5 (5, 10, 15, 20, 25)	7.4 (185) [.6]

Thus we see that in this instance the estimated mean, total, and proportion are unbiased estimates of the corresponding population parameters.

The standard errors of $\bar{x}$, x', and p_y are given next (see Box 2.3).

$$
\begin{aligned}
\text{SE}(\bar{x}) &= \sqrt{\frac{1}{5}\sum[\bar{x} - E(\bar{x})]^2} \\
&= \left\{\frac{1}{5}[(2.6 - 5.08)^2 + (4.8 - 5.08)^2 + (1.4 - 5.08)^2 + (9.2 - 5.08)^2 \right. \\
&\quad \left. + (7.4 - 5.08)^2]\right\}^{1/2} = 2.90
\end{aligned}
$$

$$
\begin{aligned}
\text{SE}(x') &= \sqrt{\frac{1}{5}\sum[x' - E(x')]^2} \\
&= \left\{\frac{1}{5}[(65 - 127)^2 + (120 - 127)^2 + (35 - 127)^2 + (230 - 127)^2 \right. \\
&\quad \left. + (185 - 127)^2]\right\}^{1/2} = 72.57
\end{aligned}
$$

$$SE(p_y) = \sqrt{\frac{1}{5}\sum[p_y - E(p_y)]^2}$$
$$= \left\{\frac{1}{5}[(.4 - .56)^2 + (.6 - .56)^2 + (.4 - .56)^2 + (.8 - .56)^2 \right.$$
$$\left. + (.6 - .56)^2]\right\}^{1/2} = .15$$

The means and standard errors of $\bar{x}$, x', and p_y in this example are compared in Table 4.3 to the means and standard errors that would have been obtained under simple random sampling. Examining the table, we see that for both sampling schemes the estimates are unbiased. However, the standard errors of the estimates are not the same. In fact, in this example, the systematic sampling standard errors are smaller than those for simple random sampling. □

In general, the estimated mean, total, and proportion under systematic sampling as described above are unbiased estimates of the corresponding population parameters only if the ratio N/k is an integer. In the previous example, $N = 25$, $k = 5$, and hence, $N/k = 25/5$, which is an integer. Thus, as was shown above, $\bar{x}$, x', and p_y are unbiased estimates.

If, on the other hand, N/k is not an integer, then the systematic sample estimates may be biased. Let us explore this situation in an example.

Illustrative Example.   Suppose we specify a one in six systematic sample of physicians from the list in Table 2.1. Then we would have the possible samples shown in Table 4.4. Since each of the six possible samples is equally likely, the means of the sampling distributions of $\bar{x}$, x', and p_y are

Table 4.3   Comparison of Means and Standard Errors for Simple Random Sampling and for Systematic Sampling*

	Estimate	$\bar{x}$	x'	p_y
Mean				
	Simple random sampling	5.08	127	.56
	Systematic sampling	5.08	127	.56
Standard error				
	Simple random sampling	3.36	84.11	.20
	Systematic sampling	2.90	72.57	.15

*$n = 5$ in all instances.

Table 4.4   Possible Samples of One in Six Physicians Chosen (from Table 2.1)

Random Number Chosen (Physicians in Sample)	Estimated Mean (Total) [Proportion]
1 (1, 7, 13, 19, 25)	12.0 (300) [.8]
2 (2, 8, 14, 20)	1.0 (25) [.25]
3 (3, 9, 15, 21)	4.25 (106.25) [.75]
4 (4, 10, 16, 22)	6.5 (162.5) [.5]
5 (5, 11, 17, 23)	3.5 (87.5) [.5]
6 (6, 12, 18, 24)	1.5 (37.5) [.5]

$$E(\bar{x}) = \frac{1}{6}(12 + 1 + 4.25 + 6.5 + 3.5 + 1.5) = 4.79 \neq \bar{X}$$

$$E(x') = \frac{1}{6}(300 + 25 + 106.25 + 162.5 + 87.5 + 37.5) = 119.79 \neq X$$

$$E(p_y) = \frac{1}{6}(.8 + .25 + .75 + .5 + .5 + .5) = .55 \neq P_y$$

Thus we see that in this instance systematic sampling does not lead to unbiased estimates.   □

The reason the estimates in the preceding example are not unbiased is that although each element has the same chance (e.g., $1/k$) of being selected, the impact made on the estimates is not the same for each element. Physician 1, for example, has less impact than physician 2 since physician 1 appears with four other physicians in the sample, whereas physician 2 appears in the sample with only three other physicians. Thus, physician 1's measurements are diluted more than those of physician 2 in obtaining the estimate. In the previous example, when N/k was an integer, each physician appeared with the same number of other physicians in the sample, and all physicians had the same impact on the resulting estimates.

If the number of elements N in the population is large, the biases in the estimates from systematic samples will, in general, be quite small and will be of little concern. A slight modification of the method of choosing the initial random number, however, will result in estimates that are unbiased. This modification will be discussed later in this chapter (Section 4.5).

4.4 VARIANCE OF ESTIMATES

Let us now consider the variances of estimates from systematic sampling. As discussed earlier, the variance of an estimate is important because it is a measure of the reliability of the estimate.

In the discussion of variances of estimates from systematic sampling, let us assume for simplicity that N/k is an integer denoted by n. Systematic sampling of one in k elements would then yield a total of k possible samples, each containing N/k elements. The possible samples are shown in Table 4.5.

In examining the systematic samples shown in Table 4.5, we see that each sample is a "cluster" of n (equal to N/k) elements with the elements being k "units" apart from each other. Thus, systematic sampling is operationally equivalent to grouping the N elements into k clusters, each containing N/k elements that are k units apart on the list, and then taking a random sample of one of these clusters. To illustrate this idea, let us look at an example.

Illustrative Example. Let us suppose that a systematic sample of one in five workers from Table 3.8 is taken. For purposes of illustration the 40 workers in Table 3.8 will be considered to be a population rather than a sample from a larger population. Then $N = 40$, $k = 5$, and $N/k = n = 40/5 = 8$. The five clusters defined by the sampling design are shown in Table 4.6. These clusters represent the five possible samples of one in five workers chosen from the list in Table 3.8. □

Table 4.5   Possible Samples of 1 in k Elements (N/k Is an Integer)

Random Number Chosen	Elements in Sample	Value of Variable $\mathcal{X}$
1	$1, 1 + k, 1 + 2k, \ldots, 1 + (n-1)k$	$X_1, X_{1+k} X_{1+2k}, \ldots, X_{1+(n-1)k}$
2	$2, 2 + k, 2 + 2k, \ldots, 2 + (n-1)k$	$X_2, X_{2+k}, \ldots, X_{2+(n-1)k}$
$\vdots$		
j	$j, j + k, j + 2k, j + (n-1)k$	$X_j, X_{j+k}, X_{j+2k}, \ldots, X_{j+(n-1)k}$
k	$k, 2k, 3k, \ldots, nk$	$X_k, X_{2k}, X_{3k}, \ldots, X_{nk}$

Table 4.6   Cluster Samples Based on Data of Table 3.8

Cluster	Workers in Cluster	Forced Vital Capacity of Workers in Cluster
1	1, 6, 11, 16, 21, 26, 31, 36	81, 97, 71, 76, 70, 96, 84, 69
2	2, 7, 12, 17, 22, 27, 32, 37	64, 82, 88, 62, 64, 62, 89, 80
3	3, 8, 13, 18, 23, 28, 33, 38	85, 99, 84, 67, 72, 67, 89, 98
4	4, 9, 14, 19, 24, 29, 34, 39	91, 96, 85, 91, 72, 95, 65, 65
5	5, 10, 15, 20, 25, 30, 35, 40	60, 91, 77, 99, 95, 87, 67, 84

The variance of estimates from systematic sampling can be understood more easily if we label the elements with double subscripts to denote the particular cluster. For example, the elements in the first cluster, elements 1, $1 + k$, $1 + 2k, \ldots,$ $1 + (n - 1)k$ would be relabeled with double subscripts as follows:

Original Label	New Label	Value of Variable $\mathscr{X}$
1	$1,1$	X_{11}
$1 + k$	$1,2$	X_{12}
$1 + 2k$	$1,3$	X_{13}
$1 + (n - 1)k$	$1, n$	X_{1n}

The elements in the jth cluster would be relabled similarly:

Original Label	New Label	Value of Variable $\mathscr{X}$
j	$j, 1$	X_{j1}
$j + k$	$j, 2$	X_{j2}
$j + 2k$	$j, 3$	X_{j3}
$j + (n - 1)k$	j, n	X_{jn}

With this new labeling, the variances of estimated means, totals, and proportions obtained from systematic sampling are given in Box 4.2.

The expressions shown in Box 4.2 are equal to those of estimates obtained from simple random sampling multiplied by the factor $[1 + \delta_x(n - 1)]$. The parameter δ_x is called the *intraclass correlation coefficient* and is a measure of the homogeneity of elements *within* the k possible systematic samples, or clusters, that could theoretically have been selected from a population of $N = nk$ elements. Calculation of δ_x involves, for each cluster, the establishing of $\binom{n}{2}$ pairs of values (X_{ij}, X_{il}), which play the same role as do the pairs (X, Y) in the usual product moment correlation coefficient. The difference is that deviations are computed about $(\bar{X}, \bar{X})$ where $\bar{X}$ is the mean of the X_{ij} over *all* observations in all possible systematic samples (i.e., the population mean). The summation in the numerator of Equation (4.5) involves the cross product

---

BOX 4.2   VARIANCES OF POPULATION ESTIMATES UNDER SYSTEMATIC SAMPLING

Total, x'

$$\text{Var}(x') = \left(\frac{N^2\sigma_x^2}{n}\right)[1 + \delta_x(n-1)] \tag{4.2}$$

Mean, $\bar{x}$

$$\text{Var}(\bar{x}) = \left(\frac{\sigma_x^2}{n}\right)[1 + \delta_x(n-1)] \tag{4.3}$$

Proportion, p_y

$$\text{Var}(p_y) = \left(\frac{P_y(1-P_y)}{n}\right)[1 + \delta_x(n-1)] \tag{4.4}$$

where $n = N/k$ and

$$\delta_x = \frac{2\sum_{i=1}^{k}\sum_{j=1}^{n}\sum_{l<j}(X_{ij}-\bar{X})(X_{il}-\bar{X})}{nk(n-1)\sigma_x^2} \tag{4.5}$$

In these equations, N is the population size, n is the sample size, k is the sampling interval, X_{ij} is the jth element from the ith cluster, X_{il} is another element from the ith cluster ($l \neq j$), and the population notation is as defined in Box 2.1

---

of these deviations over all pairs of points for each of the k possible systematic samples. This intraclass correlation coefficient can range from very small negative values, when the elements within each cluster tend to be very diverse or representative of the population of elements (this is called "heterogeneity"), to a maximum of unity when the elements within each cluster are similar but different from elements in other clusters (this is called "homogeneity").

It is clear from expressions (4.2), (4.3) and (4.4) that when δ_x is large, the variance of the total, mean, or the proportion will be large. This can occur when the population's elements are arranged in a list demonstrating a high degree of periodicity. When δ_x equals zero, the resulting variances are the same as those of simple random sampling. This usually occurs when the population's elements are arranged in random order with respect to the variable under consideration.

Finally, when δ_x is small and negative, the resulting variances will be smaller than those of simple random sampling. This can occur when the elements in the population are ordered with respect to the variable under study.

Let us now see what this all means by considering an example.

Illustrative Example. Suppose that a list of appointments for a nurse practitioner is available to us and that we will take a sample of one in four of the patients seen by this nurse on a given day for purposes of estimating the average time spent per patient. Suppose that on the day in which the sample was to be taken, the nurse saw a total of 12 patients in the order shown in Table 4.7.

Since we specify a one in four sample, the four possible samples are shown in Table 4.8.

The mean time $\bar{X}$ spent with the 12 patients is 29.583 min (minutes) with variance $\sigma_x^2 = 153.08$. The variance over all possible samples of the estimated mean time spent per patient is (see Box 2.3)

$$\text{Var}(\bar{x}) = \frac{1}{4}[(17 - 29.583)^2 + (32.33 - 29.583)^2 + (39 - 29.583)^2 + (30 - 29.583)^2] = 63.6$$

Table 4.7   Data for Nurse Practitioner's Visits (Unordered List)

Order of Visit	Time Spent with Patient (min.)	Order of Visit	Time Spent with Patient (min.)
1	15	7	49
2	34	8	40
3	35	9	25
4	36	10	46
5	11	11	33
6	17	12	14

Table 4.8   Four Possible Samples for Data of Table 4.7

Patient	Time Spent (min.)	Patient	Time Spent (min.)	Patient	Time Spent (min.)	Patient	Time Spent (min.)
1	15	2	34	3	35	4	36
5	11	6	17	7	49	8	40
9	25	10	46	11	33	12	14
Total	51		97		117		90
Mean	17		32.33		39		30

To show that this is equal to the expression given in relation (4.3), we will compute the necessary parameters. The intraclass correlation coefficient is (from Box 4.2)

$$\delta_x = \frac{\begin{matrix}2[(15 - 29.583)(11 - 29.583) + (15 - 29.583)(25 - 29.583) \\ + (11 - 29.583)(25 - 29.583) + (34 - 29.583)(17 - 29.583) \\ + \cdots + (40 - 29.583)(14 - 29.583)]\end{matrix}}{3 \times 4 \times (3 - 1) \times 153.08}$$

$$= .1241$$

Then, from Equation (4.3) with $\sigma_x^2 = 153.08$, $n = 3$, and $\delta_x = .1241$, we have

$$\mathrm{Var}(\bar{x}) = \left(\frac{153.08}{3}\right)[1 + .1241(3 - 1)] = 63.6$$

which agrees with what was found empirically.

Suppose now that the nurse scheduled appointments in such a way that the difficult patients requiring the most time would be seen first and the easier ones requiring less time would be seen later in the day. The list of appointments for the same patients discussed above might appear as shown in Table 4.9.

If we were to take a systematic sample of one in four patients from the list of appointments in Table 4.9, we would obtain the four possible samples shown in Table 4.10.

Since the procedure by which the sample was taken is a systematic sample of one in four elements, and since $N/k = 12/4 = 3$ is an integer, the sample mean is, as before, an unbiased estimate of the population mean; that is, $E(\bar{x}) = \bar{X} = 29.583$. The variance of the estimated mean $\bar{x}$ is

Table 4.9   Data for Nurse Practitioner's Visits (Monotonically Ordered List)

Order of Visit	Time Spent with Patient (min.)	Order of Visit	Time Spent with Patient (min.)
1	49	7	33
2	46	8	25
3	40	9	17
4	36	10	15
5	35	11	14
6	34	12	11

Table 4.10   Four Possible Samples for Data of Table 4.9

Sample 1		Sample 2		Sample 3		Sample 4	
Patient	Time Spent (min.)	Patient	Time Spent (min.)	Patient	Time Spent (min.)	Patient	Time Spent (min.)
1	49	2	46	3	40	4	36
5	35	6	34	7	33	8	25
9	17	10	15	11	14	12	11
Total	101		95		87		72
Mean	33.67		31.67		29		24

$$\text{Var}(\bar{x}) = \left(\frac{1}{4}\right)[(33.67 - 29.583)^2 + (31.67 - 29.583)^2$$
$$+ (29 - 29.583)^2 + (24 - 29.583)^2]$$
$$= 13.13$$

Thus we see that in this situation — when the list of appointments is ordered — the systematic sampling procedure yields an estimated mean having a lower variance than that obtained from the same systematic sampling procedure when the list was not ordered. This makes sense intuitively, because the process of sampling systematically from a list that is ordered according to the level of the variable being measured ensures that every sample will have some elements having high values of the variable, some having low values, and some having moderate values. In other words, it would not be possible for any one particular sample to have a concentration of atypically high or atypically low values.

The intraclass correlation coefficient in this instance is equal to −.371, which is a negative number and considerably lower than that obtained when the sampling was from the unordered list.

Let us now suppose that the nurse scheduled an easy patient followed by two moderately difficult patients followed by a very difficult patient (in terms of time required). The appointment list containing the same 12 patients might then appear as shown in Table 4.11.

If we were to sample systematically one in four patients from the list in Table 4.11, we would obtain the four possible samples listed in Table 4.12.

Again, the estimated mean is an unbiased estimate of the population mean. The variance of the distribution of estimated means is

$$\text{Var}(\bar{x}) = \left(\frac{1}{4}\right)[(13.33 - 29.583)^2 + (25.33 - 29.583)^2 + (34.67 - 29.583)^2$$
$$+ (45 - 29.583)^2] = 136.41$$

Table 4.11 Data for Nurse Practitioner's Visits (Periodicity in List)

Order of Visit	Time Spent with Patient (min.)	Order of Visit	Time Spent with Patient (min.)
1	11	7	35
2	17	8	46
3	36	9	15
4	49	10	25
5	14	11	33
6	34	12	40

Table 4.12 Four Possible Samples for Data of Table 4.11

Patient	Time Spent	Patient	Time Spent	Patient	Time Spent	Patient	Time Spent
1	11	2	17	3	36	4	49
5	14	6	34	7	35	8	46
9	15	10	25	11	33	12	40
Total	40		76		104		135
Mean	13.33		25.33		34.67		45

The intraclass correlation coefficient, δ_x, in this situation is equal to .837. Thus, in this situation, the estimated mean has a much larger variance than it had previously. The results we have obtained are summarized in Table 4.13

In the third systematic sampling situation — namely that in which the nurse scheduled an easy patient followed by two moderately difficult patients followed by a very difficult one, in a continuing pattern — the variance of the estimated mean was very high. The reason for this high variance is that the nurses scheduling pattern involved a 1 in 4 periodicity that coincided with the periodicity in the sample selection, with the result that all the difficult patients were in the same sample and all the easy ones were in the same sample. Thus

Table 4.13 Summary of Results for Four Types of Sampling

Sample Design	Var($\bar{x}$)	Intraclass Correlation Coefficient
Systematic sampling: unordered list	63.6	.124
Systematic sampling: monotonically ordered list	13.1	−.371
Systematic sampling: periodicity in list	136.4	.837
Simple random sampling	41.7	—

the sampling variability of estimated means was very high. This high variance contrasted with the low variance found when the appointments were made in order of increasing difficulty. As noted before, systematic sampling of this ordered list resulted in every possible sample having its share of difficult, moderate, and easy patients, so that the samples did not differ very much in the distribution of the variable being measured.   □

To generalize, systematic sampling from a list that is ordered in the variable being measured often results in estimates having small sampling variance. On the other hand, if the list has periodicities in it that coincide with the periodicity in the sampling, the estimates could have very high sampling variance and the survey estimates would have little relation to the corresponding population parameters.

When a list is in "random order" — that is, there is no particular ordering or periodicity in the list — the variance in the estimated total, mean, or proportion obtained in systematic sampling is approximately that appropriate for simple random sampling. In other words,

$$\text{Var}(x') \approx \left(\frac{N^2}{n}\right)(\sigma_x^2)\left(\frac{N-n}{N-1}\right)$$

$$\text{Var}(\bar{x}) \approx \left(\frac{\sigma_x^2}{n}\right)\left(\frac{N-n}{N-1}\right)$$

$$\text{Var}(p_y) \approx \left[\frac{P_y(1-P_y)}{n}\right]\left[\frac{N-n}{N-1}\right]$$

Note that in the previous example the intraclass correlation coefficient, δ_x, was highest in the situation in which there was a periodicity in the list. The result is understandable in light of the fact that δ_x measures homogeneity of elements with respect to the variable being measured. When the periodicity in the nurse's appointment list coincided with the periodicity in the sampling interval (e.g., when $k = 4$), all the difficult patients were in one sample and all the easy ones in another. This situation produced a homogeneity of patients within the same cluster, large differences between patients in different samples, a high intraclass correlation coefficient, and a high variance for the estimated mean.

4.5   A MODIFICATION THAT ALWAYS YIELDS UNBIASED ESTIMATES

We demonstrated earlier that systematic sampling of 1 in k elements does not yield unbiased estimates when the ratio N/k is not an integer, although the bias is likely to be small when N and k are reasonably large. In this section, we present a method of taking a systematic sample of 1 in k elements that will *always* lead to unbiased estimates of population means, totals, and proportions. This method, however, requires prior knowledge of the population size, and therefore is only useful in those situations where N is known. We illustrate the method with an example.

Illustrative Example.   Suppose that we wish to take a 1 in 6 sample from the list of 25 physicians in Table 2.1, and that we know in advance of the sampling that there are 25 physicians on the list. Instead of taking a random number between 1 and 6 to start the systematic sampling, let us take a random number j between 1 and 25. We then divide j by 6 and determine the remainder. For example, if the random number were 9, then $9/6 = 1\frac{3}{6}$; the remainder is 3, and we begin with the third physician. If the remainder were 1, we would begin with the first physician, and so on. When there is no remainder, we begin with element k (e.g., $k = 6$, in this case).

Let us examine the distribution (shown in Table 4.14) of remainders and samples for the 25 possible random numbers. It is apparent that each sample does not have the same probability of being selected. For example, a remainder of 1 has a 5/25 chance of occurring, since it occurs whenever random numbers 1, 7, 13, 19, and 25 are chosen. The other remainders have a 4/25 chance of occurring (e.g., the remainder 5 occurs whenever random number 5, 11, 17, and 23 are chosen).

With this in mind, we examine the distribution of estimated means shown in Table 4.15.

The mean $E(\bar{x})$ of the distribution of estimated mean household visits from this modified systematic sampling plan is (see Box 2.4)

$$
\begin{aligned}
E(\bar{x}) &= (12) \times (5/25) + (1) \times (4/25) + (4.25) \times (4/25) \\
&\quad + (6.5) \times (4/25) + (3.5) \times (4/25) + (1.5) \times (4/25) \\
&= 5.08 = \bar{X}
\end{aligned}
$$

Thus we see that this method, unlike the previously described method, leads to an unbiased estimate of the population mean even when N/k is not an integer. Similarly, it leads to an unbiased estimate of population totals and proportions.   □

To generalize from this example, the modified method can be put into operation as follows:

1. Choose a random number between 1 and N, where N is the number of elements in the population.

2. Compute the quotient j/k, where j is the random number selected and k is the sampling interval. Express this quotient as an integer plus a remainder (e.g., $23/6 = 3\frac{5}{6}$, and the remainder is 5).

Table 4.14   Distribution of Remainders and Samples for 25 Possible Random Numbers

Random Number j	j/k	Remainder	Elements in Sample
1	1/6	1	1, 7, 13, 19, 25
2	2/6	2	2, 8, 14, 20
3	3/6	3	3, 9, 15, 21
4	4/6	4	4, 10, 16, 22
5	5/6	5	5, 11, 17, 23
6	6/6	0	6, 12, 18, 24
7	7/6	1	1, 7, 13, 19, 25
8	8/6	2	2, 8, 14, 20
9	9/6	3	3, 9, 15, 21
10	10/6	4	4, 10, 16, 22
11	11/6	5	5, 11, 17, 23
12	12/6	0	6, 12, 18, 24
13	13/6	1	1, 7, 13, 19, 25
14	14/6	2	2, 8, 14, 20
15	15/6	3	3, 9, 15, 21
16	16/6	4	4, 10, 16, 22
17	17/6	5	5, 11, 17, 23
18	18/6	0	6, 12, 18, 24
19	19/6	1	1, 7, 13, 19, 25
20	20/6	2	2, 8, 14, 20
21	21/6	3	3, 9, 15, 21
22	22/6	4	4, 10, 16, 22
23	23/6	5	5, 11, 17, 23
24	24/6	0	6, 12, 18, 24
25	25/6	1	1, 7, 13, 19, 25

Table 4.15   Sampling Distribution of Estimated Means from Data of Tables 4.14 and 2.1

Elements in Sample	Estimated Mean No. of Visits $\bar{x}$	Chance of Selection, π
1, 7, 13, 19, 25	12.00	5/25
2, 8, 14, 20	1.00	4/25
3, 9, 15, 21	4.25	4/25
4, 10, 16, 22	6.50	4/25
5, 11, 17, 23	3.50	4/25
6, 12, 18, 24	1.50	4/25

3. If the remainder is 0, take a systematic sample of 1 in k elements in the usual way, beginning with element k. If the remainder is nonzero (e.g., m), take a systematic sample of 1 in k elements, beginning with element m.

4.6 ESTIMATION OF VARIANCES

As with all sampling methods, in order to construct confidence intervals, estimates of standards errors of the estimated population parameters are needed. In this section we demonstrate how estimates of standard errors are obtained in practice under systematic sampling.

The variance of an estimated mean $\bar{x}$ from a systematic sample of 1 in k elements (assuming that N/k is an integer) is the average squared deviation over the k possible samples of the estimated mean from the true population mean (since the estimate is unbiased when N/k is an integer). In other words, if $\bar{x}_i$ represents the mean value of $\mathscr{X}$ for the elements $i, i+k, i+2k, \ldots, i+(n-1)k$, then the *variance of an estimated mean* $\bar{x}$ from a systematic sample of 1 in k elements is given by

$$\text{Var}(\bar{x}) = \frac{\sum_{i=1}^{k}(\bar{x}_i - \bar{X})^2}{k} \tag{4.6}$$

Let us compare this expression with the variance of the estimated mean under simple random sampling, which is defined as

$$\text{Var}(\bar{x}) = \frac{\sum_{i=1}^{M}(\bar{x}_i - \bar{X})^2}{M}$$

where M is the total number of possible samples. It is a marvelous property of simple random sampling that this variance can be expressed simply in terms of σ_x^2, the variance of the original observations, using the following formula:

$$\text{Var}(\bar{x}) = \left(\frac{N-n}{N-1}\right)\left(\frac{\sigma_x^2}{n}\right)$$

Of greater importance to the statistician is that, by estimating the variance σ_x^2 with the statistic s_x^2 computed from the observations in the sample, the variance of $\bar{x}$ can be estimated as follows:

$$\widehat{\text{Var}}(\bar{x}) = \left(\frac{N-n}{N}\right)\left(\frac{s_x^2}{n}\right)$$

Hence, simply by knowing the variance of the observations in a *particular* sample, we can estimate the variance of the sampling distribution of the estimated mean under simple random sampling.

Unfortunately, the same cannot be said of systematic sampling. In order to estimate the variance given in Equation (4.6), it is necessary to have two or more of these $\bar{x}_i$ available to us. However, in our systematic sample, the estimated mean $\bar{x}$ is simply one of the $\bar{x}_i$, with the particular one depending on which random number was chosen to start the sampling. We have no information from our sample concerning the variability of estimated means over all possible samples.

In practice, if we can assume that the list from which the systematic sample was taken represents a random ordering of the elements with respect to the variable being measured, then we can assume that the systematic sample is equivalent to a simple random sample. Therefore, the procedures developed for estimating the variances of estimates from simple random samples can be used. In other words, we estimate the population variance σ_x^2 by $\hat{\sigma}_x^2$, as given by

$$\hat{\sigma}_x^2 = \left(\frac{N-1}{N}\right)(s_x^2)$$

where

$$s_x^2 = \frac{\sum_{i=1}^{n}(x_i - \bar{x})^2}{n-1}$$

and where the x_i are the sample observations and $n = N/k$. The *estimated variance* of the estimated mean $\bar{x}$ from a systematic sample is then given by

$$\widehat{\mathrm{Var}}(\bar{x}) = \left(\frac{\hat{\sigma}_x^2}{n}\right)\left(\frac{N-n}{N-1}\right) \tag{4.7}$$

Using this expression, we can then obtain confidence intervals for the population mean, $\bar{X}$, in the usual way.

Illustrative Example. Suppose we take a 1 in 5 systematic sample of physicians from the list given in Table 2.1 and that the initial random number chosen is 3. Table 4.16 lists the physicians in the sample along with their household visits.

Using the data in Table 4.16, we have the following calculations (see Box 2.2 and the equations given above):

Table 4.16   Systematic One in Five Sample Taken from Table 2.1

Physician in Sample	Number of Visits x_i
3	1
8	0
13	6
18	0
23	0

$$\bar{x} = 1.4 \qquad n = 5 \qquad N = 25$$

$$s_x^2 = \frac{1}{4}[(1 - 1.4)^2 + (0 - 1.4)^2 + (6 - 1.4)^2$$

$$+ (0 - 1.4)^2 + (0 - 1.4)^2] = 6.8$$

$$\hat{\sigma}_x^2 = \frac{24}{25} \times 6.8 = 6.528$$

$$\widehat{\text{Var}}(\bar{x}) = \left(\frac{6.528}{5}\right)\left(\frac{25 - 5}{24}\right) = 1.088$$

The upper and lower confidence intervals for a 95% confidence interval are given by

$$\bar{x} + (1.96)\sqrt{\widehat{\text{Var}}(\bar{x})} = 1.4 + (1.96)\sqrt{1.088} = 3.44$$

and

$$\bar{x} - (1.96)\sqrt{\widehat{\text{Var}}(\bar{x})} = 1.4 - (1.96)\sqrt{1.088} = -.64 = 0$$

(We use 0 for the lower limit since negative numbers make no sense in this example.) Thus, the 95% confidence interval for the mean number of visits is 0 to 3.44.   □

If, in fact, the list were not in random order, the assumption of random ordering could lead to estimated variance of estimates that are either too low or too high, and the resulting confidence intervals could be misleading.

4.7   REPEATED SYSTEMATIC SAMPLING

We discussed in previous sections how, with systematic sampling, the variances and standard errors of statistics as estimated from formulas shown in Box 4.1 can be either too small or too large if there is a relationship between the level of the particular variable and its position on the sampling frame. Also, the sample data themselves provide no insight into the nature of any ordering or periodicity in the sampling frame. It is possible, however, with a modified approach to systematic sampling to produce estimates of variances for estimated totals, means, and proportions that are unbiased no matter what kind of ordering or periodicity exists in the frame from which the sample was drawn. This modification is known as *repeated systematic sampling* and is demonstrated in the following example.

Illustrative Example. For this example, we will use the data shown in Table 4.17.

Let us suppose that we wish to take a systematic sample of approximately 18 workers from the list of 162 workers for purposes of estimating the mean number of work days lost per worker from acute illness. Since $n = 18$ and $N = 162$, a systematic sample of 1 in 9 workers would accomplish this. However, $18 = 6 \times 3$, and therefore, we can obtain a sample of 18 workers by taking 6 systematic samples, each containing 3 workers. In this case, the sampling interval $162/3 = 54$, and we would take 6 systematic samples of 1 in 54 workers. To do this, we first choose 6 random numbers between 1 and 54 (e.g., 2, 31, 46, 13, 34, 53), and then we choose systematic samples of 1 in 54 beginning with each random number. Our 6 samples are shown in Table 4.18.

If we denote $\bar{x}_i$ as the estimated mean number of work days lost due to acute illness from the ith sample and m as the number of samples taken, then our *estimated mean* is

$$\bar{\bar{x}} = \frac{\sum_{i=1}^{m} \bar{x}_i}{m} = \frac{5.00 + 4.33 + 4.00 + 3.33 + 7.00 + 3.33}{6} = 4.5$$

Since the estimated mean $\bar{\bar{x}}$ was obtained by taking a simple random sample of $m = 6$ means, $\bar{x}_i$, from a population of $M = 54$ such means, we can use the theory of simple random sampling to obtain the estimate $\widehat{\text{Var}}(\bar{\bar{x}})$ of the variance of $\bar{\bar{x}}$:

$$\widehat{\text{Var}}(\bar{\bar{x}}) = \left(\frac{1}{m}\right) \times \frac{\sum_{i=1}^{m}(\bar{x}_i - \bar{\bar{x}})^2}{m-1} \times \left(\frac{M-m}{M}\right)$$

where m is the number of samples taken and M is the total number of possible systematic samples. For this example, we have

$$\frac{\sum_{i=1}^{m}(\bar{x}_i - \bar{\bar{x}})^2}{m-1} = \frac{1}{5}[(5 - 4.5)^2 + (4.33 - 4.5)^2 + (4 - 4.5)^2$$
$$+ (3.33 - 4.5)^2 + (7 - 4.5)^2 + (3.33 - 4.5)^2] = 1.9$$

Table 4.17 Days Lost from Work Because of Acute Illness in One Year Among 162 Employees in a Plant

Employee ID	Days Lost	Employee ID	Days Lost	Employee ID	Days Lost	Employee ID	Days Lost
1	7	42	5	83	3	123	6
2	6	43	3	84	5	124	3
3	10	44	6	85	4	125	9
4	11	45	11	86	0	126	9
5	3	46	6	87	11	127	6
6	8	47	5	88	3	128	5
7	0	48	5	89	4	129	4
8	5	49	0	90	11	130	1
9	8	50	8	91	0	131	1
10	4	51	1	92	6	132	11
11	7	52	10	93	1	133	3
12	13	53	7	94	9	134	5
13	4	54	9	95	6	135	9
14	5	55	8	96	0	136	5
15	2	56	2	97	3	137	1
16	0	57	9	98	6	138	15
17	7	58	9	99	0	139	2
18	17	59	8	100	12	140	10
19	5	60	6	101	11	141	8
20	6	61	5	102	6	142	2
21	1	62	3	103	1	143	6
22	7	63	9	104	3	144	14
23	9	64	6	105	2	145	10
24	3	65	3	106	5	146	8
25	8	66	3	107	3	147	7
26	9	67	4	108	12	148	9
27	4	68	9	109	1	149	1
28	8	69	5	110	7	150	2
29	4	70	8	111	9	151	6
30	17	71	5	112	6	152	4
31	6	72	11	113	6	153	6
32	9	73	5	114	3	154	3
33	9	74	9	115	4	155	1
34	5	75	8	116	2	156	8
35	8	76	7	117	5	157	0
36	5	77	6	118	10	158	3
37	8	78	4	119	10	159	2
38	5	79	3	120	15	160	8
39	8	80	9	121	5	161	0
40	0	81	5	122	5	162	15
41	3	82	5				

Table 4.18 Data for Six Systematic Samples Taken from Table 4.17

Random Number	Elements of Sample	Days Lost	Estimated Mean, $\bar{x}$
2	2	6	
	56	2	5.00
	110	7	
13	13	4	
	67	4	4.33
	121	5	
31	31	6	
	85	4	4.00
	139	2	
34	34	5	
	88	3	3.33
	142	2	
46	46	6	
	100	12	7.00
	154	3	
53	53	7	
	107	3	3.33
	161	0	

and

$$\widehat{\text{Var}}(\bar{\bar{x}}) = \left(\frac{1}{6}\right)(1.9)\left(\frac{54-6}{54}\right) = .2814$$

The 95% confidence interval is

$$\bar{\bar{x}} - 1.96\sqrt{\widehat{\text{Var}}(\bar{\bar{x}})} \leqslant \bar{X} \leqslant \bar{\bar{x}} + 1.96\sqrt{\widehat{\text{Var}}(\bar{\bar{x}})}$$
$$4.5 - (1.96)\sqrt{.2814} \leqslant \bar{X} \leqslant 4.5 + (1.96)\sqrt{.2814}$$
$$3.46 \leqslant \bar{X} \leqslant 5.54 \qquad \qquad \square$$

A summary of the formulas needed for estimation procedures involving the sample mean under repeated systematic sampling is shown in Box 4.3. Expressions similar to those in Box 4.3 can be constructed for population totals and proportions. In such expressions, $\bar{x}_i$ and $\bar{\bar{x}}$ of Equation (4.9) would be replaced by x_i' and $\bar{x}'$ or by p_{yi} and $\bar{p}_y$, respectively.

The advantage of repeated systematic sampling over systematic sampling is that the variance and standard errors of the estimates can be estimated directly from the data. Its disadvantage is that it is necessary to go down the list more than once, whereas in systematic sampling one chooses the sample in one pass

BOX 4.3 ESTIMATION PROCEDURES FOR POPULATION MEANS UNDER REPEATED SYSTEMATIC SAMPLING

Point Estimate of the Population Mean

$$\bar{\bar{x}} = \frac{\sum_{i=1}^{m} \bar{x}_i}{m} \tag{4.8}$$

Estimated Variance

$$\widehat{\mathrm{Var}}(\bar{\bar{x}}) = \left(\frac{1}{m}\right) \times \frac{\sum_{i=1}^{m}(\bar{x}_i - \bar{\bar{x}})^2}{m-1} \times \left(\frac{M-m}{M}\right) \tag{4.9}$$

100(1 − α)% Confidence Intervals

$$\bar{\bar{x}} - z_{(1-\alpha/2)}\sqrt{\widehat{\mathrm{Var}}(\bar{\bar{x}})} \leqslant \bar{X} \leqslant \bar{\bar{x}} + z_{(1-\alpha/2)}\sqrt{\widehat{\mathrm{Var}}(\bar{\bar{x}})} \tag{4.10}$$

In these equations m is the number of systematic samples taken, each of size n'; M is the total number of possible systematic samples and is equal to N/n', where N is the population size; $\bar{x}_i$ is the mean of observations in the ith systematic sample; $\bar{X}$ is the population mean; and $z_{1-(\alpha/2)}$ is the $100[1 - (\alpha/2)]$th percentile of the standard normal distribution.

through the list. Also, in most instances periodicity will not be present in the data, and then simple random sampling will provide appropriate confidence intervals.

USE OF STATA FOR ESTIMATION IN REPEATED SYSTEMATIC SAMPLING. The analysis shown above could have been performed by use of STATA. As just discussed, the repeated systematic sample resulting in the 18 workers shown above actually came from a simple random sample of "clusters" from a population of 54 clusters, where each cluster contains 3 workers separated from each other on the list by 54 other workers. The STATA data file, *workloss.dta*, consists of 6 records, one for each cluster and contains the following data:

cluster	xi	wt1	xibar	M
2	15	9	5	54
13	13	9	4.33	54
31	12	9	4.00	54
34	10	9	3.33	54
46	21	9	7	54
53	10	9	3.33	54

The variable, *cluster*, is a number from 1 to 54 identifying the position on
the sampling frame of the first element in the particular sample cluster.

The variable, *xi*, is the total, x_i, of the work-loss days for the three workers
in the *i*th cluster.

The variable, *wt1*, is the ratio of total clusters, M, to sample clusters, m, and
equals $54/6 = 9$.

The variable, *xibar*, is the mean number of work-loss days, $\bar{x}_i$, among the
three workers in the *i*th cluster.

The variable, M, is the total number of clusters of 3 workers in the population of 162 workers and equals $162/3 = 54$.

The following STATA commands are used to estimate the mean number of
days lost from work and the standard error of the estimated mean

```
.use" A:workloss.dta",clear
.svyset pweight wt1
.svyset fpc M
.svymean xibar
```

The first command indicates the STATA data file to be used (i.e.,
workloss.dta located on the A drive).

The second command indicates that the sampling weight is located in the
variable, *wt1*. Since this repeated systematic design is equivalent to a
simple random sample of 6 clusters from a population of 54 clusters,
the variable, *wt1*, would be equal to 9 for each of the sample clusters.

The third command indicates that the total number of clusters in the population (equal to 54 in this instance) is located in the variable called M.
The finite population correction (fpc) is calculated from this variable,

The fourth command indicates that the mean of the variable, *xibar*, is to be
estimated. The variable, *xibar*, is the mean number of work-loss days
among individuals within each cluster. The mean of that variable is the
estimated mean number of work-loss days per individual.

The STATA output for this illustrative example is shown below:

Survey mean estimation					
pweight: wt1			Number of obs		= 6
Strata: < one >			Number of strata		= 1
PSU: < observations >			Number of PSUs		= 6
FPC: M			Population size		= 54
Mean	Estimate	Std. Err.	[95% Conf.	Interval]	Deff
xibar	4.5	.5305483	3.136182	5.863818	1

Finite population correction (FPC) assumes simple random sampling without replacement of PSUs within each stratum with no subsampling within PSUs.

The estimated population total and its estimated standard error can be obtained with the additional command, svytotal xi. This generates the output shown below:

Survey total estimation					
pweight: wt1			Number of obs		= 6
Strata: < one >			Number of strata		= 1
PSU: < observations >			Number of PSUs		= 6
FPC: M			Population size		= 54
Total	Estimate	Std. Err.	[95% Conf.	Interval]	Deff
xi	729	85.94882	508.0615	949.9385	1

Finite population correction (FPC) assumes simple random sampling without replacement of PSUs within each stratum with no subsampling within PSUs.

Use of SUDAAN for Estimation in Repeated Systematic Sampling. SUDAAN (an acronym for *su*rvey *da*ta *an*alysis) is a software package that was developed at the Research Triangle Institute initially in the 1970s under a different name. In contrast to STATA, which is a general-purpose statistical package, SUDAAN was developed for the sole purpose of analyzing data from complex sample surveys. A PC DOS version of SUDAAN has been available since the mid-1980s, and has found wide use among survey research professionals. It is our opinion at this time that SUDAAN is more difficult to learn and use than the survey commands in STATA, but can handle a wider variety of sample designs and estimation methods. We feel that both are important tools and, as mentioned earlier, we will throughout this book show commands and output from both STATA and SUDAAN. The particular versions of SUDAAN that we used in this book are the DOS Version 6.40 and the WINDOWS Version 7.50 (which became available during the course of our revision). The presentation in this book is appropriate for both versions.

In the illustrative example of repeated systematic sampling shown above in which we used STATA for the computations, the data file consisted of one record for each sample cluster (six records in all), and the variables of interest were aggregates over each of the sample clusters. In contrast, SUDAAN can analyze data for a repeated systematic sample using a data file consisting of the original sample records. In other words, it is not necessary to construct a data file consisting of the aggregated data.

For this illustrative example, the data file used by SUDAAN is shown below:

record	cluster	element	M	WT1	Xi
1	2	2	54	9	6
2	2	56	54	9	2
3	2	110	54	9	7
4	13	13	54	9	4
5	13	67	54	9	4
6	13	121	54	9	5
7	31	31	54	9	6
8	31	85	54	9	4
9	31	139	54	9	2
10	34	34	54	9	5
11	34	88	54	9	3
12	34	142	54	9	2
13	46	46	54	9	6
14	46	100	54	9	12
15	46	154	54	9	3
16	53	53	54	9	7
17	53	107	54	9	3
18	53	161	54	9	0

Note that the data on the 18 sample records consist of 6 variables: the record number, *record*; the cluster identification number, *cluster*; the location of the record on the sampling frame, *element*; the number of clusters in the sampling frame, M; the sampling weight, $WT1$; and the number of work-loss days for each individual in the sample, Xi.

Estimation of the mean and total number of work-loss days and their standard errors by SUDAAN can be accomplished by the following set of commands.

```
1  PROC DESCRIPT DATA = WLOSS2 FILETYPE = SAS DESIGN = WOR MEANS
      TOTALS;
2  NEST _ONE_ CLUSTER;
3  WEIGHT WT1;
4  TOTCNT M _ZERO_;
5  VAR XI;
6  SETENV COLWIDTH = 15;
7  SETENV DECWIDTH = 3;
```

The first command calls *PROC DESCRIPT*, a SUDAAN module used primarily for estimation of means and totals and their standard errors. It indicates that the data are in the SAS data file named *WLOSS2.SSD* (consisting of the 18 sample records shown above), and that the sample design is of a type recognized by SUDAAN as *WOR* (for *without replacement*). Essentially this means that the first stage of sampling is simple random sampling without replacement. Finally, it indicates that means and totals are to be estimated.

The second command is the "nest" statement. In this statement, the term _ONE_ indicates that there is no stratification; and the term CLUSTER, indicates that the primary or first stage sampling units are identified by the variable, *cluster*.

The third command indicates that the sampling weight is located in the variable, *WT1*. In this instance, it is equal to the number M of clusters in the population divided by the number m of clusters in the sample, or $54/6 = 9$.

In the fourth command, the term *TOTCNT* indicates that the total number of clusters in the population is found in the variable, M, and the term _ZERO_ indicates that there is no further subsampling after the first stage of sampling (i.e., all elements within each sample cluster are selected and there is no variance component in this design due to variation between elements within the same cluster).

The fifth command indicates the estimation is to be performed for the variable, Xi (which indicates work-loss days).

The sixth and seventh commands indicate the column width and number of decimal places to appear in the output.

The set of commands described above will yield the following SUDAAN output:

Number of observations read :	18	Weighted count :	162
Number of observations skipped :	0		
(WEIGHT variable nonpositive)			
Denominator degrees of freedom :	5		

Date : 07-10-97   Research Triangle Institute   Page:1

Time : 14 : 25 : 90   Table:1

by : Variable, One.

Variable		One 1
XI	Sample Size	18.000
	Weighted Size	162.000
	Total	729.000
	SE Total	85.949
	Mean	4.500
	SE Mean	0.531

4.8 HOW LARGE A SAMPLE DO WE NEED?

If we assume that the list from which the systematic sample is to be taken is in random order, we can assume that the situation is approximately that of simple random sampling. In such instances, the methods for determining sample size that were developed in Chapter 3 can be used.

If we were not, however, willing to assume that the list is in random order, then the determination of sample size becomes a formidable problem. The reason for this is that the variance of an estimate obtained from systematic sampling depends on the sampling interval. For example, a 1 in 4 systematic sample from a list of 100 enumeration units yields a sample of 25 enumeration units, whereas a 1 in 5 systematic from the same list yields a sample of 20 enumeration units. However, the periodicity in the list may be such that the first sample yields estimates having larger variance than those obtained from the second sample, even though the first sample contains more enumeration units than the second sample. Since we will not usually know characteristics of the list before taking the sample, it will be difficult for us to determine an appropriate sampling interval and hence, to determine the appropriate sample size beforehand.

In repeated systematic sampling it is possible to obtain some idea of the required sample size by taking a preliminary set of m' repeated systematic samples from the list, estimating the parameters on the basis of the preliminary sample, and determining the required number m of samples on the basis of the following formula:

$$m = \frac{z_{1-(\alpha/2)}^2 \times \dfrac{\sum_{i=1}^{m'}(\bar{x}_i - \bar{\bar{x}})^2/(m'-1)}{\bar{\bar{x}}^2} \times \left(\dfrac{N}{n}\right)}{\left(\dfrac{N}{n}-1\right) \times \varepsilon^2 + z_{1-(\alpha/2)}^2 \times \dfrac{\sum_{i=1}^{m'}(\bar{x}_i - \bar{\bar{x}})^2/(m'-1)}{\bar{\bar{x}}^2}}$$

(4.11)

where ε, $z_{1-(\alpha/2)}$, N, and n are as defined before.

Illustrative Example. Suppose we wish to sample the list of employees shown in Table 4.17 for purposes of estimating the mean number of days lost from work due to acute illnesses, and that to do so we will take repeated systematic samples of 1 in 81 employees. Suppose further we wish to be virtually certain of estimating the mean number of days lost from work to within 20% of the true value, and that we wish to determine how many systematic samples m of 1 in 81 workers are needed. Let us take a preliminary sample of six such samples for purposes of estimating m. We first choose six random numbers between 1 and 81 (e.g., 22, 48, 27, 61, 53, 10) and obtain the six samples given in Table 4.19.

We then have the following calculations:

$$\bar{\bar{x}} = \frac{2+4+8+4.5+6+3.5}{6} = 4.67$$

$$\frac{\sum_{i=1}^{m'}(\bar{x}_i - \bar{\bar{x}})^2}{m'-1} = \left(\frac{1}{6-1}\right)[(2-4.67)^2 + (4-4.67)^2 + (8-4.67)^2$$

$$+ (4.5-4.67)^2 + (6-4.67)^2 + (3.5-4.67)^2$$

$$= 4.367$$

$$\varepsilon = .2 \qquad N = 162 \qquad n = 2 \qquad N/n = 81$$

Table 4.19   Six Samples Taken from Table 4.17

Random Number	Workers in Sample	Estimated Mean Days Lost, $\bar{x}_i$
10	10, 91	2.0
22	22, 103	4.0
27	27, 108	8.0
48	48, 129	4.5
53	53, 134	6.0
61	61, 142	3.5

From relation (4.11), we have

$$m = \frac{9 \times \left[\dfrac{4.367}{(4.67)^2}\right] \times 81}{(.2)^2(81 - 1) + 9 \times \left[\dfrac{4.367}{(4.67)^2}\right]} = 29.18 \approx 30$$

Thus, we would need approximately 30 systematic samples of 1 in 81 workers from the list to meet the specifications of the problem. □

The formula for the required sample size in repeated systematic sampling is based on the fact that repeated systematic sampling of 1 in N/n elements from a list is equivalent to simple random sampling from a population of N/n elements, where the estimates obtained from each of the N/n samples are considered as the basic variables.

4.9 USING FRAMES THAT ARE NOT LISTS

So far we have discussed systematic sampling primarily from the viewpoint of taking a 1 in k sample from a list of elements. The list may either be available beforehand or be compiled during the sampling process. An example of the latter type of list would be the situation in which we may be sampling one in every five patients entering the emergency room of a hospital. There would be no list of patients available beforehand in this situation. An advantage of systematic sampling over other sampling schemes is that the sampling can be done while the frame is being constructed.

Systematic sampling also can be done when no list is available. For example, if a set of records is located in 12 file drawers, each having a depth of 26 in. (inches), and if a sample of 100 records is needed, we could take a systematic sample in the following way:

1. Compute the total length of filed records (e.g., $26 \times 12 = 312$ in.).
2. Divide the total length by the total number of records to be sampled; denote the ratio by k (e.g., $k = 312/100 = 3.12$ in).
3. Take a random number j between 1 and k (e.g., between 0.00 and 3.12; suppose that the number chosen is 1.19).
4. Using some kind of measuring device, take the record that is j units from the front of the first file drawer. Next, take the record that is a length of k units from the first record taken (it might be necessary to go to the next file drawer to choose the record). Continue this process until the end of the last file drawer is reached.

(In our example, we first take the record that is 1.19 in. from the front of the first file drawer. Then we take as our next record the one that is 3.12 in. from the first one we took, and we continue taking records every 3.12 in. until we come to the end of the last drawer.)

Another instance in which systematic sampling could be used without the existence of a list is in the sampling of geographical areas from a map. For example, suppose that we wish to estimate the average phosphate concentration of a river that is 250 miles long by taking a sample of 100 specimens from the river. A simple method would be to divide the length of the river (250 miles) by the number of specimens needed (100) to obtain the sampling interval (2.5 miles). We could then choose a random number between 0 and 2.5 (e.g., 2.1) and locate the first sampling point 2.1 miles from the source of the river. (A second random number might be chosen corresponding to each point, indicating the distance from the shore at which the sample should be taken). The second sample point would be 4.6 miles from the source (2.1 + 2.5); the third would be 7.1 miles from the source, etc. This procedure could be done quite easily with the use of a good map. An intuitively appealing advantage of systematic sampling in this instance is that it leads to samples being taken along the entire length of the river, so that it would be difficult to miss any spots having unusually high (or low) phosphate levels.

4.10 SUMMARY

In this chapter, we discussed systematic sampling, which may be the most widely used of all sampling procedures. Systematic sampling, unlike most sampling procedures, does not require knowledge of the total number of sampling units in the population, and so the sampling can be performed at the same time that the sampling frame is being compiled.

Three methods of systematic sampling were discussed. One method leads to unbiased estimates only when the ratio N/k of the number of elements in the population to the sampling interval is an integer. The second method always leads to unbiased estimates, but is of limited utility since it requires prior knowledge of N, the number of elements in the population. The third method, repeated sytematic sampling, allows variances of the estimates, and hence confidence intervals, to be obtained.

Methodology for obtaining required sample sizes was developed and issues were discussed relating to the use of systematic sampling when lists are not available.

EXERCISES

4.1 Suppose the local Childhood Lead Poisoning Prevention Council in a metropolitan area in western Tennessee undertakes the responsibility of determining the proportion of homes in a certain development of 120 homes with unsafe lead levels. Because of the great expense involved in performing spectrometric testing of interior walls, ceilings, floors, baseboards, cabinets, and other obvious lead hazards such as crib bars, as well as of exterior sidings, porches and porch rails, it was decided to select a sample of the homes under study. A good up-to-date frame exists for sampling purposes. This frame is a street listing containing the address and owner of each home for each of the streets in the target area. It was decided to select a 1 in 3 sample of homes. Let us assume that the only houses with serious lead hazard problems are the 26th, 27th, 28th, and 29th on the list.

a. Suppose the random number 2 was chosen to start the sequence. Estimate the proportion of homes with lead hazards from the   sample.

b. Obtain a 95% confidence interval for the proportion of homes with lead hazards. What assumptions did you make?

c. What is the true variance of the distribution of the estimated proportion of homes with lead hazards? How does this compare with the variance estimated in part (b)?

d. Suppose that a simple random sample of 40 homes had been selected instead. What is the variance of the distribution of the estimated proportion of lead hazardous homes in this case? How does this value compare with the variance from a 1 in 3 systematic sample?

4.2 From the 120 homes of Exercise 1, suppose a 1 in 5 systematic sample was taken and supose that the initial random number was 5.

a. Estimate the proportion of homes with lead hazards from this   sample.

b. Obtain a 95% confidence interval for the proportion of homes with lead hazards.

c. What is the true variance of the distribution of the estimated proportion of lead hazardous homes? Compare this result with the estimated variance you used in part (b).

d. Suppose that instead of a 1 in 5 systematic sample, a simple random sample of the same number of homes is taken. What is the variance of the sampling distribution of the estimated proportion of lead hazardous homes obtained from this sampling scheme? How does it compare to that obtained from a 1 in 5 systematic sample?

4.3 Refer again to Exercise 4.1. Suppose that instead of a 1 in 5 systematic sample, a total of 24 sample homes are obtained by repeated systematic sampling of 1 in 40 homes.

a. Suppose that the random numbers chosen are 3, 7, 12, 26, 31, 33, 38, and 40. Estimate the proportion of homes with lead hazards and obtain a confidence interval for the estimated proportion.

b. What is the estimated variance of the distribution of the estimated proportion of lead hazardous homes obtained from these eight systematic samples of 1 in 40 households? Compare this to the actual variance that arises from a 1 in 5 systematic sample, which you calculated in part (c) of Exercise 4.2.

4.4 From the list of 162 workers in Table 4.17, use repeated systematic sampling to take a total sample of 18 workers for purposes of estimating the total number of work days lost due to acute illnesses by all workers and the proportion of workers having eight or more work days lost due to acute illnesses. Obtain 95% confidence intervals for each of these estimates. (Suppose that the random numbers you chose were 4, 44, 29, 20, 27, and 5.)

4.5 Suppose that a study is planned of the level of the pesticide dieldrin, which is believed to be a carcinogen, in a 7.5 mile stretch of a particular river. To assure representativeness, a map of the river is divided into 36 zones, (see the following figure) and a 1 in 4 systematic sample of these zones is to be selected. Water samples will be drawn by taking a boat out to the geographic center of the designated zone, and drawing a grab

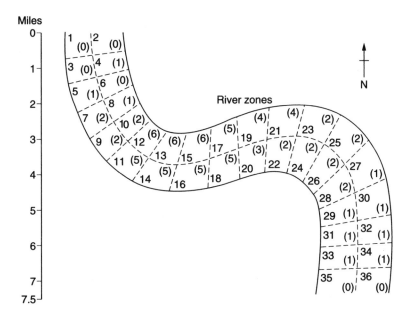

sample of water from a depth of several centimeters below the surface level. The levels of dieldrin, in micrograms per liter, for each of these zones are shown in parentheses.

a. Compute the 90% confidence interval for the average level of dieldrin in this stretch of the river.

b. What advantages can you identify for this method of sampling the river over simple random sampling?

4.6 During a specific year, 200 cardiac catheterization procedures were performed on persons over 70 years of age at a large university hospital. From a list of these patients, 4 systematic samples of 1 in 50 patients yielded the following data relating to pulmonary artery pressure:

Sample	Individual	Mean Pulmonary Artery Pressure
1	30	16
	80	25
	130	15
	180	17
2	17	14
	67	19
	117	18
	167	20
3	22	19
	72	27
	122	30
	172	11
4	43	10
	93	33
	143	17
	193	13

Based on these preliminary data, how many repeated systematic samples of 1 in 50 persons would have to be taken in order to estimate the mean pulmonary artery pressure in this population to within 10% of the true mean?

4.7 The following represents a week of scheduled appointments for the staff dentist at a small community health center characterized by major activity (B = Basic Care; C = Comprehensive Care):

Week 1	Mon	Tue	Wed	Thur	Fri
9:00	B	B	B	B	B
10:00	B	C	C	C	B
11:00	B	C	B	C	B
1:00	C	C	C	B	C
2:00	C	C	B	C	B
3:00	B	B	B	B	B
4:00	B	B	B	B	B

It is desired to estimate the proportion of visits devoted to comprehensive care during a particular 52-week period by use of a sampling plan involving systematic sampling. A 1 in 7 systematic sample is proposed. Is this a good sampling plan in this situation? Why or why not?

4.8 During a 52-week period there are 1820 (35 × 52) appointment slots in the situation described in Exercise 4.7. A repeated systematic sampling design of 1 in 26 appointment slots is to be used to estimate the proportion of appointments devoted to comprehensive care during that 52-week period. A pilot study of 3 such 1 in 26 samples yielded the following results:

Sample	Proportion Comprehensive
1	12/70
2	23/70
3	18/70

Based on the above results, how many replicated 1 in 26 samples would be required in order to be 95% certain of estimating this proportion to within 10% of the true value?

4.9 Which of the following is *not* true about systematic sampling?
a. Variances of estimates are large when the sampling ratio coincides with a periodicity in the frame.
b. Variances of estimates are related to the size of the intraclass correlation coefficient.
c. Unlike simple random sampling, one does not need to know the number of elements in the population in order to perform systematic sampling.
d. Estimated means, totals, and proportions are always unbiased under systematic sampling.

4.10 Systematic sampling works best under which of the following scenarios?

    a. The sampling frame (or list) is ordered with respect to a variable that is directly related to and highly correlated with the variable of interest.

    b. The sampling frame is neither ordered nor has any periodicity with respect to any variable of interest.

    c. The sampling frame has a periodicity in it that is congruent with the sampling fraction.

    d. The sampling frame is not a list.

4.11 Suppose that in the scenario of Exercise 4.1, it is decided to take a sample of 18 homes according to a repeated systematic sampling design which specifies 6 replications of a systematic sample of 3 homes.

    a. In the notation developed in this chapter for repeated systematic sampling, specify N, M, n, and m. What is the numerical value of the sampling weight?

    b. Suppose that the 6 random numbers chosen for the sampling design specified in part a are: 3, 15, 20, 27, 34, and 39. Which households appear in the sample?

    c. (For those having access to SUDAAN or STATA) From the sample taken in part b, use SUDAAN or STATA to estimate the number and proportion of homes having lead hazards and the standard errors of these estimates.

4.12 A data file contains 100,000 records on 2012 members of a health maintenance organization (HMO). Records are labeled beginning with "1" and ending with "100,000," and a random number is selected between 1 and 1000. The random number selected is 253, and all records ending with 253 are sampled (e.g., 253, 1253, 2253, 3253, etc.). For each record selected, the HMO member corresponding to each sample record is queried concerning his/her risk factors for coronary heart disease. An estimate of the proportion of persons at high risk for coronary heart disease (CHD) is then constructed by use of the sample proportion (number of persons at high risk divided by number of persons in the sample).

    a. The sample proportion described above is a biased estimate of the true population proportion. Show why this is true.

    b. Construct an unbiased estimate for this sample design.

4.13 The sample described in Exercise 4.12 yields the following data on the 100 HMO enrollees selected as described above. From these data estimate the proportion of persons in the HMO population at high risk for coronary heart disease.

Record Number	Number of Records per HMO Member	CHD High Risk	Record Number	Number of Records per HMO Member	CHD High Risk
253	50	0	50253	50	0
1253	36	0	51253	47	0
2253	45	0	52253	55	0
3253	61	0	53253	56	0
4253	50	0	54253	44	0
5253	77	0	55253	36	0
6253	70	0	56253	46	0
7253	41	0	57253	64	0
8253	63	0	58253	59	0
9253	43	0	59253	55	0
10253	53	0	60253	10	1
11253	17	1	61253	12	1
12253	44	0	62253	62	0
13253	54	0	63253	34	0
14253	70	0	64253	48	0
15253	46	0	65253	27	1
16253	62	0	66253	43	0
17253	48	0	67253	23	1
18253	37	0	68253	36	0
19253	53	0	69253	52	0
20253	38	0	70253	55	0
21253	39	0	71253	19	1
22253	53	0	72253	35	0
23253	25	1	73253	19	1
24253	54	0	74253	50	0
25253	39	0	75253	40	0
26253	41	0	76253	37	0
27253	56	0	77253	70	0
28253	24	1	78253	56	0
29253	59	0	79253	33	0
30253	68	0	80253	28	1
31253	65	0	81253	36	0
32253	63	0	82253	54	0
33253	63	0	83253	48	0
34253	70	0	84253	57	0
35253	45	0	85253	55	0
36253	18	1	86253	41	0
37253	21	1	87253	50	0
38253	46	0	88253	64	0
39253	48	0	89253	54	0
40253	57	0	90253	33	0
41253	40	0	91253	63	0
42253	57	0	92253	51	0
43253	27	1	93253	55	0
44253	48	0	94253	36	0
45253	51	0	95253	36	0
46253	59	0	96253	51	0
47253	48	0	97253	31	0
48253	74	0	98253	28	1
49253	46	0	99253	35	0

BIBLIOGRAPHY

The sampling texts cited in Chapters 1 and 2 all develop the concepts of systematic sampling discussed in this chapter, each in its own way. As had been stated earlier, systematic sampling is widely used in practice since it is considerably easier to sample systematically from a list than to take a simple random sample.

The module, SAMPLE, written for the statistical package, SYSTAT, gives several methods for taking systematic samples.

1. Frankel, M. R., and Spencer, B. D., *SAMPLE: A Supplementary Module for SYSTAT*, SYSTAT, Inc, Evanston, Ill. 1990.

Bellhouse has written two review articles on systematic sampling that contain many valuable cross references to methodological articles and substantive applications.

2. Bellhouse, D. R., Systematic sampling. In *Sampling, Handbook of Statistics*, Vol. 6, Krishniah, P. R., and Rao, C. R., Eds., Amsterdam, Elsevier, 1988.

3. Bellhouse, D. R., Systematic sampling methods. In *Encyclopedia of Biostatistics*, Armitage, P. A. and Colton, T., Eds., Wiley, Chichester, U.K., 1998.

CHAPTER 5

Stratification and Stratified Random Sampling

Simple random sampling and systematic sampling, the two types of sampling discussed up to this point, each involve taking a sample from the population as a whole; neither requires identification of subdomains or subgroups before the sample is taken. Sometimes, however, the sampling frame can be partitioned into groups or *strata*, and the sampling can be performed separately within each stratum. The resulting sampling design is called *stratified sampling*. If simple random sampling is used to select the sample within each of the strata, the sample design is called *stratified random sampling*.

In this chapter, we introduce some "basics" of stratification and stratified random sampling. This includes discussion of methods of taking samples, definition of terms and notation for population and sample characteristics used in discussing sample designs having stratification, and basic estimates of population characteristics. In the next chapter, we discuss in some detail methods of using stratification designs in ways that are most likely to produce the most reliable estimates.

5.1 WHAT IS A STRATIFIED RANDOM SAMPLE?

A *stratified random sample*, as indicated above, is a sampling plan in which a population is divided into L mutually exclusive and exhaustive strata, and a simple random sample of n_h elements is taken within each stratum h. The sampling is performed *independently* within each stratum. In essence, we can think of a stratified random sampling scheme as being L separate simple random samples.

Operationally, a stratified random sample is taken in the same way as a simple random sample, but the sampling is done separately and independently within each stratum. If we let $N_1, N_2, \ldots, N_L$ represent the number of sampling units within each stratum, and $n_1, n_2, \ldots, n_L$ represent the number of randomly

121

selected sampling units within each stratum, then the total number of possible stratified random samples is equal to

$$\binom{N_1}{n_1} \times \binom{N_2}{n_2} \times \cdots \times \binom{N_L}{n_L}$$

which is less than or equal to $\binom{N}{n}$, the total number of possible simple random samples.

For example, if we have three strata and $N_1 = 3$, $N_2 = 5$, and $N_3 = 6$, the total number of possible samples of $n_1 = 1$ element from stratum 1, $n_2 = 2$ elements from stratum 2, and $n_3 = 4$ elements from stratum 3 is

$$\binom{3}{1} \times \binom{5}{2} \times \binom{6}{4} = 450$$

The total number of simple random samples of 7 elements from the 14 elements in the population is

$$\binom{14}{7} = 3432$$

The probability of an element being selected in the sample depends on the particular stratum into which the element is grouped and can be shown to be equal to n_h/N_h (if the element is in stratum h). In the example we just discussed, the probability of an element being selected is equal to 1/3 for elements in stratum 1, 2/5 for elements in stratum 2, and 4/6 for elements in stratum 3.

5.2   HOW TO TAKE A STRATIFIED RANDOM SAMPLE

As described above, one takes a stratified random sample simply by taking independently within each stratum simple random samples of n_h elements ($h = 1, \ldots, L$). The actual taking of the sample can be accomplished by any of the methods described earlier for taking a simple random sample.

For example, if one is taking a sample of records that are stored in a data file on computer, one can use an algorithm for taking a stratified random sample described in a SAS manual [7]. Also, the supplementary SYSTAT module, *SAMPLE* [6], can be used to take a stratified random sample.

5.3   WHY STRATIFIED SAMPLING?

Stratified sampling is used in certain types of surveys because it combines the conceptual simplicity of simple random sampling with potentially significant gains in reliability. It is a convenient technique to use whenever we wish to obtain separate estimates for population parameters for each subdomain within an overall population and, in addition, wish to ensure that our sample is representative of the population. For example, suppose we wish to estimate the total number of beds in the hospitals of a certain state. We know that the majority of the hospitals are small or middle sized and that there are only a few very large hospitals. We also know that these very large hospitals account for a substantial portion of the total number of beds.

Now suppose we decide to select a simple random sample of the hospitals in the state, determine the number of beds in each one so selected and, using the methods of Chapter 3, estimate the total number of beds among all hospitals in the entire state. The problem with this procedure is that there is a good chance that our sample may contain either too many or too few of the very large hospitals. As a result, the sample may not adequately represent the population.

Our solution to this problem is to stratify the sampling units (hospitals) prior to sampling, into three groups on the basis of size (i.e., small, middle, large), and then select, using simple random sampling techniques, certain numbers of hospitals from each of the three groups. An estimate of the total number of beds can then be obtained from the combined results of the three strata. This is the essence of stratified sampling.

To illustrate the ideas and advantages of stratification, let us look at an example.

Illustrative Example. Suppose that a road having a length of 24 miles traverses areas that can be classified as urban and rural and that the road is divided into eight segments, each having a length equal to 3 miles. A sample of three segments is taken, and on each segment sampled, special equipment is installed for purposes of counting the number of total motor vehicle miles traveled by cars and trucks on the segment during a particular year. In addition, a record of all accidents occurring on each sample segment is kept.

The number of truck miles and the number of accidents in which a truck was involved during a certain period are given in Table 5.1 for each of the eight segments in the population.

Suppose that we take a simple random sample of three segments for purposes of estimating the total number of truck miles traveled on the road. There are 56 possible samples of three segments from the population of eight segments. The sampling distribution of the number of truck miles traveled on the road is given in Table 5.2.

Estimates of the total number of truck miles obtained in this way range from 15,026.67 to 60,938.67 with the mean of the sampling distribution of x' equal to 34,054, the population total, and the standard error of x' equal to 10,536.9.

Now suppose that instead of taking a simple random sample of three segments from the population of eight segments, we first group the segments into two strata, one consisting of urban segments, the other consisting of rural segments, as shown in Table 5.3.

Table 5.1   Truck Miles and Number of Accidents Involving Trucks by Type of Road Segment

Segment	Type	Number of Truck Miles ($\times 100$)	Number of Accidents Involving Trucks
1	Urban	6327	8
2	Rural	2555	5
3	Urban	8691	9
4	Urban	7834	9
5	Rural	1586	5
6	Rural	2034	1
7	Rural	2015	9
8	Rural	3012	4

Table 5.2   Sampling Distribution of x' for 56 Possible Samples of Three Segments

Segments in Sample	x'	Segments in Sample	x'
(1, 2, 3)	46,861.33	(2, 4, 7)	33,077.33
(1, 2, 4)	44,576	(2, 4, 8)	35,736
(1, 2, 5)	27,914.67	(2, 5, 6)	16,466.67
(1, 2, 6)	29,109.33	(2, 5, 7)	16,416
(1, 2, 7)	29,058.67	(2, 5, 8)	19,074.67
(1, 2, 8)	31,717.33	(2, 6, 7)	17,610.67
(1, 3, 4)	60,938.67	(2, 6, 8)	20,269.33
(1, 3, 5)	44,277.33	(2, 7, 8)	20,218.67
(1, 3, 6)	45,472	(3, 4, 5)	48,296
(1, 3, 7)	45,421.33	(3, 4, 6)	49,490.67
(1, 3, 8)	48,080	(3, 4, 7)	49,440
(1, 4, 5)	41,992	(3, 4, 8)	52,098.67
(1, 4, 6)	43,186.67	(3, 5, 6)	32,829.33
(1, 4, 7)	43,136	(3, 5, 7)	32,778.67
(1, 4, 8)	45,794.67	(3, 5, 8)	35,437.33
(1, 5, 6)	26,525.33	(3, 6, 7)	33,973.33
(1, 5, 7)	26,474.67	(3, 6, 8)	36,632
(1, 5, 8)	29,133.33	(3, 7, 8)	36,581.33
(1, 6, 7)	27,669.33	(4, 5, 6)	30,544
(1, 6, 8)	30,328	(4, 5, 7)	30,493.33
(1, 7, 8)	30,277.33	(4, 5, 8)	33,152
(2, 3, 4)	50,880	(4, 6, 7)	31,688
(2, 3, 5)	34,218.67	(4, 6, 8)	34,346.67
(2, 3, 6)	35,413.33	(4, 7, 8)	34,296
(2, 3, 7)	35,362.67	(5, 6, 7)	15,026.67
(2, 3, 8)	38,021.33	(5, 6, 8)	17,685.33
(2, 4, 5)	31,933.33	(5, 7, 8)	17,634.67
(2, 4, 6)	33,128	(6, 7, 8)	18,829.33

Table 5.3 Two Strata for Data of Table 5.1

Stratum 1 (Urban Segments)		Stratum 2 (Rural Segments)	
Segment	Truck Miles ×1000	Segment	Truck Miles ×1000
1	6327	2	2555
3	8691	5	1586
4	7834	6	2034
		7	2015
		8	3012

We might now take a sample of one segment from stratum 1 and two segments from stratum 2 and estimate the total number of truck miles by the estimate x'_{str} given by

$$x'_{str} = x'_1 + x'_2$$

where

$x'_1 =$ estimated number of truck miles in the three segments composing stratum 1

$x'_2 =$ estimated number of truck miles in the five segments composing stratum 2

Conceptually, we consider each stratum as a subpopulation, sample independently within each subpopulation, and obtain an estimate for the population as a whole by aggregating the individual stratum estimates over all subpopulations or strata. Therefore, if we take a simple random sample of one segment from stratum 1 and two segments from stratum 2, we obtain a total of $\binom{3}{1} \times \binom{5}{2} = 30$ possible samples. If we then use the estimation procedure given by the equation above for x'_{str}, we obtain the sampling distribution of x'_{str} shown in Table 5.4.

The mean, $E(x'_{str})$, of the sampling distribution of x'_{str} is equal to 34,054 (see Box 2.3), which is the true population total. The standard error, $SE(x'_{str})$, of the estimated total x'_{str} is equal to 3297.6 which is much lower than the standard error of x', the equivalent estimate of the population total under simple random sampling. These results are summarized in Table 5.5.

Intuitively, we can see why the sampling plan based on stratification yielded an estimate having a lower standard error than the corresponding estimate based on simple random sampling. There are 56 possible values of the estimated total x' that can be obtained by simple random sampling, whereas stratification yields only 30 values of x'_{str}. Also, examination of the ranges of

Table 5.4 Sampling Distribution of x'_{str} for 30 Possible Samples of Three Segments

Stratum 1	Stratum 2	x'_1 $(= 3\bar{x}_1)$	x'_2 $(= 5\bar{x}_2)$	x'_{str} $= (x'_1 + x'_2)$
1	(2, 5)	18,981	10,352.5	29,333.5
1	(2, 6)	18,981	11,472.5	30,453.5
1	(2, 7)	18,981	11,425	30,406
1	(2, 8)	18,981	13,917.5	32,898.5
1	(5, 6)	18,981	9,050	28,031
1	(5, 7)	18,981	9,002.5	27,983.5
1	(5, 8)	18,981	11,495	30,476
1	(6, 7)	18,981	10,122.5	29,103.5
1	(6, 8)	18,981	12,615	31,596
1	(7, 8)	18,981	12,567.5	31,548.5
3	(2, 5)	26,073	10,352.5	36,425.5
3	(2, 6)	26,073	11,472.5	37,545.5
3	(2, 7)	26,073	11,425	37,498
3	(2, 8)	26,073	13,917.5	39,990.5
3	(5, 6)	26,073	9,050	35,123
3	(5, 7)	26,073	9,002.5	35,075.5
3	(5, 8)	26,073	11,495	37,568
3	(6, 7)	26,073	10,122.5	36,195.5
3	(6, 8)	26,073	12,615	38,688
3	(7, 8)	26,073	12,567.5	38,640.5
4	(2, 5)	23,502	10,352.5	33,854.5
4	(2, 6)	23,502	11,472.5	34,974.5
4	(2, 7)	23,502	11,425	34,927
4	(2, 8)	23,502	13,917.5	37,419.5
4	(5, 6)	23,502	9,050	32,552
4	(5, 7)	23,502	9,002.5	32,504.5
4	(5, 8)	23,502	11,495	34,997
4	(6, 7)	23,502	10,122.5	33,624.5
4	(6, 8)	23,502	12,615	36,117
4	(7, 8)	23,502	12,567.5	36,069.5

the two distributions shows that stratification eliminated those samples that resulted in either extremely high or extremely low estimates of the total. The three urban segments had high values and the five rural segments had low values of the characteristic being measured (truck miles). Stratification ensured that at least one urban and one rural segment would be selected in the sample, thus eliminating the possibility of extremely high and extremely low estimates of the total.   □

There are three major advantages of stratification over simple random sampling.

Table 5.5   Comparison of Results for Simple Random Sampling and Stratification

	Sampling Design	
	Simple Random Sampling	Stratification
Number of elements in sample	3	3*
Number of possible samples	56	30
Mean of distribution of estimated totals	34,054[†]	34,054[†]
Standard error of estimated total	10,536.9	3,297.6
Range of distributions of estimated totals	45,912	12,007

*One element from stratum 1, two from stratum 2.
[†]This is also the population total.

1. Given certain conditions, precision may be increased over simple random sampling (i.e., lower standard errors may result from the estimation procedure).

2. It is possible to obtain estimates for each of the strata that have specified precision.

3. It may be just as easy, for either political or administrative reasons, to collect information for a stratified sample as is possible for a simple random sample. If such is the case, there is little to lose by taking a stratified sample, since the resulting standard errors will rarely exceed those of simple random sampling.

The strategy employed for constructing strata involves two steps. First we determine the population parameter we are interested in estimating. Then we stratify the population with respect to another variable that is thought to be associated with the variable of interest. If our assumption of association is correct, this second step ensures that the strata are homogeneous with respect to the variable under consideration.

For example, if we wish to estimate the number of beds in all hospitals in the state, we may wish to stratify the hospitals with respect to floor space (which is information readily available for reasons of taxation), reasoning that hospitals with more space will have more beds. On the other hand, if we are interested in the average daily cost of a hospital bed to the patient, we might choose to stratify the hospitals according to their geographical location, reasoning that hospitals in economically thriving parts of the state can charge their patients more than can hospitals in economically depressed parts of the state.

In most practical situations, it is difficult to stratify the population with respect to the variable under consideration, primarily for reasons of cost and practicality. More often the population is stratified in the most convenient manner by use of administrative criteria (e.g., voting districts), geographical criteria (e.g., north, south, east, or west), or other natural criteria (e.g., sex or age). Stratification by convenience is not unreasonable, since it is not common for a modern survey to estimate a single parameter. Instead, much information is collected on each sampling unit and many parameters are of interest. Clearly, what might be an optimal stratification strategy for one variable, providing relatively homogeneous strata may provide very heterogeneous strata with respect to another variable. It is important for the statistician to consider the scope of the data to be collected before deciding on an appropriate criterion for stratification. Such issues are sometimes discussed in reports of health surveys that use stratification [1]–[3].

The major disadvantage of stratified sampling is that it requires that every enumeration unit be identified by stratum in advance of the sampling. If such information were not readily available, this method would be rarely feasible.

You may wish to compare stratification to the strategy of cluster sampling (Chapters 8–11) where major savings in time and cost may be possible. Nevertheless, because of the advantages discussed above, stratification is a very powerful and widely used technique.

5.4 POPULATION PARAMETERS FOR STRATA

Population parameters for strata can be defined with the same type of notation that we used to define parameters of a population in general. In this section we introduce notation that will be used throughout our discussion of sampling plans based on stratification.

Let us consider a population containing N elementary units that are grouped exclusively and exhaustively into L strata in such a way that stratum 1 contains N_1 elementary units, stratum 2 contains N_2 elementary units, ..., and stratum L contains N_L elementary units. In other words,

$$N = \sum_{h=1}^{L} N_h$$

is the *population size*.

Suppose we are considering a variable or characteristic $\mathscr{X}$ in the population. We use the notation $X_{h,i}$ to represent the *value of the characteristic* $\mathscr{X}$ for the ith elementary unit within stratum h. In other words, the elementary units within any particular stratum h are labeled from 1 to N_h.

Illustrative Example. Suppose we are interested in estimating the average daily pharmaceutical cost per patient at a hospital. We decide to stratify the hospital into services (medical, surgical, ob-gyn, all other services combined), and we define the elementary units as patients on any given day.

Suppose that on a designated day, there are 250 patients in the hospital, of which 100 are medical, 75 surgical, 50 ob-gyn, and 25 other services. Then using the notation introduced above we have

$$N = 250 \qquad N_1 = 100 \qquad N_2 = 75 \qquad N_3 = 50 \qquad N_4 = 25$$

If $X_{h,i}$ designates the value of the variable $\mathcal{X}$ for the ith elementary unit within stratum h, then, for example, in stratum 2 we have

$X_{2,1} =$ the value of variable $\mathcal{X}$ for element 1 within stratum 2

$X_{2,2} =$ the value of variable $\mathcal{X}$ for element 2 within stratum 2

and so on, up to

$X_{2,75} =$ the value of variable $\mathcal{X}$ for element 75 within stratum 2

Elements within the other strata would be defined in a similar manner. □

We define population parameters for strata in a way that is similar to the way we defined general population parameters.

The *total* or aggregate amount of a variable $\mathcal{X}$ *within a stratum h* is defined by X_{h+} as given by

$$X_{h+} = \sum_{i=1}^{N_h} X_{h,i}$$

The *total for the whole population* is given by the sum of the stratum totals, or

$$X = \sum_{h=1}^{L} \sum_{i=1}^{N_h} X_{h,i} = \sum_{h=1}^{L} X_{h+}$$

The *mean* level of a characteristic $\mathcal{X}$ for a stratum h is denoted by $\bar{X}_h$ and is given by

$$\bar{X}_h = \frac{\sum_{i=1}^{N_h} X_{h,i}}{N_h} = \frac{X_{h+}}{N_h}$$

The *mean* $\bar{X}$ of a variable $\mathscr{X}$ for the entire population is given by

$$\bar{X} = \frac{X}{N}$$

or its algebraic equivalent

$$\bar{X} = \frac{\sum_{h=1}^{L} N_h \bar{X}_h}{N} = \sum_{h=1}^{L} W_h \bar{X}_h$$

where

$$W_h = \frac{N_h}{N}$$

In other words, the mean $\bar{X}$ for the entire population is a *weighted average* of the individual stratum means $\bar{X}_h$, with weights $(W_h = N_h/N)$ proportional to the number of elements in each stratum.

The *variance* σ_{hx}^2 of the distribution of a variable $\mathscr{X}$ within a particular stratum h is defined as the average squared deviation about the stratum mean and is given by

$$\sigma_{hx}^2 = \frac{\sum_{i=1}^{N_h} (X_{h,i} - \bar{X}_h)^2}{N_h}$$

Coefficients of variation and rel–variances are defined for each stratum in the same way as they were defined for a population that is not grouped into strata. The *coefficient of variation* for the distribution within a particular stratum is given by

$$V_{hx} = \frac{\sigma_{hx}}{\bar{X}_h}$$

and the *rel–variance* is simply the square of the coefficient of variation.

For convenience in later reference, the population parameters for stratified sampling are summarized in Box 5.1.

Now let us see how these formulas can be used in practice.

Illustrative Example.　　Consider a population of 14 families living on three city blocks. If we consider the families as elementary units, the blocks as strata, and family size as the characteristic $\mathscr{X}$, we might have the situation shown in Table 5.6.

BOX 5.1   POPULATION AND STRATA PARAMETERS FOR STRATIFIED SAMPLING

	Within Stratum	Entire Population

Total

$$X_{h+} = \sum_{i=1}^{N_h} X_{h,i} \qquad\qquad X = \sum_{h=1}^{L} \sum_{i=1}^{N_h} X_{h,i} = \sum_{h=1}^{L} X_{h+} \qquad (5.1)$$

Mean

$$\bar{X}_h = \frac{\sum_{i=1}^{N_h} X_{h,i}}{N_h} = \frac{X_{h+}}{N_h} \qquad\qquad \bar{X} = \frac{\sum_{h=1}^{L} N_h \bar{X}_h}{N} = \sum_{h=1}^{L} W_h \bar{X}_h = \frac{X}{N} \quad (5.2)$$

Proportion

$$P_{hy} = \frac{\sum_{i=1}^{N_h} Y_{h,i}}{N_h} \qquad\qquad P_y = \frac{\sum_{h=1}^{L} N_h P_{hy}}{N} = \sum_{h=1}^{L} W_h P_{hy} \quad (5.3)$$

Variance

$$\sigma_{hx}^2 = \frac{\sum_{i=1}^{N_h} (X_{h,i} - \bar{X}_h)^2}{N_h} \qquad\qquad\qquad\qquad (5.4)$$

Relative Variance

$$V_{hx}^2 = \frac{\sigma_{hx}^2}{\bar{X}_h^2} \qquad\qquad\qquad\qquad (5.5)$$

In these definitions, L is the number of strata, N_h is the number of elements in stratum h, N is the total number of elements, $X_{h,i}$ is the value of $\mathcal{X}$ for the ith element in stratum h, $Y_{h,i}$ indicates the presence or absence of some dichotomous attribute $\mathcal{Y}$ for the ith element in stratum h, and $W_h = N_h/N$ is the proportion of the total population belonging to stratum h.

Table 5.6 Strata for a Population of 14 Families

Block	Family	Family Size
1	1	4
	2	3
	3	4
2	1	4
	2	6
	3	4
	4	7
	5	8
3	1	2
	2	3
	3	2
	4	2
	5	2
	6	3

In terms of the notation introduced above, we have the following values of $\mathscr{X}$ for each stratum:

Stratum 1 $(N_1 = 3)$	Stratum 2 $(N_2 = 5)$	Stratum 3 $(N_3 = 6)$
$X_{1,1} = 4$	$X_{2,1} = 4$	$X_{3,1} = 2$
$X_{1,2} = 3$	$X_{2,2} = 6$	$X_{3,2} = 3$
$X_{1,3} = 4$	$X_{2,3} = 4$	$X_{3,3} = 2$
	$X_{2,4} = 7$	$X_{3,4} = 2$
	$X_{2,5} = 8$	$X_{3,5} = 2$
		$X_{3,6} = 3$

The totals of the variable $\mathscr{X}$ within each stratum h, using Equation (5.1), are as follows:

$$X_{1+} = 4 + 3 + 4 = 11$$
$$X_{2+} = 4 + 6 + 4 + 7 + 8 = 29$$
$$X_{3+} = 2 + 3 + 2 + 2 + 2 + 3 = 14$$

The total for the entire population, again using Equation (5.1), is

$$X = 11 + 29 + 14 = 54$$

The population means for the strata, from Equation (5.2), are as follows:

$$\bar{X}_1 = \frac{11}{3} = 3.67 \qquad \bar{X}_2 = \frac{29}{5} = 5.8 \qquad \bar{X}_3 = \frac{14}{6} = 2.33$$

The population mean for the entire population, from Equation (5.2), is given by

$$\bar{X} = \frac{3}{14} \times 3.67 + \frac{5}{14} \times 5.8 + \frac{6}{14} \times 2.33 = 3.857$$

The variances for the strata, using Equation (5.4), are

$$\sigma_{1x}^2 = \frac{(4 - 3.67)^2 + (3 - 3.67)^2 + (4 - 3.67)^2}{3} = .222$$

$$\sigma_{2x}^2 = \frac{(4 - 5.8)^2 + (6 - 5.8)^2 + \cdots + (8 - 5.8)^2}{5} = 2.56$$

$$\sigma_{3x}^2 = \frac{(2 - 2.33)^2 + (3 - 2.33)^2 + \cdots + (3 - 2.33)^2}{6} = .222$$

The relative variances for the strata, from Equation (5.5), are given by

$$V_{1x}^2 = \frac{0.222}{(3.67)^2} = .0165 \qquad V_{2x}^2 = \frac{2.56}{(5.8)^2} = .0761 \qquad V_{3x}^2 = \frac{.222}{(2.33)^2} = .0409$$

$\square$

5.5 SAMPLE STATISTICS FOR STRATA

Within a particular stratum h, let us suppose we have selected in some way a sample of n_h elements from the N_h elements in the stratum and that each sample element is measured with respect to some variable $\mathscr{X}$. For convenience we label the sample elements from 1 to n_h, and we let $x_{h,1}$ denote the value of the variable $\mathscr{X}$ for the sample element labeled "1," we let $x_{h,2}$ denote the value of $\mathscr{X}$ for the sample element labeled "2," and we let x_{h,n_h} denote the value of $\mathscr{X}$ for the element labeled "n_h." If a sample of n_h elements is taken within each stratum h, then the total sample size n is given by

$$n = \sum_{h=1}^{L} n_h$$

where L is the number of strata into which the population's elements have been grouped.

For instance, in the previous example, if we select one element from stratum 1, two elements from stratum 2, and four elements from stratum 3, we have

$$n_1 = 1 \qquad n_2 = 2 \qquad n_3 = 4$$

and

$$n = 1 + 2 + 4 = 7$$

If the values of the four elements selected from stratum 3 are $X_{3,1}, X_{3,3}, X_{3,4}$, and $X_{3,6}$, then we have

$$x_{3,1} = X_{3,1} = 2 \qquad x_{3,3} = X_{3,4} = 2$$
$$x_{3,2} = X_{3,3} = 2 \qquad x_{3,4} = X_{3,6} = 3$$

Sample totals and *sample means for a particular stratum* are given by

$$x_{h+} = \sum_{i=1}^{n_h} x_{h,i}$$

and

$$\bar{x}_h = \frac{\sum_{i=1}^{n_h} x_{h,i}}{n_h} = \frac{x_{h+}}{n_h}$$

5.6   ESTIMATION OF POPULATION PARAMETERS FROM STRATIFIED RANDOM SAMPLING

If the selection of sample elements is done independently within each stratum by simple random sampling, then the design is that of *stratified random sampling*, and the appropriate estimates of population parameters are shown in Box 5.2, along with their standard errors.

In these definitions, L is the number of strata, N_h is the number of elements in stratum h, N is the total number of elements, $x_{h,i}$ is the value of $\mathcal{X}$ for the ith element in stratum h, $y_{h,i}$ indicates the presence or absence of some dichotomous attribute, $\mathcal{Y}$, for the ith sample element in stratum h.

Also, s_{hx}^2 is the estimated variance of the distribution of $\mathcal{X}$ for stratum h, and is given by

$$s_{hx}^2 = \frac{\sum_{i=1}^{n_h}(x_{h,i} - \bar{x}_h)^2}{n_h - 1} \tag{5.9}$$

BOX 5.2 ESTIMATES OF POPULATION PARAMETERS AND STANDARD ERRORS OF THESE ESTIMATES FOR STRATIFIED SAMPLING

Parameter	Stratum Specific Estimate	Estimate for Entire Population	Standard Error of Estimate for Entire Population	
Total	$x_h' = N_h \bar{x}_h$	$x_{str}' = \sum_{h=1}^{L} x_h'$	$\widehat{SE}(x_{str}') = \sqrt{\sum_{h=1}^{L} \dfrac{N_h^2 s_{hx}^2}{n_h}\left(\dfrac{N_h - n_h}{N_h}\right)}$	(5.6)
Mean	$\bar{x}_h = \dfrac{\sum_{i=1}^{n_h} x_{h,i}}{n_h}$	$\bar{x}_{str} = \dfrac{\sum_{h=1}^{L} N_h \bar{x}_h}{N}$	$\widehat{SE}(\bar{x}_{str}) = \sqrt{\sum_{h=1}^{L} \left(\dfrac{N_h}{N}\right)^2 \dfrac{s_{hx}^2}{n_h}\left(\dfrac{N_h - n_h}{N_h}\right)}$	(5.7)
Proportion	$p_{hy} = \dfrac{\sum_{i=1}^{n_h} y_{hi}}{n_h}$	$p_{y,str} = \dfrac{\sum_{h=1}^{L} y_{hi}}{N}$	$\widehat{SE}(p_{y,str}) = \sqrt{\sum_{h=1}^{L} \left(\dfrac{N_h}{N}\right)^2 \dfrac{p_{hy}(1 - p_{hy})}{n_h - 1}\left(\dfrac{N_h - n_h}{N_h}\right)}$	(5.8)

Illustrative Example Using STATA. One hundred fifty-eight (158) hospitals in a region are grouped into 3 strata according to the level of their obstetric services which is designated by the variable, *oblevel*. Of the 158 hospitals in the region, 42 were in stratum 1 (basic), 99 in stratum 2 (intermediate), and 17 in stratum 3 (tertiary). A stratified random sample of 15 hospitals is taken from this population: 4 hospitals in stratum 1; 5 hospitals in stratum 2; and 6 hospitals in stratum 3. The particular sample of 15 hospitals with the relevant variables for estimation are in the STATA datafile, *hospsamp.dta*. This file is shown overleaf.

Hospno	oblevel	weighta	tothosp	births
15	1	10.50	42	480
80	1	10.50	42	426
86	1	10.50	42	342
136	1	10.50	42	174
7	2	19.80	99	2022
26	2	19.80	99	576
62	2	19.80	99	1999
90	2	19.80	99	482
101	2	19.80	99	836
28	3	2.83	17	3108
34	3	2.83	17	4674
39	3	2.83	17	2539
102	3	2.83	17	1610
119	3	2.83	17	4618
149	3	2.83	17	1781

The meanings of the variables are as follows:

hospno = the identification code for the particular hospital.

oblevel = the level of the obstetrics service for each hospital.

weighta = the sampling weight, N_h/n_h, associated with the particular hospital.

tothosp = the population total number of hospitals in the stratum in which the sample hospital resides.

births = the number of births occurring in the hospital during the previous year.

The following commands can be used to obtain estimates of the total number of births and standard errors of the estimates:

```
. use "a:\hospsamp.dta", clear
. svyset pweight weighta
. svyset strata oblevel
. svyset fpc tothosp
. svytotal births
. svytotal births, by (oblevel)
```

The first command indicates that the data are contained in the STATA datafile, *hospsamp.dta.*

The second command indicates that the sampling weight for the hospital is in the variable, *weighta.*

The third command indicates that the stratum indicator variable is located in the variable, *oblevel.*

The fourth command indicates that the number, N_h, of stratum hospitals is in the variable, *tothosp.* Again, this is the same for records belonging to the same stratum, but is not the same for hospitals in different strata. The finite population correction is calculated from this variable.

The fifth command indicates that the total number of births is to be estimated from the sample data.

The sixth command indicates that the total number of births for each stratum is to be estimated from the data.

The STATA output generated by the above commands is shown below:

Survey total estimation

pweight:	weighta	Number of obs	= 15
Strata:	oblevel	Number of strata	= 3
PSU:	< observations >	Number of PSUs	= 15
FPC:	tothosp	Population size	= 158

Total	Estimate	Std. Err.	[95% Conf. Interval]		Deff
births	183983	34014.35	109872.1	258093.9	.7035476

Finite population correction (FPC) assumes simple random sampling without replacement of PSUs within each stratum with no subsampling within PSUs.

Survey total estimation

pweight:	weighta	Number of obs	= 15
Strata:	oblevel	Number of strata	= 3
PSU:	< observations >	Number of PSUs	= 15
FPC:	tothosp	Population size	= 158

Total Subpop.	Estimate	Std. Err.	[95% Conf. Interrval]		Deff
births					
oblevel = = 1	14931	2669.857	9113.882	20748.12	.1564799
oblevel = = 2	117117	33067.68	45068.7	189165.3	1.089406
oblevel = = 3	51935	7508.403	35575.6	68294.4	.0330073

Finite population correction (FPC) assumes simple random sampling without replacement of PSUs within each stratum with no subsampling within PSUs.

Illustrative Example Using SUDAAN.   Let us consider again the example used in which 158 hospitals in a region were grouped into 3 strata according to level of obstetrics service, and we took a stratified random sample of 4 hospitals from stratum 1, 5 hospitals from stratum 2, and 6 hospitals from stratum 3. The particular sample of 15 hospitals is shown above in the discussion of the use of STATA for analysis of these data. Let us now assume that the data file *hospsamp* is a SAS PC data file (*hospsamp.ssd*). We will show below how the statistical package, SUDAAN, can produce estimates and standard errors for this stratified random sampling design.

Again, assuming that *hospsamp* has been exported to a SAS data file, we can use the following command file to obtain estimates of total births for each stratum, and for the 158 hospitals making up the universe.

```
PROC DESCRIPT DATA = HOSPSAMP FILETYPE=SAS DESIGN = WOR TOTALS;
NEST OBLEVEL;
WEIGHT WEIGHTA;
TOTCNT TOTHOSP;
VAR BIRTHS;
SUBGROUP OBLEVEL;
LEVELS 3;
SETENV COLWIDTH = 20;
SETENV DECWIDTH = 3;
```

The first line gives information on the data file and indicates that the sampling is without replacement and that estimated totals are to be obtained.

The second line indicates that the sample records are nested within the stratum variable, *oblevel*.

The third line specifies the variable that is to be used as the sampling weight. In this instance, it is called *weighta* and is the reciprocal of the stratum specific sampling fraction.

The fourth line indicates the variable, *tothosp*, contains the total population number of hospitals (42 for stratum 1; 99 for stratum 2; 17 for stratum 3).

The fifth line indicates that estimation is for the total number of births.

Lines 6 and 7 indicate that estimated total births are to be obtained for each stratum.

Lines 8 and 9 specify the format of the output.

The following output is generated from the SUDAAN commands shown above:

```
1 PROC DESCRIPT DATA = HOSPSAMP FILETYPE = SAS DESIGN = WOR TOTALS;
2 NEST OBLEVEL;
3 WEIGHT WEIGHTA;
4 TOTCNT TOTHOSP;
5 VAR BIRTHS;
6 SUBGROUP OBLEVEL;
7 LEVELS 3;
8 SETENV COLWIDTH = 20;
9 SETENV DECWIDTH = 3;
```

Number of observations read : 15 Weighted count: 158
Number of observations skipped: 0
(WEIGHT variable nonpositive)
Denominator degrees of freedom: 12

by: Variable, OBLEVEL.

Variable		OBLEVEL Total	1
BIRTHS	Sample Size	15.000	4.000
	Weighted Size	158.00	42.000
	Total	183982.904	14931.000
	SE Total	34014.329	2669.857
	Mean	1164.449	355.500
	SE Mean	215.281	63.568

by: Variable, OBLEVEL.

Variable		OBLEVEL 2	3
BIRTHS	Sample Size	5.000	6.000
	Weighted Size	99.000	17.000
	Total	117116.928	51934.977
	SE Total	33067.664	7508.399
	Mean	1183.000	3055.000
	SE Mean	334.017	441.671

The estimates obtained from SUDAAN and STATA agree with each other, and the reader can verify that they agree with what would be computed using the formulas in Box 5.2.   □

5.7 SUMMARY

In this chapter we presented an overview of stratification. We introduced the concept of strata, and we defined what is meant by a stratified random sample. We discussed instances in which stratification might be appropriate and the advantages stratification has over simple random sampling as well as its major disadvantages. We presented the expressions that are used to characterize the population parameters and the sample statistics under simple random sampling. Finally, we illustrated how estimates from stratified random sampling can be obtained along with their standard errors by use of two software packages, SUDAAN and STATA.

EXERCISES

5.1 From a simple random serological sample of 1000 runners selected from 10,000 who completed the 1995 Chicago Marathon, 35 were found to be positive for steroids and other performance-enhancing drugs. When categorized by completion time, the results were as follows:

Completion Time (h)	No. in Sample	No. Positive for Drugs	Percentage Positive
Under 2.5	100	25	25.00
2.5–4.0	500	7	1.40
Over 4.0	400	3	0.75
Total	1000	35	3.50

   a. What is the standard error of the estimated proportion positive?
   b. From inspection (without making calculations) of the rates given above, would you feel that stratification may have resulted in a substantially better estimate? Why or why not?

5.2 Suppose that in the situation of Exercise 5.1, of the 10,000 completing the marathon, 2000 completed the event in less than 2.5 h; 6000 completed the event in 2.5–4.0 h; and 2000 completed the event in more than 4 h. Comment on the results of the sampling as given in Exercise 5.1.

5.3 If a stratified random sample of 333 persons in each of the three groups had been taken, what would likely be the resulting estimated percentage positive?

5.4 An additional 2000 runners entered the race but did not complete it. Of these runners, a mail questionnaire was sent to a random sample of 600 and completed by 500. One of the items in this questionnaire asked the respondent to estimate the average number of miles run weekly during the 8 weeks preceding the marathon. The mean, $\bar{x}$, of the number of miles run was 32.4 with standard deviation, s_x, equal to 7.3. A simple random sample of 500 of the 10,000 runners completing the marathon yielded 400 respondents who averaged 46.8 miles weekly with standard deviation equal to 6.2 miles. What is the average weekly miles run in that period among all those who entered the marathon?

5.5 The following data are available for 1988 for 6 health maintenance organizations (HMOs) in a medium-size city:

Number of personnel providing patient care and number of patient encounters during 1988 among six HMOs

HMO	No. of Physicians Providing Patient Care	No. of Patient Encounters
1	10	22,000
2	6	14,000
3	4	10,200
4	30	70,000
5	7	15,000
6	3	5,000

As a time- and cost-sharing device, it is proposed that a sample of two of these HMOs be taken for purposes of estimating the total number of patient encounters in 1988 among these six HMOs.
  a. Enumerate all simple random samples of size 2 and estimate the total number of patient encounters in 1988 among the 6 HMOs.
  b. What is the standard error of the estimated total from the sample design specified above?
  c. Group HMOs 1, 2, 3, 5, and 6 into 1 stratum and HMO 4 into another (by itself). From these two strata, enumerate all stratified random samples of size 2. What is the standard error of the estimated total as obtained by this sampling plan?
  d. Comment on the utility of using stratification in this situation as opposed to simple random sampling.

5.6 Suppose that in the situation given in Exercise 5.5 it is desired to estimate the number of encounters per physician in 1988. Repeat parts (a)–(d) in Exercise 5.5 for this estimation situation. Is stratified random sampling superior to simple random sampling in this situation? Why is it or why is it not?

5.7 In a large clinic located in an inner city hospital, 56 patients with non-symptomatic HIV infection have been treated with an experimental drug believed to have the capability of restoring certain immune system functions associated with HIV infection. Of these patients, 12 had CD4 cell counts below 250 at the initial visit; 20 had counts between 250 and 400; and 24 had counts above 400. (The lower the count, the worse the prognosis.) It is desired to take a stratified random sample of 30 patients, 10 from each of the three groups described above, for purposes of estimating the 12-month incidence of AIDS-defining events among these patients.

a. How many samples of 30 patients taken as described above are possible?

b. Assuming that a patient can have more than one AIDS-defining event during this period, show algebraically how you would estimate the 12-month incidence of AIDS-defining events from the sample.

c. How many samples of size 30 are possible under simple random sampling without stratification.

5.8 The results of the sample survey described in Exercise 5.7 are shown below:

	Number of Persons		
Number of Events	**CD4 < 250**	**250 ≤ CD4 < 400**	**CD4 ≥ 400**
0	5	7	9
1	1	2	1
2	2	1	0
3	2	0	0

From these data, estimate the incidence of AIDs defining events in the target population. What is the standard error of the estimated incidence rate? (You have to derive the formula for the standard error from "first principles.")

5.9 From the data in Exercise 5.8, estimate the proportion of patients having one or more AIDS-defining events. What is the standard error of this estimated proportion?

5.10 A simple random sample (without stratification) of 30 of these 56 patients yielded the following data:

| | **Number of Persons** | | |
Number of Events	CD4 < 250	250 ≤ CD4 < 400	CD4 ≥ 400
0	3	8	12
1	1	2	0
2	0	1	1
3	2	0	0

Estimate the incidence of AIDS-defining events from these data and the standard error of this estimate. Compare this to the results obtained from the stratified sampling design. Which design produces the more reliable estimate? Why does it?

BIBLIOGRAPHY

The following articles present sample surveys in which stratification is used.

1. Hemphill, F. M., A sample survey of home injuries, *Public Health Reports*, 67: 1026, 1952.

2. Horvitz, D. G., Sampling and field procedures of the Pittsburgh morbidity survey, *Public Health Reports*, 67: 1003, 1952.

3. Goldberg, J., Levy, P. S., Mullner, R., Gelfand, H., Iverson, N., Lemeshow, S., and Rothrock, J., Factors affecting trauma center utilization in Illinois, *Medical Care* 19: 547, 1981.

4. Stasny, E. A., Toomey, B. G., and First, R. J., Estimating the rate of rural homelessness: A study of nonurban Ohio, *Survey Methodology*, 20: 87, 1994.

5. Barner, B. M., and Levy, P. S., State-wide shoulder belt usage by type of roadway and posted speed limit: A three year comparison, *38th Annual Proceedings Association for the Advancement of Automotive Medicine*, Association for the Advancement of Automotive Medicine, Des Plaines Ill., 1994.

The following software programs have the capability of taking stratified samples.

6. Frankel, M. R., and Spencer, B. D., *SAMPLE, A Supplementary Module for SYSTAT*, SYSTAT, Inc., Evanston, Ill., 1990.

7. SAS Institute Inc., *SAS Language and Procedures*, Usage 2, Version 6, 1st ed., Cary, N.C., SAS Institute Inc., 1991, pp. 649.

In addition, there is material on stratification in virtually every text on sampling theory and survey methodology, including those listed in the bibliography sections of earlier chapters.

CHAPTER 6

Stratified Random Sampling: Further Issues

In the previous chapter we introduced the concept of stratification and discussed the reasons why stratification is used as a strategy in designing sample surveys. We also introduced notation commonly used by statisticians in discussing population characteristics and estimation procedures appropriate for stratified sampling. In this chapter we will discuss one type of stratified sampling in considerable detail, namely stratified random sampling.

6.1 ESTIMATION OF POPULATION PARAMETERS

Estimates of population means, proportions, and totals under stratified random sampling are obtained by computing weighted averages of the individual stratum-specific estimates and aggregating them across strata. The formulas for these estimates were given in Box 5.2. Now let us see how these formulas can be used by looking at an example.

Illustrative Example. Consider the population of 14 families shown in Table 5.6. Suppose we decide to take a sample of two families from stratum 1, two families from stratum 2, and four families from stratum 3. Then we have $n_1 = 2$, $n_2 = 2$, $n_3 = 4$, $N_1 = 3$, $N_2 = 5$, $N_3 = 6$, and $N = 14$. Suppose we select elements $X_{1,2}$ and $X_{1,3}$ from stratum 1 (i.e., $x_{1,1} = 3$ and $x_{1,2} = 4$), $X_{2,2}$ and $X_{2,5}$ from stratum 2 (i.e., $x_{2,1} = 6$ and $x_{2,2} = 8$), and we select $X_{3,1}, X_{3,2}, X_{3,4}$, and $X_{3,6}$ from stratum 3 (i.e., $x_{3,1} = 2, x_{3,2} = 3, x_{3,3} = 2$, and $x_{3,4} = 3$).

Using Equation (5.6), we obtain the total number of individuals in Block 1:

$$x_1' = \frac{3 \times (3+4)}{2} = 10.5.$$

Similarly, we obtain $x_2' = 35$ and $x_3' = 15$. Then, by Equation (5.6), the estimated total number of people in the population is given by

$$x'_{str} = 10.5 + 35 + 15 = 60.5$$

Using Equation (5.7), we obtain the estimated mean number of individuals per family in block 1:

$$\bar{x}_1 = \frac{3 + 4}{2} = 3.5$$

Similarly, $\bar{x}_2 = 7$ and $\bar{x}_3 = 2.5$. Then, by Equation (5.7), the estimated mean number of individuals per family is

$$\bar{x}_{str} = \frac{3 \times 3.5}{14} + \frac{5 \times 7}{14} + \frac{6 \times 2.5}{14} = 4.32$$

By Equation (5.9), the variance for family size in stratum 1 is given by

$$s_{1x}^2 = \frac{(3 - 3.5)^2 + (4 - 3.5)^2}{1} = 0.5$$

Similarly, $s_{2x}^2 = 2$ and $s_{3x}^2 = 0.33$.

If we let

$$y_{h,i} = \begin{cases} 0 & \text{if family size is 4 or more} \\ 1 & \text{if family size is less than 4} \end{cases}$$

Then by equation (5.8) we have

$$p_{1y} = \frac{0 + 1}{2} = 0.5$$

Similarly, $p_{2y} = 1$ and $p_{3y} = 0$.   □

6.2 SAMPLING DISTRIBUTIONS OF ESTIMATES

Since a stratified random sample consists of L simple random samples, which are drawn separately and independently within each stratum, and since the estimated population mean, total, or proportion is a linear combination of the estimated individual stratum means, totals, or proportions obtained from the sample, it follows that the mean of the sampling distribution of any of these estimated values is equal to the corresponding linear combination of population parameters. In other words, population totals, means, and proportions, when estimated as indicated in relations (5.6), (5.7), and (5.8), are, under stratified random sampling, unbiased estimates of the corresponding population means, totals, and proportions.

Means and standard errors of population estimates are given in Box 6.1.

BOX 6.1   MEANS AND STANDARD ERRORS OF POPULATION ESTIMATES UNDER STRATIFIED RANDOM SAMPLING

Mean

$$E(x'_{\text{str}}) = \sum_{h=1}^{L} E(x'_h) = \sum_{h=1}^{L} X_{h+} = X$$

$$\text{SE}(x'_{\text{str}}) = N[\text{SE}(\bar{x}_{\text{str}})] = \left[\sum_{h=1}^{L} (N_h^2) \left(\frac{\sigma_{hx}^2}{n_h} \right) \left(\frac{N_h - n_h}{N_h - 1} \right) \right]^{1/2} \tag{6.1}$$

Total

$$E(\bar{x}_{\text{str}}) = \frac{\sum_{h=1}^{L} (N_h) E(\bar{x}_h)}{N} = \frac{\sum_{h=1}^{L} N_h \bar{X}_h}{N} = \bar{X}$$

$$\text{SE}(\bar{x}_{\text{str}}) = \left[\frac{1}{N^2} \sum_{h=1}^{L} (N_h^2) \left(\frac{\sigma_{hx}^2}{n_h} \right) \left(\frac{N_h - n_h}{N_h - 1} \right) \right]^{1/2} \tag{6.2}$$

Proportion

$$E(p_{y,\text{str}}) = \frac{\sum_{h=1}^{L} N_h P_{hy}}{N} = \frac{\sum_{h=1}^{L} Y_{h+}}{N} = P_y$$

$$\text{SE}(p_{y,\text{str}}) = \left\{ \frac{1}{N^2} \sum_{h=1}^{L} (N_h^2) \left[\frac{P_{hy}(1 - P_{hy})}{n_h} \right] \left(\frac{N_h - n_h}{N_h - 1} \right) \right\}^{1/2} \tag{6.3}$$

The population notation used in these formulas is defined in Box 5.1, and n_h is the sample size for stratum h.

Let us see how these formulas are used by looking at an example.

Illustrative Example.   In the example used earlier, strata are three city blocks (Table 5.6), the elementary units are families, and the variable $\mathcal{X}$ is family size. We took a stratified random sample of two families from stratum 1, two from stratum 2, and four from stratum 3. Thus, we have $n_1 = 2, n_2 = 1, n_3 = 4, N_1 = 3, N_2 = 5, N_3 = 6$. $\sigma_{1x}^2 = .222, \sigma_{2x}^2 = 2.56, \sigma_{3x}^2 = .222, P_1 = .67,$

$P_2 = 1.00$, and $P_3 = 0$, where P_i is the proportion of families in the ith stratum with four or more persons. Using Equation (6.2), we have

$$
\mathrm{SE}(\bar{x}_{\mathrm{str}}) = \left\{ \frac{1}{14^2} \left[3^2 \times \left(\frac{.222}{2} \right) \left(\frac{3-2}{3-1} \right) + 5^2 \times \left(\frac{2.56}{2} \right) \left(\frac{5-2}{5-1} \right) \right. \right.
$$
$$
\left. \left. + 6^2 \times \left(\frac{.222}{4} \right) \left(\frac{6-4}{6-1} \right) \right] \right\}^{1/2}
$$
$$
= .359
$$
$$
\mathrm{SE}(x'_{\mathrm{str}}) = 14 \times 0.359 = 5.03
$$

From relation (6.3) we have

$$
\mathrm{SE}(p_{y,\mathrm{str}}) = \left\{ \frac{1}{14^2} \left[3^2 \times \left(\frac{.67 \times (1 - .67)}{2} \right) \left(\frac{3-2}{3-1} \right) \right. \right.
$$
$$
+ 5^2 \times \left(\frac{1 \times (1-1)}{2} \right) \left(\frac{5-2}{5-1} \right)
$$
$$
\left. \left. + 6^2 \times \left(\frac{0 \times (1-0)}{4} \right) \left(\frac{6-4}{6-1} \right) \right] \right\}^{1/2}
$$
$$
= .0504
$$

where $\mathcal{Y}$ is the attribute of having a family size of four or more persons. □

6.3   ESTIMATION OF STANDARD ERRORS

Under stratified random sampling the standard errors of estimated means, totals, and proportions can be estimated by substituting into relations (6.1), (6.2), and (6.3) $\hat{\sigma}_{hx}^2$ for σ_{hx}^2, or p_{hy} for P_{hy}, where

$$
\hat{\sigma}_{hx}^2 = \frac{(N_h - 1)s_{hx}^2}{N_h} \tag{6.4}
$$

$$
s_{hx}^2 = \frac{\sum_{i=1}^{n_h}(x_{h,i} - \bar{x}_h)^2}{n_h - 1} \tag{6.5}
$$

and p_{hy} is the observed proportion of elements in the stratum having attribute $\mathcal{Y}$. The resulting standard errors were presented in Box 5.2 and are repeated again in Box 6.2.

Now let us see how we can use some of these formulas.

BOX 6.2   ESTIMATED STANDARD ERRORS UNDER STRATIFIED RANDOM SAMPLING

Total

$$\widehat{SE}(\bar{x}_{str}) = \sqrt{\sum_{h=1}^{L} \frac{N_h^2 s_{hx}^2}{n_h} \left(\frac{N_h - n_h}{N_h} \right)} \tag{6.6}$$

Mean

$$\widehat{SE}(\bar{x}_{str}) = \sqrt{\sum_{h=1}^{L} \left(\frac{N_h}{N} \right)^2 \frac{s_{hx}^2}{n_h} \left(\frac{N_h - n_h}{N_h} \right)} \tag{6.7}$$

Proportion

$$\widehat{SE}(p_{y,str}) = \sqrt{\left(\frac{N_h}{N} \right)^2 \frac{p_{hy}(1 - p_{hy})}{n_h - 1} \left(\frac{N_h - n_h}{N_h} \right)} \tag{6.8}$$

where N is the population size; N_h is the number of elements in stratum h; s_{hx} is defined in Equation (5.9); and p_{hy} is the observed proportion of elements in stratum h having attribute $\mathcal{Y}$.

Illustrative Example.   For the illustrative example considered in Section 6.1, we have the following:

$$\begin{array}{llll}
\bar{x}_1 = 3.5 & x_1' = 10.5 & s_{1x}^2 = 0.5 & \hat{\sigma}_{1x}^2 = .33 \\
\bar{x}_2 = 7 & x_2' = 35 & s_{2x}^2 = 2 & \hat{\sigma}_{2x}^2 = 1.6 \\
\bar{x}_3 = 2.5 & x_3' = 15 & s_{3x}^2 = 0.33 & \hat{\sigma}_{3x}^2 = .275
\end{array}$$

The last column was obtained by using Equation (6.4).

As shown in the example of Section 6.1, the estimate x_{str}' of the total number of persons X on the three blocks is, from Equation (5.6),

$$x_{str}' = 10.5 + 35 + 15 = 60.5$$

with standard error, from relation (6.6), estimated by

$$\widehat{SE}(x'_{str}) = \left[(3)^2 \left(\frac{.5}{2}\right)\left(\frac{3-2}{3}\right) + (5)^2 \left(\frac{2}{2}\right)\left(\frac{5-2}{5}\right) + (6)^2 \left(\frac{.33}{4}\right)\left(\frac{6-4}{6}\right)\right]^{1/2} = 4.09$$

Thus, a 95% confidence interval for X, the population total is given by

$$x'_{str} - 1.96 \times \widehat{SE}(x'_{str}) \leqslant X \leqslant x'_{str} + 1.96 \times \widehat{SE}(x'_{str})$$
$$60.5 - 1.96 \times 4.09 \leqslant X \leqslant 60.5 + 1.96 \times 4.09$$
$$52.48 \leqslant X \leqslant 68.52$$

Clearly, this interval covers the true population total $X = 54$. □

In a manner similar to that in the example above, estimates may be obtained for standard errors of estimated means and proportions, which can be used in obtaining approximate confidence intervals.

6.4 ESTIMATION OF CHARACTERISTICS OF SUBGROUPS

In Chapter 3, we showed that under simple random sampling, estimated means, totals, and proportions for subgroups are unbiased estimates of the corresponding population means, totals, and proportions for the subgroups. This is not necessarily true in stratified random sampling, as is shown in the next example.

Illustrative Example. Let us consider the data given in Table 6.1. If we let $\bar{X}_1$ denote the average price among the five independent pharmacies in the combined two communities, we see that $\bar{X}_1 = \$11.60$. Suppose we take a stratified random sample of six pharmacies from stratum 1 and three pharmacies from stratum 2 for purposes of estimating $\bar{X}_1$. Suppose also that we do not know before the sampling whether a given pharmacy is an independent or an affiliate of a chain.

Our estimate $\bar{x}_{1,str}$ of $\bar{X}_1$ is given by

$$\bar{x}_{1,str} = \frac{\sum_{h=1}^{2} N_h \bar{x}_{1_h}}{N}$$

where $\bar{x}_{1_h}$ is the estimated mean for the independent pharmacies obtained from the sample taken in stratum h.

There are seven possible samples of six pharmacies that can be taken in stratum 1, and there are four possible samples of three pharmacies that can be taken in stratum 2. These samples and the estimated mean for each sample are listed in Table 6.2.

Table 6.1 Retail Prices of 20 Capsules of a Tranquilizer in All Pharmacies in Two Communities (Strata)

Community	Pharmacy	Type*	Price of Drug ($)
1	1	C	10.00
	2	I	9.00
	3	I	12.00
	4	I	11.00
	5	C	9.00
	6	C	9.50
	7	C	9.90
2	1	I	13.50
	2	I	12.50
	3	C	12.00
	4	C	11.00

*I = independent; C = chain.

Table 6.2 Possible Samples for the Stratified Random Sample

Stratum 1		Stratum 2	
Pharmacies in Sample	$\bar{x}_{I_1}$ ($)	Pharmacies in Sample	$\bar{x}_{I_2}$ ($)
1, 2, 3, 4, 5, 6	10.67	1, 2, 3	13.00
1, 2, 3, 4, 5, 7	10.67	1, 2, 4	13.00
1, 2, 3, 4, 6, 7	10.67	1, 3, 4	13.50
1, 2, 3, 5, 6, 7	10.50	2, 3, 4	12.50
1, 2, 4, 5, 6, 7	10.00		
1, 3, 4, 5, 6, 7	11.50		
2, 3, 4, 5, 6, 7	10.67		

There are $\binom{7}{6} \times \binom{4}{3} = 28$ possible values of $\bar{x}_{I,\text{str}} = (7\bar{x}_{I_1} + 4\bar{x}_{I_2})/11$. The sampling distribution of $\bar{x}_{I,\text{str}}$ is shown in Table 6.3.

The mean $E(\bar{x}_{I,\text{str}})$ of the distribution of $\bar{x}_{I,\text{str}}$ over the 28 samples is equal to \$11.52, which is not equal to \$11.60, the value of $\bar{X}_I$, the mean price over the five independent pharmacies in the two communities. □

In the example above, we have demonstrated empirically that for stratified random sampling, the estimate $\bar{x}_{I,\text{str}}$ of the population mean $\bar{X}_I$ for a subgroup within the population is not necessarily an unbiased estimate of $\bar{X}_I$. The reason for this lies in the fact that the individual stratum sample means $\bar{x}_{I_h}$ for the subgroup I are weighted in the construction of $\bar{x}_{I,\text{str}}$ by N_h/N, the proportion of all elements in the population belonging to stratum h, rather than by the proportion of all elements in subgroup I belonging to stratum h. If N_{I_h} denotes the number of elements in stratum h belonging to subgroup I, and if N_I denotes

Table 6.3 Sampling Distribution for $\bar{x}_{\text{I,str}}$

$\bar{x}_{\text{I,str}}$ ($)	f	$\bar{x}_{\text{I,str}}$ ($)	f
11.510	8	12.046	2
11.692	4	11.590	1
11.330	4	11.228	1
11.410	2	11.272	1
11.090	2	12.228	1
10.910	1	11.864	1
Total			28

the total number of elements in the population belonging to subgroup I (i.e., $N_{\text{I}} = \sum_{h=1}^{L} N_{\text{I}_h}$), then it is not necessarily true that $N_{\text{I}_h}/N_{\text{I}}$ is equal to N_h/N. That is, the elements in subgroup I are not necessarily represented in the various strata in the same proportions as are the elements in the population as a whole. It is for this reason that the estimate $\bar{x}_{\text{I,str}}$ is not necessarily an unbiased estimate of $\bar{X}_{\text{I}}$. If the proportions $N_{\text{I}_h}/N_{\text{I}}$ were known, then they would be used as weights in constructing an unbiased estimate of $\bar{X}_{\text{I}}$. Generally, however, they are not known.

For the same reason as given above, the sample proportion $p_{\text{I}_y,\text{str}}$ and the estimated total $x'_{\text{I,str}}$ are not, in general, unbiased estimates of P_{I_y} and X_{I} for subgroups under stratified random sampling.

Estimation of characteristics of subgroups of a population under stratified random sampling is generally done by *ratio estimation* procedures, which are discussed in the next chapter.

6.5 ALLOCATION OF SAMPLE TO STRATA

Once we decide to use stratified sampling, and once we specify the strata and the total number, n, of sample elements, the next important decision we must make is that of *allocation* or specification of how many elements are to be taken from each stratum under the constraint that a total of n elements is to be taken over all strata. As we will see in this section, the standard errors of the estimated population parameters may be reduced considerably if careful thought is given to allocation.

6.5.1 Equal Allocation

In equal allocation, the same number of elements are sampled from each stratum. In other words, for each stratum, h, the *sample size* is given by

$$n_h = \frac{n}{L}$$

Equal allocation would be the allocation of choice if the primary objective of the sample survey is to test hypotheses about differences among the strata with respect to levels of variables of interest, under the assumption that within stratum variances were equal. If this assumption could not be made, then the allocation of choice for testing such hypotheses would be given by

$$n_h = \frac{\sigma_{hx}}{\sum_{h=1}^{L} \sigma_{hx}} \times n$$

In other words, for testing hypotheses concerning differences among strata with respect to levels of variables, sample sizes for each stratum should be proportional to the standard deviation of the variable of interest within that stratum. If there are no differences among the strata with respect to within stratum standard deviations, then this would reduce to equal allocation. Since, in this text, our primary interest is estimation rather than hypothesis testing, we will not discuss this type of allocation further.

6.5.2 Proportional Allocation: Self-Weighting Samples

In proportional allocation, the sampling fraction n_h/N_h is specified to be the same for each stratum, which implies also that the overall sampling fraction n/N is the fraction taken from each stratum. In other words, the *number of elements* n_h taken from each stratum is given by

$$n_h = N_h \times \frac{n}{N} \tag{6.9}$$

Under proportional allocation, the estimated population mean, $\bar{x}_{str}$, as given in Relation (5.7) reduces to the form

$$\bar{x}_{str} = \frac{\sum_{h=1}^{L} \sum_{i=1}^{n_h} x_{h,i}}{n} \tag{6.10}$$

which is a considerably simpler expression than the one given in Equation (5.7).

Let us compare the formula for $\bar{x}_{str}$ under proportional allocation with the general formula for an estimated population mean under stratified random sampling. We see that in the general formula [relation (5.7)], the value $x_{h,i}$ of characteristic $\mathscr{X}$ for a sample element is multiplied by the ratio $N_h/(n_h N)$, which is not necessarily the same for each stratum. Thus, in order to obtain $\bar{x}_{str}$, it is necessary to keep track of the stratum to which each element belongs. On the other hand, relation (6.10) indicates that for proportional allocation, each sample element is multiplied by the same constant, $1/n$, irrespective of the stratum to which the element belongs. Estimates of this type are known as *self-weighting estimates*.

This technique of proportional allocation greatly simplifies the amount of bookkeeping involved in the data processing, and hence reduces computational expenses. In large surveys in which much information is collected on each sample individual, proportional allocation is often used because of its simplicity, even if it is not the optimal design in terms of precision of estimates.

We note that a stratified sample with proportional allocation will be self-weighting only if the proportion of sampled individuals *who respond* is the same within each stratum. Nonresponse, particularly where the nonresponse rate differs from stratum to stratum, can drastically affect the validity of the estimate given in expression (6.10). For this reason, methods of handling nonresponse, as discussed in Chapter 13, are critically important.

Now let us look at an example of proportional allocation.

Illustrative Example. Consider the data in Table 6.4, which shows the number of general hospitals located in four strata, where a stratum is composed of one or more geographical regions within Illinois.

Suppose we wish to take a stratified random sample of 51 hospitals from among the 255 hospitals in the universe, and we wish to use proportional allocation. Then letting $N = 255$ and $n = 51$, we have from relation (6.9),

$$n_1 = (44)\left(\frac{51}{255}\right) = 8.8 \approx 9$$

$$n_2 = (116)\left(\frac{51}{255}\right) = 23.2 \approx 23$$

$$n_3 = (48)\left(\frac{51}{255}\right) = 9.6 \approx 10$$

$$n_4 = (47)\left(\frac{51}{255}\right) = 9.4 \approx 9$$

Table 6.4 General Hospitals in Illinois by Geographical Stratum, 1971 [3]

Stratum	No. of General Hospitals
1	44
2	116
3	48
4	47
Total	255

Thus, we would take 9 elements (hospitals) from stratum 1; 23 from stratum 2; 10 from stratum 3; and 9 from stratum 4.

The sampling fractions within each stratum are

$$\frac{n_1}{N_1} = \frac{9}{44} = .2045 \qquad \frac{n_2}{N_2} = \frac{23}{116} = .1983$$

$$\frac{n_3}{N_3} = \frac{10}{48} = .2083 \qquad \frac{n_4}{N_4} = \frac{9}{47} = .1915$$

Note that $\sum_{h=1}^{4} n_h = n$.

The slight differences in sampling fractions among the strata are due to the fact that the required allocation given by relation (6.9) does not necessarily yield integer values. Thus, the n_h taken are those specified by Equation (6.9), but rounded up or down to the nearest integer. These minor differences among sampling fractions are generally ignored in constructing the estimates, and the sample is generally treated as if it were exactly a self-weighting sample. □

In proportional allocation, the *variance*, $\text{Var}(\bar{x}_{\text{str}})$, of an estimated mean, $\bar{x}_{\text{str}}$, obtained from relation (6.10) with n_h set equal to $N_h(n/N)$ becomes

$$\text{Var}(\bar{x}_{\text{str}}) = \left(\frac{N-n}{N^2}\right) \sum_{h=1}^{L} \left(\frac{N_h^2}{N_h - 1}\right) \left(\frac{\sigma_{hx}^2}{n}\right) \tag{6.11}$$

If all the N_h are reasonably large, the expression reduces to the approximation given by

$$\text{Var}(\bar{x}_{\text{str}}) \approx \left(\frac{\sigma_{w.x}^2}{n}\right) \left(\frac{N-n}{N}\right) \tag{6.12}$$

where

$$\sigma_{w.x}^2 = \frac{\sum_{h=1}^{L} N_h \sigma_{hx}^2}{N} \tag{6.13}$$

The *sample estimate* of $\text{Var}(\bar{x}_{\text{str}})$ is given by

$$\widehat{\text{Var}}(\bar{x}_{\text{str}}) = \left(\frac{N-n}{N^2}\right) \sum_{h=1}^{L} N_h \left(\frac{s_{hx}^2}{n}\right)$$

Note that relation (6.12) has a form that is very similar to the formula for the variance of an estimated mean $\bar{x}$ under simple random sampling. The formula for the standard error was given in Box 3.1, and the square of this quantity, the variance, is given as

$$\text{Var}(\bar{x}) = \left(\frac{\sigma_x^2}{n}\right)\left(\frac{N-n}{N-1}\right) \tag{6.14}$$

The difference between the two formulas is that for proportional allocation in stratified random sampling, the population variance σ_x^2 is replaced by $\sigma_{w\cdot x}^2$, which is a weighted average of the individual variances σ_{hx}^2 of the distribution of $\mathscr{X}$ among elements within each stratum. The weights in $\sigma_{w\cdot x}^2$ are proportional to N_h, the number of elements in each stratum.

Comparison of relations (6.12) and (6.14) indicates that stratified random sampling with proportional allocation will yield an estimated mean having lower variance than that obtained from simple random sampling whenever $\sigma_{w\cdot x}^2$ is less than σ_x^2. But note that, as in analysis of variance methodology, the population variance σ_x^2 may be partitioned into the two components σ_{bx}^2 and $\sigma_{w\cdot x}^2$

$$\sigma_x^2 = \sigma_{bx}^2 + \sigma_{w\cdot x}^2$$

where

$$\sigma_{bx}^2 = \frac{\sum_{h=1}^{L} N_h(\bar{X}_h - \bar{X})^2}{N} \tag{6.15}$$

and $\sigma_{w\cdot x}^2$ is as given in relation (6.13). Thus the ratio of the variance of the estimated mean $\bar{x}$ under simple random sampling to that of $\bar{x}_{\text{str}}$, the estimated mean under stratified random sampling with proportional allocation, is given by

$$\frac{\text{Var}(\bar{x})}{\text{Var}(\bar{x}_{\text{str}})} = \frac{\sigma_{bx}^2 + \sigma_{w\cdot x}^2}{\sigma_{w\cdot x}^2} = 1 + \frac{\sigma_{bx}^2}{\sigma_{w\cdot x}^2} \tag{6.16}$$

This ratio is always greater than or equal to unity, and the extent to which it differs from unity depends on the size of the ratio $\sigma_{bx}^2/\sigma_{w\cdot x}^2$. When this ratio is large, the estimated mean under stratified random sampling with proportional allocation will have a smaller variance than the corresponding estimate under simple random sampling. The component σ_{bx}^2 represents the *variance among the stratum means*, whereas the component $\sigma_{w\cdot x}^2$ represents the *variance among the elements* within the same stratum.

If the stratum means $\bar{X}_h$ are of the same order of magnitude, then little or nothing is gained by using stratified random sampling rather than simple random sampling. On the other hand, if the stratum means are very different, it is likely that considerable reduction in the variance of an estimated mean can be obtained by use of stratified random sampling rather than simple random sampling. This makes sense intuitively because the purpose of stratification is to group the elements, in advance of the sampling, into strata on the basis of their similarity with respect to the values of a variable or a set of variables. If the elements within each stratum have very similar values of the variable being measured, then it would be difficult to obtain a "bad" sample, since each stratum is represented in the sample. A reliable estimate could then be obtained by sampling a small number of elements within each stratum. On the other hand, if the stratum means are very similar, then there is no point to stratification, and the extra effort required to take a stratified sample would not result in an improved estimate.

For convenience, formulas for estimates of population parameters under proportional allocation are summarized in Box 6.3.

Now let us look at an example that investigates whether stratified random sampling is likely to have lower variance than one obtained from simple random sampling.

Illustrative Example. Let us suppose that we wish to estimate the average number of hospital admissions for major trauma conditions per county among 82 counties in Illinois having general hospitals. A sample of counties will be taken, and the admission records of all hospitals in the sample counties will be reviewed for major trauma admissions. If it is reasonable to assume that there may be a strong correlation between the number of hospital beds among general hospitals within a county and the total number of admissions for major trauma conditions, then it would make sense to stratify by number of hospital beds. So this is the sampling plan that is chosen. In Table 6.5, counties in Illinois are grouped into two strata on the basis of number of hospital beds. Stratum 1 consists of those counties having 1–399 beds, and stratum 2 consists of those having 400 beds or more.

From Table 6.5 we calculate the following:

$$\bar{X}_1 = 123.91 \qquad \sigma_{1x}^2 = 6{,}131.63 \qquad N_1 = 65$$
$$\bar{X}_2 = 871.59 \qquad \sigma_{2x}^2 = 77{,}287.92 \qquad N_2 = 17$$
$$\bar{X} = 278.92 \qquad \sigma_x^2 = 112{,}751.93 \qquad N = 82$$

where $\mathscr{X}$ = the number of beds.

From relations (6.15) and (6.13) we have

$$\sigma_{bx}^2 = \frac{65 \times (123.91 - 278.92)^2 + 17 \times (871.59 - 278.92)^2}{82}$$
$$= 91{,}868.39$$
$$\sigma_{wx}^2 = \frac{65 \times 6{,}131.63 + 17 \times 77{,}287.92}{82} = 20{,}883.54$$

Thus, from relation (6.16), the ratio of the variances $\text{Var}(\bar{x})/\text{Var}(\bar{x}_{\text{str}})$ are given by

---

BOX 6.3   ESTIMATES OF POPULATION PARAMETERS UNDER STRATIFIED RANDOM SAMPLING WITH PROPORTIONAL ALLOCATION

Under proportional allocation [i.e., $n_h = (N_h/N)n$] the following formulas are used for estimating population parameters.

Total

$$x'_{str} = N \times \frac{\sum_{h=1}^{L} \sum_{i=1}^{n_h} x_{h,i}}{n}$$

$$\widehat{Var}(x'_{str}) = N^2 \times \left(\frac{N-n}{N^2}\right) \sum_{h=1}^{L} N_h \times \left(\frac{s_{hx}^2}{n}\right)$$

Mean

$$\bar{x}_{str} = \frac{\sum_{h=1}^{L} \sum_{i=1}^{n_h} x_{h,i}}{n}$$

$$\widehat{Var}(\bar{x}_{str}) = \left(\frac{N-n}{N^2}\right) \sum_{h=1}^{L} N_h \times \left(\frac{s_{hx}^2}{n}\right)$$

Proportion

$$p_{y,str} = \frac{\sum_{h=1}^{L} \sum_{i=1}^{n_h} y_{h,i}}{n}$$

$$\widehat{Var}(p_{y,str}) = \left(\frac{N-n}{N^2}\right) \sum_{h=1}^{L} N_h \times \left[\frac{p_{hy}(1-p_{hy})}{n-1}\right]$$

All quantities in these expressions are as defined in Box 5.2.

$$\frac{Var(\bar{x})}{Var(\bar{x}_{str})} = 1 + \frac{91,868.39}{20,883.54} = 5.40$$

Therefore, we conclude that in terms of reduction of the variance of an estimated mean, stratification is likely to be of great benefit in this situation if, in fact, admissions for multiple trauma and number of beds are related, since the variance under stratification is less than 20% of the variance under simple random sampling.   □

Table 6.5 Strata for Number of Hospital Beds by County Among Counties in Illinois (Excluding Cook County) Having General Hospitals

Stratum 1 (1–399 Beds)				Stratum 2 (400+ Beds)	
County	No. of Beds	County	No. of Beds	County	No. of Beds
1	216	34	113	1	823
2	170	35	64	2	1343
3	252	36	100	3	908
4	38	37	58	4	648
5	170	38	54	5	1043
6	179	39	82	6	1325
7	31	40	35	7	1123
8	40	41	204	8	690
9	295	42	42	9	519
10	336	43	72	10	1118
11	166	44	39	11	522
12	121	45	144	12	715
13	280	46	210	13	851
14	188	47	160	14	552
15	35	48	204	15	470
16	134	49	200	16	1187
17	63	50	195	17	980
18	280	51	140		
19	75	52	96		
20	142	52	108		
21	293	54	121		
22	152	55	61		
23	103	56	63		
24	262	57	104		
25	105	58	150		
26	80	59	48		
27	54	60	48		
28	66	61	69		
29	54	62	79		
30	50	63	75		
31	50	64	32		
32	165	65	39		
33	200				

6.5.3 Optimal Allocation

Often proportional allocation is not the type of allocation that would result in an estimated total, mean, or proportion having the lowest variance among all possible ways of allocating a total sample of n elements among the L strata. It can be shown that the allocation of n sample units into each stratum that will yield an estimated total, mean, or proportion for a variable $\mathfrak{X}$ having minimum variance is given by

$$n_h = \left(\frac{N_h \sigma_{hx}}{\sum_{h=1}^{L} N_h \sigma_{hx}}\right)(n) \tag{6.17}$$

Illustrative Example. Let us use the data in Table 6.5 and assume a close relationship between number of beds and number of admissions for major trauma. From relation (6.17), the following allocation of 25 sample elements will produce the estimated mean having the lowest variance:

$$n_1 = \left(\frac{65\sqrt{6131.63}}{65\sqrt{6131.63} + 17\sqrt{77,287.92}}\right) \times 25 = 12.96 \approx 13$$

$$n_2 = \left(\frac{17\sqrt{77,287.92}}{65\sqrt{6131.63} + 17\sqrt{77,287.92}}\right) \times 25 = 12.04 \approx 12$$

Thus, the optimal allocation of the 25 sample elements is 13 elements from stratum 1 and 12 elements from stratum 2. Proportional allocation would have specified that 20 elements be taken from stratum 1 and 5 elements from stratum 2.

The standard error of an estimated mean under stratified random sampling with optimal allocation is given by relation (6.2), which is valid in general for any type of allocation under stratified random sampling. For the data in Table 6.5, using number of beds as the characteristic of interest, we have for optimal allocation from Equation (6.1),

$$\text{SE}(\bar{x}_{\text{str}}) = \left\{ \left(\frac{1}{82^2}\right) \left[(65)^2 \left(\frac{6131.63}{13}\right) \left(\frac{65-13}{65-1}\right) \right. \right.$$
$$\left. \left. + (17)^2 \left(\frac{77,287.92}{12}\right) \left(\frac{17-12}{17-1}\right) \right] \right\}^{1/2}$$
$$= 18.09$$

For proportional allocation we have, taking the square root of the expression in Equation (6.11),

$$\text{SE}(\bar{x}_{\text{str}}) = \left[\left(\frac{82-25}{82^2}\right) \left\{ \left(\frac{65^2}{64}\right) \left(\frac{6131.63}{25}\right) \right. \right.$$
$$\left. \left. + \left(\frac{17^2}{16}\right) \left(\frac{77,287.92}{25}\right) \right\} \right]^{1/2} = 24.71$$

Thus we see that for these data the estimated mean under optimal allocation has a standard error considerably lower than that under proportional allocation. □

From relation (6.17) we see that the optimal number of sample elements to be taken from a given stratum is proportional to N_h, the total number of elements in the stratum, and to σ_{hx}, the standard deviation of the distribution of $\mathcal{X}$ among all elements in the stratum. This makes sense intuitively. The population mean $\bar{X}$, which we are trying to estimate is equal to $\sum_{h=1}^{L} N_h \bar{X}_h / N$, or, in other words, $\bar{X}$ is a weighted average of the individual stratum means, $\bar{X}_h$, with weights that are proportional to the total number of elements in the stratum. Since the strata that have the largest number of elements are the most important in determining the population mean, it makes sense that they also be the most important in estimating it from a sample. If the distribution of characteristic $\mathcal{X}$ among elements in a particular stratum has a small standard deviation, then only a small number of sample elements are required to yield a reliable estimate of a stratum parameter relative to the number required to estimate a parameter in a stratum in which the distribution of $\mathcal{X}$ has a large standard deviation. This fact is taken into consideration in the formula for optimal allocation, since the sample allocation, as given by relation (6.17), is proportional to the size of the standard deviation, σ_{hx}. Also note that if the distribution of $\mathcal{X}$ within each stratum has the same standard deviation, then optimal allocation, as given by relation (6.17), reduces to proportional allocation, as given by relation (6.9).

6.5.4 Optimal Allocation and Economics

Suppose now that the cost of sampling an elementary unit is not the same for each stratum. Then the *total cost* C, of taking a sample of n_1 elements from stratum 1, n_2 elements from stratum 2, and so forth, is given by

$$C = \sum_{h=1}^{L} n_h C_h$$

where C_h is the cost of sampling an elementary unit in stratum h.

For a given sample size n, the allocation that will yield an estimate having the lowest variance per unit cost is given by

$$n_h = \frac{N_h \sigma_{hx} / \sqrt{C_h}}{\sum_{h=1}^{L} (N_h \sigma_{hx} / \sqrt{C_h})} \times n \qquad (6.18)$$

Similarly, if the total cost of taking the sample is fixed at C, the allocation that will yield the estimated mean having the lowest standard error at fixed cost C is given by

$$n_h = \frac{N_h \sigma_{hx} / \sqrt{C_h}}{\sum_{h=1}^{L} N_h \sigma_{hx} \sqrt{C_h}} \times C \qquad (6.19)$$

Both relations (6.18) and (6.19) choose samples sizes n_h that are directly proportional to N_h and σ_{hx} and inversely proportional to the cost C_h of sampling an element in a particular stratum.

Now let us look at an example of optimum allocation, taking cost into consideration.

Illustrative Example. Let us suppose that a corporation has 260,000 accident reports available over a period of time and that a sample survey is being contemplated for purposes of estimating the average number of days of work lost per accident. Of the 260,000 accident reports, 150,000 are coded and 110,000 are uncoded. The coded forms could be processed on the computer directly, whereas the uncoded forms must first be coded before processing. Approximately $10,000 is available for selecting the sample and coding and processing the data. With this in mind, it is desired to find the best way of allocating the sample elements among coded and uncoded forms.

In the terminology of stratified sampling we have

$$N_1 = 150,000 \text{ coded forms (stratum 1)}$$
$$N_2 = 110,000 \text{ uncoded forms (stratum 2)}$$
$$C = \$10,000$$

Let us suppose that the cost of sampling and processing sample forms is equal to $0.32 for a coded form and $0.98 for an uncoded form; that is,

$$C_1 = \$0.32 \quad \text{and} \quad C_2 = \$0.98$$

If we assume that the standard deviation of the distribution of days lost from work is twice as large among uncoded reports as among coded reports (i.e., $\sigma_{1x} = \sigma_{2x}/2$), then from relation (6.19) we have

$$n_1 = \frac{\dfrac{150,000 \times (\sigma_{2x}/2)}{\sqrt{0.32}}}{150,000 \times (\sigma_{2x}/2) \times \sqrt{0.32} + 110,000 \times \sigma_{2x} \times \sqrt{0.98}} \times 10,000 \approx 8,762$$

$$n_2 = \frac{\dfrac{110,000 \times \sigma_{2x}}{\sqrt{0.98}}}{150,000 \times (\sigma_{2x}/2) \times \sqrt{0.32} + 110,000 \times \sigma_{2x} \times \sqrt{0.98}} \times 10,000 \approx 7,343$$

Thus we would take a sample of 8762 coded reports and 7343 uncoded reports.

We can verify that the total cost of the sampling is equal to $10,000 by substituting the values for C_1, C_2, n_1, and n_2 into the relation for C:

$$C = 8762 \times 0.32 + 7343 \times 0.98 = \$10,000 \qquad \square$$

We note that in order to obtain the optimal allocation, it is not necessary to know the actual values of the σ_{hx}. If we can express each σ_{hx} in terms of one of them (e.g., σ_{rx}), as was done in the example discussed above, then σ_{rx} appears as a common factor in both the numerator and denominator and therefore can be canceled.

One problem often encountered in optimal allocation, either with or without costs being taken into consideration, is that the optimal sample size n_h may be greater than N_h, the total number of elements in the stratum. When this occurs, we set n_h equal to N_h for each stratum having optimal allocation greater than N_h. Then we reallocate the remaining sample to other strata as specified by the algorithm of obtaining optimal allocation.

For example, let us consider the summary data from three strata:

Stratum	N_h	σ_{hx}
1	100	50
2	110	10
3	120	5

If we wish to allocate a total sample of 140 elements to each stratum by using optimal allocation, we have, by relation (6.17),

$$n_1 = 104 \qquad n_2 = 23 \qquad n_3 = 13$$

We would then take $n_1 = N_1 = 100$ and allocate the four remaining elements to strata 2 and 3 according to relation (6.17) as follows:

$$n_2 = \left[\frac{110 \times 10}{110 \times 10 + 120 \times 5}\right](4) = 2.6 \approx 3$$

$$n_3 = \left[\frac{120 \times 5}{110 \times 10 + 120 \times 5}\right](4) = 1.4 \approx 1$$

Thus the final optimum allocation is

$$n_1 = 100 \qquad n_2 = 26 \qquad n_3 = 14$$

In the planning of a sample survey for which stratified random sampling is indicated, it is often a good strategy to calculate the optimal allocation for the most important variables in the survey. If the allocation differs among the variables, some compromise allocation might be considered (such as the mean of the optimal n_h over all variables of importance). Also, proportional allocation should be given some consideration. If the standard errors anticipated under proportional allocation are not much higher than those anticipated under optimal allocation, then the simplicity and convenience of proportional allocation may offset the small reduction in standard error under optimal allocation, and proportional allocation may be the best choice.

Illustrative Example: Case Study. This example from a recent study of elderly twins [4] illustrates the use of optimal allocation in stratified random sampling. The objective of this study was to test a method for identifying elderly twins (65 years and older) from lists of living Medicare beneficiaries. Studies on monozygotic and dizygotic twins are extremely useful in providing insight into the relative contribution of genetic and nongenetic influences on health and disease, and twins so identified would be placed in a registry for possible participation in future medical investigations.

Since approximately 1 in every 100 deliveries results in a multiple birth, any attempt at screening unselected lists of individuals for identification of twins would be prohibitively expensive. The following characteristics of twins, however, might be used to obtain modified lists that have a higher prevalence of twins:

1. Both members of a twin pair (with very rare exceptions) are born in the same place and have the same date of birth.
2. They are also of the same race.
3. Both members of a male–male twin pair will have the same last name and a different first name.
4. It was hypothesized that members of a twin pair are very likely to have Social Security numbers (SS#) that are very close to each other.

With this in mind, the following data set was extracted from a file containing approximately 10 million living Medicare beneficiaries:

- From living male beneficiaries, pairs were constructed consisting of individuals having the same date of birth, the same state of birth, the same last name, and a different first name. The pairs so obtained were then assigned a number representing the difference in their SS#. This difference (called *sequence difference*) was obtained by a complex algorithm [47]; the size of this sequence difference being proportional to the length of time separating the issuance dates of the SS card to each member of the pair.
- From living female beneficiaries, female–female pairs were constructed from records that had the same date and state of birth and the same first seven digits of the SS#. (Surnames could not be used as was done with the males because of name change upon marriage.)
- Male–female pairs were constructed by the same algorithm used to construct female–female pairs.

The data set constructed as described above consisted of 255,848 paired records categorized into six classes according to race (white/African-American) and sex (M–M, M–F, F–F). Each of these six groups was further subdivided into three classes based on the size of the sequence difference in SS# (first quartile/second and third quartiles/fourth quartile). Those pairs having sequence differences in the first quartile represent SS#'s issued relatively close in time, and so on. Table 6.6 indicates the number of pairs that were obtained in each of the 18 "strata" defined above.

A pilot survey of approximately 1000 pairs was to be conducted, having as its objective the estimation in each of the six race–sex groups of the proportion of pairs in this database that are truly twins. This was considered important as a test of whether or not this methodology would produce a database that has a high prevalence of twins. A sample of pairs was to be taken, and each individual sampled was to be queried on his/her twin status. The design of the sample for this pilot survey was to be that of stratified random sampling with optimal allocation applied separately to each of the six race–sex groups. With this in mind, the formula for allocation of sample into the three SS# sequence difference groups is given by Equation (6.17), where $\sigma_{hx} = \sqrt{p_{hx}(1 - p_{hx})}$, and p_{hx} is the proportion of twins in stratum h ($h = 1, 2, 3$).

The proportions, p_{hx}, are not known, and it is necessary to make some "educated" guesses concerning their values. The overall prevalence rate of twins in the master file of Medicare beneficiaries is likely to be about 1%, the rate in the population as a whole. We would then expect that the algorithms used to construct the set of pairs would yield a very much higher prevalence of twins—let us assume a 10-fold higher prevalence—which would be a rate of 10%. We further assume that the prevalence of twins in the first sequence difference quartile is four times that in the middle two quartiles and eight times that in the fourth quartile. From these assumptions, using white M–M

Table 6.6 Number of Pairs Available in Each of 18 Sex–Race-Sequence Difference Quantiles

Race	Sequence Difference Quantile	Sex		
		M–M	M–F	F–F
White	1	39,872	11,263	10,024
	2–3	79,727	22,501	20,031
	4	39,872	11,263	10,024
African-American	1	2,546	99	153
	2–3	5,076	299	300
	4	2,546	99	153

pairs as an example, we can then determine the prevalence of twins in the fourth quartile from the following relation:

$$\frac{\sum_{h=1}^{3} N_h p_{hx}}{\sum_{h=1}^{3} N_h} = .10$$

where N_h = the total number of pairs in stratum h.

Setting $p_{1x} = 8p_{3x}$ and $p_{2x} = 2p_{3x}$, we obtain the following:

$$\frac{8 \times p_{3x} \times 39{,}872 + 2 \times p_{3x} \times 79{,}727 + p_{3x} \times 39{,}872}{39{,}872 + 79{,}727 + 39{,}872} = .10$$

or

$$p_{3x} = 0.0308$$

It then follows that

$$p_{2x} = 0.0615 \qquad \text{and} \qquad p_{1x} = .2461$$

We can now obtain the σ_{hx}

$$\sigma_{3x} = [(0.0308)(1 - 0.0308)]^{0.5} = 0.1728$$
$$\sigma_{2x} = [(0.0615)(1 - 0.0615)]^{0.5} = 0.2402$$
$$\sigma_{1x} = [(0.2461)(1 - 0.2461)]^{0.5} = 0.4307$$

Optimal allocation based on relation (6.17) is as follows:

$$n = 1000/6 \approx 167 \qquad \text{(1000 total sample/6 sex–race strata)}$$

$$n_1 = \frac{39{,}872 \times .4307}{39{,}872 \times .4307 + 79{,}727 \times .2402 + 39{,}872 \times .1728} \, 167 \approx 66$$

$$n_2 = \frac{79{,}727 \times .2402}{39{,}872 \times .4307 + 79{,}727 \times .2402 + 39{,}872 \times .1728} \, 167 \approx 74$$

$$n_3 = \frac{39{,}872 \times .1728}{39{,}872 \times .4307 + 79{,}727 \times .2402 + 39{,}872 \times .1728} \, 167 \approx 27$$

While the method shown above was used to determine allocation into each of the 18 strata shown in Table 6.6, the actual sample so obtained and shown in Table 6.7 differed slightly from the desired allocation owing to unforeseen events (inability to locate members of the sampled pairs, financial considerations, etc.).

Table 6.7 Total Pairs Available and Total Pairs Sampled

Race	Sequence Difference Quartile	M–M		M–F		F–F	
		pop.	sample	pop.	sample	pop.	sample
White	1	39,872	52	11,263	59	10,024	60
	2–3	79,727	59	22,501	66	20,031	67
	4	39,872	21	11,263	24	10,024	24
Black	1	2,546	49	99	53	153	56
	2–3	5,076	55	299	59	300	63
	4	2,546	20	99	21	153	23

Estimation of the prevalence of twins and its standard error for the entire population of pairs and for each sequence difference quartile can be accomplished using relations (5.8), which are shown in Box 5.2. We illustrate below how these estimates can be obtained by use of SUDAAN software.

The data required for the SUDAAN processing on the record of each of the 831 sampled pairs are as follows:

id: Unique number given to each pair.

stratum: One of the 18 sex-race-sequence difference quartiles listed above.

npop: Total number of pairs in the stratum.

sampwt: Total number of pairs in stratum divided by total number sampled in stratum.

twin: Dichotomous variable: "1" if twin; "0" if not.

quart1: Quartile based on SS# sequence difference: "1" if lowest quartile; "2" if middle two quartiles; "3" if highest quartile.

The data containing the variables listed above are in a SAS file labeled JACKTWIN, and the SUDAAN command file shown below is used to obtain the estimated prevalences for the population as a whole and for each of the three quartile groups based on SS# sequence difference.

```
1. PROC  DESCRIPT  DATA = JACKTWIN  FILETYPE  =  SAS  MEANS  TOTALS
      DESIGN = STRWOR;
2. NEST STRATUM;
3. WEIGHT SAMPWT;
4. TOTCNT NPOP;
5. SETENV DECWIDTH = 3;
6. SUBGROUP QUART1;
7. LEVELS        3;
8. TABLES QUART1;
9. VAR TWIN;
```

The command file listed above has the same general form as that used in an illustrative example in the previous chapter, and the reader is referred to that example for explanation of the meaning of the individual commands. The output is shown below:

Variable		Quart 1 Total	1	2	3
Twin	Sample size	831.000	329.000	369.000	133.000
	Weighted size	256,998.000	63,937.000	127,874.000	65,187.000
	Total	26,055.397	19,183.803	6,737.907	133.687
	SE Total	3,791.044	2,661.629	2,696.605	126.744
	Mean	0.101	0.300	0.053	0.002
	SE mean	0.015	0.042	0.021	0.002

The major findings are that an estimated 10% of the pairs constructed as described above are twins (as opposed to approximately 1% of all individuals in the general population). Also, if the screening is confined to the lowest SS# sequence difference quartile, the prevalence of twins in that quartile is 30% (30 times the prevalence in unselected individuals). Thus, the pilot indicates that this methodology can be used to identify twins relatively efficiently.

An equivalent analysis could be done by use of STATA from the following command file and the STATA data file *jacktwn2.dta*.

```
. use "a:\jacktwn 2.dta", clear
. svyset strata stratum
. svyset pweight sampwt
. svyset fpc npop
. svytotal twin
. svytotal twin,by (quart1)
```

The above commands would result in the following STATA output:

Survey total estimation

pweight:	sampwt	Number of obs = 831
Strata:	stratum	Number of strata = 18
PSU:	< observations >	Number of PSUs = 831
FPC:	npop	Population size = 256998

Total	Estimate	Std. Err.	[95% Conf. Interval]		Deff
twin	26055.4	3791.044	18614.01	33496.78	1.988843

Finite population correction (FPC) assumes simple random sampling without replacement of PSUs within each stratum with no subsampling within PSUs.

```
.svytotal twin,by (quart1)

Survey total estimation

pweight:  sampwt                Number of obs = 831
Strata:   stratum               Number of strata = 18
PSU:      < observations >      Number of PSUs = 831
FPC:      npop                  Population size = 256998
```

Total Subpop.	Estimate	Std. Err.	[95% Conf. Interval]		Deff
twin					
quart1 = = 1	19183.8	2661.629	13959.33	24408.28	1.293026
quart1 = = 2	6737.907	2696.605	1444.778	12031.04	3.590895
quart1 = = 3	133.687	126.7443	−115.0976	382.4715	.3895368

Finite population correction (FPC) assumes simple random sampling without replacement of PSUs within each stratum with no subsampling within PSUs.

□

6.6 STRATIFICATION AFTER SAMPLING

A sample design in which the sampling plan is that of simple random sampling but the estimation procedure is that appropriate for stratified random sampling can sometimes produce estimates having standard errors that are not much higher than those obtained by stratified random sampling. The advantage of this design is that it eliminates the inconvenience, or impossibility, of grouping the elements into strata in advance of the sampling. This type of design has been considered by Hansen et al. [10] and by Cochran [9] among others. It is known as *stratification after sampling* or *poststratification*. For example, it may be of interest to estimate the proportion of premature births in a given hospital during the past year. It is known from past experience that the prematurity rate among blacks is higher than the corresponding rate for whites. However, to stratify the entire set of hospital records by racial group would be impractical, since racial group is recorded in the records and all records would have to be inspected to do such stratification prior to the sampling. However, if the total number of blacks and the total number of whites who have entered the hospital during the year for deliveries is known (as it may well be by the hospital administration), a simple random sample may be stratified after the sampling to improve the precision of the estimate.

Let $\bar{x}_{\text{pstr}}$ and $\text{Var}(\bar{x}_{\text{pstr}})$ represent the *poststratified sample mean* and *variance of its sampling distribution*, respectively. Then

$$\bar{x}_{\text{pstr}} = \sum_{h=1}^{L} \left(\frac{N_h}{N}\right) \bar{x}_h$$

$$\text{Var}(\bar{x}_{\text{pstr}}) = \left(\frac{N-n}{nN}\right) \sum_{h=1}^{L} \frac{N_h}{N} S_{hx}^2 + \left(\frac{1}{n^2}\right) \sum_{h=1}^{L} S_{hx}^2 \left(\frac{N-n_h}{N}\right) \tag{6.20}$$

where

$$S_{hx}^2 = \sum_{i=1}^{N_h} (X_{h,i} - \bar{X}_h)^2 / (N_h - 1)$$

The first term in relation (6.20) is approximately the variance of an estimated mean under stratified sampling with proportional allocation. The second term increases the variance and reflects the fact that the n_h in the resulting sample are random variables. The second term will generally be small when the sample size n is large.

Although S_{hx}^2 is not known, it can be estimated by s_{hx}^2 [relation (5.9)] and the *sample estimate* of Var ($\bar{x}_{\text{pstr}}$) is given by

$$\hat{\text{Var}}(\bar{x}_{\text{pstr}}) = \left(\frac{N-n}{nN}\right) \sum_{h=1}^{L} \frac{N_h}{N} s_{hx}^2 + \left(\frac{1}{n^2}\right) \sum_{h=1}^{L} s_{hx}^2 \left(\frac{N-n_h}{N}\right) \tag{6.21}$$

Expressions similar to relations (6.20) and (6.21) can be derived for the variance of estimated poststratified totals and proportions, as well as the estimated variances from the sample information.

Now let us look at an example of how poststratification can be useful in reducing sampling error.

Illustrative Example. A veterinarian is interested in studying the annual veterinary costs of his clientele (who own either dogs or cats). From a separate record system, he knows that he sees 850 dogs and 450 cats regularly in his practice (these are numbers of animals, not numbers of visits). He knows that the information on type of animal (i.e., dog or cat) is contained in the medical records, but that it would take too much time to sort the records into strata defined by animal type. So he decides to select a simple random sample and then poststratify. He regards the poststratification process as necessary since he knows that, on average, it costs more to keep dogs healthy than to keep cats healthy. He samples 50 records, recording the total amount of money spent (including medication) by the owners of the animals he saw over the past two years. The sampling results are given in Table 6.8.

Now suppose that this sample of 50 animals is to be used to estimate the average annual expense of owning a dog or a cat. Then we have the following calculations (refer to Boxes 2.2 and 3.1):

Table 6.8 Sample Data of Veterinarian's Survey

Sample Animal	Animal Type	No. of Visits	Total Expenses	Sample Animal	Animal Type	No. of Visits	Total Expenses
1	Dog	4	$45.14	26	Dog	4	$48.30
2	Dog	5	50.13	27	Dog	5	54.64
3	Cat	2	27.15	28	Cat	3	21.45
4	Dog	3	45.80	29	Cat	3	10.71
5	Cat	1	23.39	30	Dog	4	60.57
6	Cat	2	8.24	31	Dog	6	53.37
7	Dog	6	61.22	32	Dog	5	40.52
8	Cat	2	29.90	33	Dog	4	50.26
9	Dog	5	56.57	34	Cat	2	15.23
10	Dog	4	42.39	35	Dog	4	42.02
11	Cat	2	27.24	36	Dog	5	32.78
12	Cat	3	22.17	37	Cat	2	30.21
13	Dog	6	39.67	38	Cat	1	27.54
14	Dog	4	40.52	39	Dog	6	52.03
15	Dog	4	39.48	40	Dog	5	54.47
16	Cat	1	7.14	41	Dog	5	46.88
17	Dog	4	61.82	42	Cat	2	23.77
18	Cat	2	39.88	43	Dog	3	52.48
19	Cat	2	16.89	44	Dog	2	60.49
20	Dog	3	55.31	45	Dog	2	53.70
21	Dog	2	63.19	46	Dog	2	46.39
22	Dog	2	45.11	47	Dog	2	53.24
23	Dog	3	66.20	48	Cat	1	14.18
24	Cat	3	17.16	49	Dog	3	41.52
25	Cat	3	28.55	50	Dog	2	39.26

$$\bar{x} = \frac{45.14 + 50.13 + \cdots + 39.26}{50} = 39.73$$

$$s_x^2 = \frac{(45.14 - 39.73)^2 + \cdots + (39.26 - 39.73)^2}{(50 - 1)} = 256.68$$

$$\widehat{SE}(\bar{x}) = \left[\left(\frac{1300 - 50}{1300}\right)\left(\frac{256.68}{50}\right)\right]^{1/2} = \sqrt{4.936} = 2.222$$

Hence the 95% confidence interval estimate of the population mean $\bar{X}$ is given by

$$\bar{x} - 1.96 \times \widehat{SE}(\bar{x}) \leqslant \bar{X} \leqslant \bar{x} + 1.96 \times \widehat{SE}(\bar{x})$$

$$39.73 - 1.96 \times 2.222 \leqslant \bar{X} \leqslant 39.73 + 1.96 \times 2.222$$

$$35.38 \leqslant \bar{X} \leqslant 44.08$$

Let us now use the known stratum totals in a poststratification process to obtain a more precise estimate of $\bar{X}$. The veterinarian knows that the number of dogs in his files is $N_1 = 850$ and the total number of cats is $N_2 = 450$. Stratifying the 50 animals in the sample given in Table 6.8 into dogs and cats yields $n_1 = 32$ dogs and $n_2 = 18$ cats in the sample. Then we have (refer to Box 2.2):

$$\bar{x}_1 = \frac{45.14 + 50.13 + \cdots + 39.26}{32} = 49.86$$

$$\bar{x}_2 = \frac{27.15 + 23.39 + \cdots + 14.18}{18} = 21.71$$

$$s_{1x}^2 = \frac{(45.14 - 49.86)^2 + \cdots + (39.26 - 49.86)^2}{31}$$

$$= 70.22$$

$$s_{2x}^2 = \frac{(27.15 - 21.71)^2 + \cdots + (14.18 - 21.71)^2}{17}$$

$$= 75.00$$

$$\bar{x}_{pstr} = \left(\frac{850}{1300}\right) \times 49.86 + \left(\frac{450}{1300}\right) \times 21.71 = 40.12$$

$$\widehat{Var}(\bar{x}_{pstr}) = \left(\frac{1300 - 50}{50 \times 1300}\right)\left[\frac{850}{1300} 70.22 + \frac{450}{1300} 75.00\right]$$

$$+ \left(\frac{1}{50^2}\right)\left[\left(\frac{1300 - 850}{1300}\right) \times 70.22 + \left(\frac{1300 - 450}{1300}\right) \times 75.00\right]$$

$$= 1.439$$

$$\widehat{SE}(\bar{x}_{pstr}) = \sqrt{1.439} = 1.20$$

Hence the 95% confidence interval estimate of the population mean, $\bar{X}$, is given, by poststratification, as

$$\bar{x}_{pstr} - 1.96 \times \widehat{SE}(\bar{x}_{pstr}) \leqslant \bar{X} \leqslant \bar{x}_{pstr} + 1.96 \times \widehat{SE}(\bar{x}_{pstr})$$

$$40.12 - 1.96 \times 1.20 \leqslant \bar{X} \leqslant 40.12 + 1.96 \times 1.20$$

$$37.77 \leqslant \bar{X} \leqslant 42.47$$

We see that by poststratifying the originally selected random sample, the veterinarian obtained a narrower confidence interval than the one calculated for the original simple random sample.

Poststratified estimates and their standard errors can be obtained by use of SUDAAN. For the illustrative example discussed above, the following set of commands can be used to obtain a poststratified estimate of the mean expenses associated with dogs and cats.

```
PROC DESCRIPT DATA = DOGSCATS FILETYPE = SAS DESIGN = WOR;
NEST _ONE_;
TOTCNT N;
WEIGHT WEIGHT;
SUBGROUP TYPE;
LEVELS 2;
VAR TOTEXP;
POSTVAR TYPE;
POSTWGT 850 450;
```

The data file *dogscats.ssd* consisting of the 50 sample animals sorted by *type* ("1" = dog, "2" = cat) is shown below:

id	type	totexp	weight	N	id	type	totexp	weight	N
35	1	42.02	26	1300	32	1	40.52	26	1300
33	1	50.26	26	1300	4	1	45.80	26	1300
50	1	39.26	26	1300	39	1	52.03	26	1300
31	1	53.37	26	1300	9	1	56.57	26	1300
10	1	42.39	26	1300	7	1	61.22	26	1300
26	1	48.30	26	1300	17	1	61.82	26	1300
20	1	55.31	26	1300	47	1	53.24	26	1300
27	1	54.64	26	1300	16	2	7.14	26	1300
41	1	46.88	26	1300	29	2	10.71	26	1300
46	1	46.39	26	1300	37	2	30.21	26	1300
15	1	39.48	26	1300	6	2	8.24	26	1300
36	1	32.78	26	1300	34	2	15.23	26	1300
22	1	45.11	26	1300	28	2	21.45	26	1300
21	1	63.19	26	1300	48	2	14.18	26	1300
43	1	52.48	26	1300	38	2	27.54	26	1300
23	1	66.20	26	1300	3	2	27.15	26	1300
45	1	53.70	26	1300	19	2	16.89	26	1300
1	1	45.14	26	1300	18	2	39.88	26	1300
13	1	39.67	26	1300	42	2	23.77	26	1300
2	1	50.13	26	1300	24	2	17.16	26	1300
40	1	54.47	26	1300	12	2	22.17	26	1300
14	1	40.52	26	1300	25	2	28.55	26	1300
30	1	60.57	26	1300	11	2	27.24	26	1300
44	1	60.49	26	1300	5	2	23.39	26	1300
49	1	41.52	26	1300	8	2	29.90	26	1300

Each record consists of the following five variables:

id: the identification number of each sample animal.

type: 1 = dog; 2 = cat.

totexp: total veterinary medical expenses incurred by the animal.

weight: $N/n = 1300/50 = 26$.

N: total number of animals in the population.

Note that the *weight* and *totcnt* variables used in the processing are the same for each record and would be appropriate for estimation from a simple random sampling design. The *postvar* command indicates the categorical variable that serves as the basis for the poststratification (type of animal in this instance), and the *postwgt* command indicates the population totals for each category. The following output would be produced by the commands

```
1   PROC DESCRIPT DATA = DOGSCATS FILETYPE = SAS DESIGN = WOR;
2   NEST _ONE_;
3   TOTCNT N;
4   WEIGHT WEIGHT;
5   SUBGROUP TYPE;
6   LEVELS 2;
7   VAR TOTEXP;
8   POSTVAR TYPE;
9   POSTWGT 850 450;
```

Number of observations read :	50	Weighted count : 1300
Number of observations skipped :	0	
(WEIGHT variable nonpositive)		
Denominator degrees of freedom :	49	

Research Triangle Institute

Page : 1
Table : 1

Post-stratified estimates
by: Variable, TYPE.

Variable		TYPE total	1
TOTEXP	Sample Size	50	32
	Weighted Size	1300.00	850.00
	Total	52149.67	42379.67
	Mean	40.12	49.86
	SE Mean	1.16	1.44

Post-stratified estimates
by: Variable, TYPE.

Variable		TYPE 2
TOTEXP	Sample Size	18
	Weighted Size	450.00
	Total	9770.00
	Mean	21.71
	SE Mean	1.97

It should be noted that the estimated standard error of the poststratified mean, $\bar{x}_{pstr}$, produced by SUDAAN differs slightly from that obtained from relation (6.21) in this text (1.16 calculated by SUDAAN as opposed to 1.20 calculated from the formula in the text). The reason is that SUDAAN uses a slightly different approximation formula.

At the time of this writing, poststratified estimates cannot be obtained directly from the survey commands in STATA.

We note that poststratification will only be profitable (in terms of smaller standard errors) when the established strata are homogeneous with respect to the variable of interest. In other words, poststratification will work well when stratification works well. In addition, the method cannot be carried out unless the stratum totals are known. However, when the sample is taken from human populations, it is often possible to use available census or other population data to obtain a good enough guess of the stratum totals to make use of the method advantageous.

6.7 HOW LARGE A SAMPLE IS NEEDED?

Suppose that we wish to determine the number of elements needed to be $100 \times (1 - \alpha)\%$ certain of obtaining from a stratified random sampling, an estimated mean, $\bar{x}_{str}$, that differs from the true mean $\bar{X}$ by no more than $100 \times \varepsilon\%$. This formulation is equivalent to that discussed earlier for simple random sampling and systematic sampling. The formula (valid for reasonably large N_h) for the required n is as follows:

$$n \approx \frac{\left(\dfrac{z^2_{1-(\alpha/2)}}{N^2}\right)\left(\displaystyle\sum_{h=1}^{L}\dfrac{N_h^2\sigma_{hx}^2}{\pi_h\bar{X}^2}\right)}{\varepsilon^2 + \left(\dfrac{z^2_{1-(\alpha/2)}}{N^2}\right)\left(\displaystyle\sum_{h=1}^{L}\dfrac{N_h\sigma_{hx}^2}{\bar{X}^2}\right)} \qquad (6.22)$$

where

$$\pi_h = \frac{n_h}{n}$$

Relation (6.22) is valid for any type of allocation. It is also valid for the estimation of a population total. The analogous sample size formula for estimation of a population proportion P_y from stratified random sampling is given by

$$
n \approx \frac{\left(\dfrac{z^2_{1-(\alpha/2)}}{N^2}\right)\left(\displaystyle\sum_{h=1}^{L}\dfrac{N_h^2 P_{hy}(1-P_{hy})}{\pi_h P_y^2}\right)}{\varepsilon^2 + \left(\dfrac{z^2_{1-(\alpha/2)}}{N^2}\right)\left(\displaystyle\sum_{h=1}^{L}\dfrac{N_h P_{hy}(1-P_{hy})}{P_y^2}\right)}
\tag{6.23}
$$

We can see from relation (6.22) that its use requires more knowledge about parameters of the distribution than is likely to be available or than can be guessed with any degree of confidence. For this reason, relation (6.22) is unlikely to be of much help in actual practice. However, if one assumes proportional allocation, then relation (6.22) reduces to the form

$$
n \approx \frac{N z^2_{1-(\alpha/2)}(\sigma_{wx}^2/\bar{X}^2)}{N\varepsilon^2 + z^2_{1-(\alpha/2)}(\sigma_{wx}^2/\bar{X}^2)}
\tag{6.24}
$$

Note that relation (6.24) is similar to expression (3.15) for the sample size required for estimation of a sample mean under simple random sampling (Box 3.4). The only difference between the two expressions is that V_x^2 (which is equal to $\sigma_x^2/\bar{X}^2$) in relation (3.15) is replaced by $\sigma_{wx}^2/\bar{X}^2$ in relation (6.24). If we have some idea of the order of magnitude of V_x^2, the relative variance of the distribution of variable $\mathcal{X}$ in the population, and if in addition we have some idea of the ratio $\gamma = \sigma_{bx}^2/\sigma_{wx}^2$, then since $\sigma_x^2 = \sigma_{bx}^2 + \sigma_{wx}^2$, relation (6.24) becomes

$$
n \approx \frac{z^2_{1-(\alpha/2)} \times \dfrac{N}{1+\gamma} \times V_x^2}{N\varepsilon^2 + z^2_{1-(\alpha/2)} \times \dfrac{V_x^2}{1+\gamma}}
\tag{6.25}
$$

Let us look at an example to see how relation (6.25) might be used in practice.

Illustrative Example.   Suppose that we are planning to take a sample of the members of a health maintenance organization (HMO) for purposes of estimating the average number of hospital episodes per person. The sample will be selected from membership lists grouped according to age (under 45 years; 45–64 years; 65 years and over). Let us suppose that the distributions of hospital episodes are available from national data (such as the National Health Interview Survey) and are as given in Table 6.9.

Suppose further that the number of HMO members in each age group is as follows:

Age group 1: $N_1 = 600$
Age group 2: $N_2 = 500$
Age group 3: $N_3 = 400$

Table 6.9   Distribution of Hospital Episodes per Person per Year

	Age Group	Average Number of Hospital Episodes	Variance of Distribution of Hospital Episodes
1.	Under 45 years	0.164	0.245
2.	45–64 years	0.166	0.296
3.	65 years and over	0.236	0.436

If we assume that the results found on the national level also are likely to be true for the HMO members, then the anticipated mean number of hospital episodes per person is, from Equation (6.1),

$$\bar{X} = \frac{600 \times .164 + 500 \times .166 + 400 \times .236}{1500} = .184$$

The anticipated variance component σ_{bx}^2 is, from Equation (6.15),

$$\sigma_{bx}^2 = \frac{600 \times (.164 - .184)^2 + 500 \times (.166 - .184)^2 + 400 \times (.236 - .184)^2}{1500}$$
$$= .0009891$$

The anticipated variance component σ_{wx}^2 is, from Equation (6.13),

$$\sigma_{wx}^2 = \frac{600 \times .245 + 500 \times .296 + 400 \times .436}{1500} = .31293$$

Finally, the anticipated values of σ_x^2, V_x^2, and γ are

$$\sigma_x^2 = .0009891 + .31293 = .31392$$
$$V_x^2 = \frac{.31392}{(.184)^2} = 9.27$$
$$\gamma = \frac{.0009891}{.31293} = .00316$$

Now, using relation (6.25), we can calculate the estimated number of subjects needed to be virtually certain of estimating the mean number of hospital episodes to within 20% of the true mean under stratified random sampling with proportional allocation:

$$n \approx \frac{[(9 \times 1500)/(1 + .00316)] \times 9.27}{[(9 \times 9.27)/(1 + .00316)] + 1500 \times (.20)^2} = 872$$

The number n_h allocated to each stratum would then be as follows:

$$n_1 = 600 \times \frac{872}{1500} = 349$$

$$n_2 = 500 \times \frac{872}{1500} = 291$$

$$n_3 = 400 \times \frac{872}{1500} = 232$$

If we wish to use optimal allocation assuming equal stratum costs, the required sample size could be estimated by first determining the optimal n_h from national estimates and then computing the required n from relation (6.22). This would be done as follows.

First, compute the optimal π_h (which is equal to $N_h \sigma_{hx} / \sum_{h=1}^{L} N_h \sigma_{hx}$) based on the national data:

$$\pi_1 = \frac{600\sqrt{.245}}{600\sqrt{.245} + 500\sqrt{.296} + 400\sqrt{.436}} = .356$$

$$\pi_2 = \frac{500\sqrt{.296}}{600\sqrt{.245} + 500\sqrt{.296} + 400\sqrt{.436}} = .327$$

$$\pi_3 = \frac{400\sqrt{.436}}{600\sqrt{.245} + 500\sqrt{.296} + 400\sqrt{.436}} = .317$$

Next, compute the required n based on relation (6.22) with $\varepsilon = .20$:

$$n \approx \frac{\left[\frac{9}{(1500)^2}\right]\left[\frac{(600)^2(.245)}{(.356)(.184)^2} + \frac{(500)^2(.296)}{(.327)(.184)^2} + \frac{(400)^2(.436)}{(.317)(.184)^2}\right]}{(.2)^2 + \left[\frac{9}{(1500)^2}\right]\left[\frac{600 \times .245}{(.184)^2} + \frac{500 \times .296}{(.184)^2} + \frac{400 \times .436}{(.184)^2}\right]} = 860$$

Finally, the sample of 860 necessary to achieve $\varepsilon = .20$ with virtual certainty is allocated to the strata by multiplying 860 by the appropriate π_h:

$$n_1 = n \times \pi_1 = 860 \times .356 = 306$$
$$n_2 = n \times \pi_2 = 860 \times .327 = 281$$
$$n_3 = n \times \pi_3 = 860 \times .317 = 273$$

Note that the required sample size (860) is smaller under optimal allocation as compared to that required under proportional allocation (872). □

It should be noted that under proportional allocation, the required sample size for estimation of a proportion [relation (6.23)] reduces to the following:

$$n \approx \frac{\left(\dfrac{z^2_{1-(\alpha/2)}}{N}\right)\left(\displaystyle\sum_{h=1}^{L} \dfrac{N_h P_{hy}(1 - P_{hy})}{P_y^2}\right)}{\varepsilon^2 + \left(\dfrac{z^2_{1-(\alpha/2)}}{N^2}\right)\left(\displaystyle\sum_{h=1}^{L} \dfrac{N_h P_{hy}(1 - P_{hy})}{P_y^2}\right)} \qquad (6.26)$$

However, since $P_{hy}(1 - P_{hy}) \leqslant .25$, relation (6.26) reduces to the following inequality:

$$n \leqslant \frac{.25 \times \dfrac{z^2_{1-(\alpha/2)}}{P_y^2}}{\varepsilon^2 + .25 \times \dfrac{z^2_{1-(\alpha/2)}}{N \times P_y^2}} \qquad (6.27)$$

From relation (6.27), one can obtain a conservative estimate of the required sample size based on knowledge of the number N of elements in the population and a "guestimate" of the proportion P_y having the attribute $\mathscr{Y}$ in the population.

6.8 CONSTRUCTION OF STRATUM BOUNDARIES AND DESIRED NUMBER OF STRATA

In many situations, stratum boundaries are determined by the availability of the population information needed for selecting a stratified sample and performing the estimation. For example, it may not be possible to stratify on postal ZIP codes within a defined target geographical area if there is no available population information on the ZIP code level and no way to construct a sampling frame within a ZIP code.

In other situations where stratification is thought to be desired, it may be possible to choose the stratum boundaries. In that case, one would want to select boundaries that would enhance the reliability of the resulting estimates. For example, the sampling frame may be a computer file containing the totality of all visits during a particular year to health professionals made by members of a particular HMO. It may be considered desirable to stratify on some characteristic of the patient such as age or blood pressure level at enrollment into the HMO. An issue to consider would be the particular choice of stratum boundaries.

One general strategy in choosing stratum boundaries is to choose these boundaries in such a way that the variance of the resulting estimate under optimum allocation is minimized. Dalenius [12] derived equations for determining these boundaries which, however, are difficult to use in practice because of dependencies among the components. An approximate method was developed by Dalenius and Hodges [13] which seems to work well in practice. This approximate method involves (1) grouping the stratification variable, $\mathscr{X}$, into a number of classes; (2) determining the frequency distribution $f(x)$ of $\mathscr{X}$ for each class; (3) cumulating the square root of $f(x)$; and (4) determining Q, the quotient of the sum over all classes of the square root of $f(x)$, and the number, L, of strata to be used. The final division points obtained in this way are Q, $2Q, \ldots, (L - 1)Q$. This method (which we will refer to as the *rootfreq* method) is illustrated in the following example.

Illustrative Example. An audit is to be performed on the records of a large medical group that treats patients on Medicaid. The purpose of the audit is to estimate the amount of money overcharged to Medicaid by this medical group during 1996. During that year, the medical group treated 2387 patients, and a frequency distribution of the total dollar amount charged to Medicaid by each patient during the year is shown in Table 6.10 (ungrouped data are in STATA file, *medaudit.dta*):

Table 6.10 Frequency Distribution of Total Amount Charged During 1996 to Medicaid for 2387 Patients Treated by a Large Medical Group

Totpaid ($)	Freq	Cumfreq	Rootfreq	Cumrootf	Stratum
0–49	39	39	6.244997998	6.244998	1
50–99	819	858	28.61817604	34.863174	1
100–149	570	1428	23.87467277	58.7378468	2
150–199	350	1778	18.70828693	77.4461337	3
200–299	314	2092	17.72004515	95.1661789	3
300–399	136	2228	11.66190379	106.828083	4
400–499	71	2299	8.426149773	115.254232	4
500–599	37	2336	6.08276253	121.336995	4
600–699	17	2353	4.123105626	125.460101	4
700–799	11	2364	3.31662479	128.776725	4
800–899	10	2374	3.16227766	131.939003	5
900–999	2	2376	1.414213562	133.353217	5
1000–1099	1	2377	1	134.353217	5
1100–1199	1	2378	1	135.353217	5
1200–1299	3	2381	1.732050808	137.085267	5
1300–1399	1	2382	1	138.085267	5
1400–1499	1	2383	1	139.085267	5
1500–1599	0	2383	0	139.085267	5
1600–1699	1	2384	1	140.085267	5
1700–1799	1	2385	1	141.085267	5
1800–1899	1	2386	1	142.085267	5
1900–1999	1	2387	1	143.085267	5

The first column in the above table shows the Medicaid dollars spent on behalf of each patient grouped into 22 categories.

The second column gives the frequency distribution for each of these categories.

The third column shows the cumulative frequency distribution of that variable.

The fourth column gives the square root of the frequency distribution of that variable.

The fifth column shows the cumulative frequency distribution of the square root of that variable. Note that the sum of this cumulative root frequency is 143.085267.

If we wish to have five strata, then the quotient $Q = 143.085267/5 = 28.6170535$, and the upper boundaries of each stratum are determined by values of the cumulative root frequency: 28.6170535, 57.23411, 85.85116, 114.4682, and 143.0853. These correspond (as indicated in Table 6.10, column 6) to the stratum boundaries on the variable *Totpaid*, the total amount paid by Medicaid for each patient.

Optimal allocation based on this stratification would yield the percentage allocation shown in column 5 of Table 6.11.

Let us now compare this stratification with the following two seemingly "reasonable" strategies for constructing strata;

1. Stratification based on dividing the range of the distribution by the number of strata (*equal range* method).
2. Stratification based on dividing the total percentage distribution by the desired number of strata (*quantile* method).

We show comparisons among the three stratification methods, *rootfreq, equal range*, and *quantile*, in Table 6.12.

Table 6.11 Optimal Allocation Based on Use of the *rootfreq* Method for Construction of Strata

Stratum	*Totpaid* ($)	Number in Stratum (N_h)	Standard Deviation, σ_{bx} of *Totpaid*	Optimal Allocation into Stratum (%n)
1	0–99	858	14.890	14.56
2	100–149	570	13.847	9.00
3	150–299	664	40.606	30.76
4	300–799	272	116.617	36.19
5	800–1999	23	360.947	9.47

Table 6.12   Results of Three Methods of Strata Construction Combined with Optimal Allocation from Data on 2387 Patients Shown in Table 6.10*

| Stratum | Stratum Boundaries (Number in Strata, N_h) Stratum Construction Method | | | Within Stratum Standard Deviation (Percentage Allocation into Stratum) Stratum Construction Method | | |
	rootfreq	*equal range*	*quantile*	*rootfreq*	*equal range*	*quantile*
1	0–99	0–398	0–71.2	14.89	78.90	7.98
	($N_1 = 858$)	($N_1 = 2225$)	($N_1 = 477$)	(14.56%)	(91.97%)	(2.93%)
2	100–149	399–780	71.3–107.5	13.85	95.77	9.75
	($N_2 = 570$)	($N_2 = 136$)	($N_2 = 478$)	(9.00%)	(6.82%)	(3.59%)
3	150–299	781–1162	107.6–150.4	40.61	93.22	11.52
	($N_3 = 664$)	($N_3 = 17$)	($N_3 = 477$)	(30.76%)	(0.83%)	(4.23%)
4	300–799	1163–1544	150.5–229.6	116.62	72.62	22.34
	($N_4 = 272$)	($N_4 = 5$)	($N_4 = 478$)	(36.19%)	(0.19%)	(8.22%)
5	800–1999	1545–1926	229.7–1926	360.95	92.81	220.78
	($N_5 = 23$)	($N_5 = 4$)	($N_5 = 477$)	(9.47%)	(0.19%)	(81.04%)

*Stratification is on variable, *Totpaid*, the total amount charged to Medicaid during 1996 for each patient.

EQUAL RANGE METHOD.   For data such as these, which are highly skewed to the right, the *equal range* method results in construction of strata that have most of the elements in the lower numbered strata and very few in the higher strata. In the present example, stratum 1, the lowest stratum, contains 2225 patients, while stratum 5 contains only 4 patients. Since the within-stratum standard deviations, σ_{hx}, among the strata are very close to each other by this construction algorithm, optimal allocation results in most of the elements allocated to the lower strata. In this example, optimal allocation would allot approximately 92% of the sample to stratum 1.

QUANTILE METHOD.   The *quantile* method of stratum construction results in each stratum having the same number of elements. Moreover, in situations such as that of the present example where the variable used in construction of the strata has high positive skewness, the quantile method would result in within-stratum standard deviations that are highest in the highest strata (see Table 6.12). Thus, optimal allocation in combination with this method of stratum construction results in a greater proportion of the sample being in the higher strata. In the present example, optimal allocation would result in more than 81% of the sample being allocated to stratum 5.

ROOTFREQ METHOD.   Finally, the rootfreq method will tend to avoid the extremes shown by the other two methods of stratum construction—the disparity in number of elements per stratum will be less than that obtained by the *equal range* method, and the disparity in within-stratum standard deviations will be less than that obtained by the *quantile* method. Optimum allocation will then tend to reduce the variability among strata with respect to the allocated sample elements. In fact, for variables that have little skewness, this method of stratum construction will result in optimal allocation yielding sample strata sizes that do not differ substantially from what would have been obtained from equal allocation. This is a great advantage in situations where there is interest in testing hypotheses concerning differences among strata with respect to levels of a variable, since for a specified total sample size, statistical power is generally highest when strata have equal sample sizes. Finally, optimal allocation in combination with the *rootfreq* method of stratum construction will generally yield estimates having the lowest standard errors over optimal allocation in combination with other methods of stratum construction. In the present example, the standard error of the estimated mean level of the variable, *totpaid*, for a hypothetical stratified random sample of $n = 500$ patients, where the stratum sample sizes were obtained by optimal allocation, is equal to $3.18 for *equal range* construction, $1.33 for *quantile* stratum construction, and $1.19 for *rootfreq* stratum construction (the lowest among the three). □

An issue related to construction of stratum boundaries is the actual number, L, of strata to be constructed. This issue is discussed in the texts by Kish [11] and Cochran [9]. Cochran [9] in particular, uses the model shown below (relation 6.28), in which stratification is based on the variable $\mathcal{X}$, and the variable to be estimated is $\mathcal{Y}$.

$$\text{Var}(\bar{y}_{\text{str}}) \approx \frac{\sigma_y^2}{n}\left[\frac{\rho^2}{L^2} + (1 - \rho^2)\right] \tag{6.28}$$

where ρ is the correlation between $\mathcal{X}$ and $\mathcal{Y}$. Clearly, the factor $(\rho^2/L^2) + (1 - \rho^2)$ represents the approximate reduction in variance over simple random sampling gained by the stratification. For correlations between $\mathcal{X}$ and $\mathcal{Y}$ existing in most situations, it can be seen from relation (6.28) that little is gained from having more than five or six strata.

6.9 SUMMARY

In this chapter we developed the concepts of stratification. In particular, we discussed estimation of population means, proportions, and totals under stratified random sampling, along with methods of allocating the sample to the strata (e.g., equal allocation, proportional allocation, optimal allocation with and without cost constraints). We discussed poststratification, which involves use of a simple random sampling plan along with an estimation procedure similar to that used in stratified random sampling. Finally, we presented methods of estimating the required sample size under stratified random sampling.

EXERCISES

6.1 A sample survey of households in a community containing 1500 households is to be conducted for the purpose of determining the total
number of persons over 18 years of age in the community who have
one or more permanent teeth (other than third molars) missing. Since
this variable is thought to be correlated with age and income, the strata
shown in the accompanying table are formed by using available population data. A stratified random sample of 100 families is to be taken.

	Stratum			
Variable	1	2	3	4
Age				
Mean	30	32	25	27
Standard deviation	15	15	10	10
Annual family income ($\times$ $1000)				
Mean	15	7	15	8
Standard deviation	5	3	3	2
No. of families	300	500	100	600

a. Specify in algebraic detail how the estimate of the total number of
persons having one or more missing teeth is to be estimated.

b. Determine the number of families to be taken from each stratum if
proportional allocation is used.

c. Determine the number of families to be taken from each stratum if
optimal allocation is used based on annual family income.

d. Determine the number of families to be taken from each stratum if
optimal allocation is used based on age.

e. How would you allocate sample to strata, taking into consideration
both age and annual family income?

f. What is the variance of the distribution of annual family income for
the entire population?

g. Suppose the number of persons over 18 years of age having missing
teeth in a family is highly correlated with family income. Is stratified
random sampling with proportional allocation likely to yield an estimate having lower variance than that obtained from a simple random sample of the same number of households?

6.2 Let us suppose that the data from Table 3.8 were obtained from a
stratified random sample of the 1200 workers in the plant in which the
working force was stratified according to pulmonary stressors (high,
medium, low) and that proportional allocation was used to allocate
the sample.

   a. How many workers are there in each stratum?
   b. Estimate the mean forced vital capacity among the workers in the plant. How does this estimate differ from the mean that would have been obtained if the sample had been taken by simple random sampling?
   c. Obtain a 95% confidence interval for the population mean.
   d. What is the gain from stratified random sampling over what would have been obtained from simple random sampling?

6.3 Let us suppose that a household survey is to be taken for the purpose of estimating characteristics of families having female household heads. Since it is not known in advance of the survey which families have female household heads, the sample households will be screened and those sample households with female heads will be given a detailed interview. It is anticipated that the cost of screening a household is $10.00 and of interviewing a household having a female head is $50.00. The population is stratified into three strata according to the latest census information on the proportion of households having female heads. The strata are shown in the accompanying table. Assume that the variance of the characteristics being measured is the same in each stratum and that a total budget of $10,000 is allowed for the field work. How many households in each stratum should be sampled?

Stratum	No. of Households	Percentage of Households Having Female Head
1	10,000	25
2	20,000	15
3	5,000	10

6.4 Consider the 40 workers presented in Table 3.8 to be a simple random sample from the 1200 workers in the plant.
   a. Compute a 90% confidence interval for the population mean forced vital capacity.
   b. Suppose it is known, prior to analyzing the data, that the 1200 workers were distributed as follows:

$$N_1 = 1000 \quad \text{(number with high exposure)}$$
$$N_2 = 100 \quad \text{(number with medium exposure)}$$
$$N_3 = 100 \quad \text{(number with low exposure)}$$

Poststratify the original sample of Table 3.8 and construct a 90% confidence interval for the population mean forced vital capacity.

c. Compare the intervals of parts (a) and (b). Which is larger? Why?

6.5 A marketing research firm specializing in the health care industry has a file containing approximately 150,000,000 names organized by ZIP codes (the file contains 65,000 ZIP codes). A stratified random sample is to be taken with ZIP codes as the strata and proportional allocation. The purpose of this survey is to estimate the proportion of persons who would be likely to purchase a new type of electric toothbrush. An intensive marketing program would be initiated if, as a result of the survey, 15% or more of the population indicate willingness to purchase the product. How many names per ZIP code should be sampled if it is desired to estimate with 95% confidence this proportion to within 5% of its true value?

6.6 Esther is an epidemiologist and a very successful amateur body builder ("Ms. Drug Free Chicago Upper Body, 1989"). She is planning a survey of Chicago area body builders to determine the proportion who have ever used anabolic steroids. Her sampling frame consists of membership lists obtained from all accredited health clubs in the six-county Chicago metropolitan area. She has stratified clubs into the following three groups on the basis of their clientele:

1. Inner city yuppie
2. Inner city blue collar
3. Suburban

She anticipates that the proportion using anabolic steroids will be twice as high in stratum 1, which contains most of the "hard-core" competitors as in stratum 2, and that the proportion in stratum 3 will be about two-thirds as high as that in stratum 2. From her membership lists, she enumerates 8345 members in stratum 1, 5286 in stratum 2, and 6300 in stratum 3. If she can sample 1000 persons, how many should be allocated to each stratum? (Assume overall proportion using steroids is 12%)

6.7 Esther (the heroine of Exercise 6.6) is able to obtain $25,000 from BBAAS (Body Builders Against Anabolic Steroids) to conduct her survey. This will be her only source of funding. She estimates that it would cost $30.00 per interview in strata 1 and 2, and $40.00 per interview in stratum 3. With this in mind, how many persons should she interview in each stratum?

6.8 Esther (the same Esther from Exercises 6.6 and 6.7) feels that it would only be worth while to do her survey if she can be 95% certain of estimating the rate to within 15% of its true value. She anticipates that the true overall rate will be about 12%. Based on her funding level indicated in Exercise 6.7, does she have enough funds to meet her specifications?

6.9 In a large population survey 15,000 persons were screened, with chest radiographs. Physicians noted possible pulmonary artery enlargement in 230 of these patients. This enlargement was confirmed by a second reading in 203 of these 230 persons. A sample of 175 of the 14,770 chest radiographs in which no enlargement of the pulmonary artery was noted yielded 12 radiographs that were actually positive for pulmonary artery enlargement.

   a. Based on these data, what is the prevalence of pulmonary artery enlargement in the population?

   b. Obtain 95% confidence intervals for this prevalence rate.

6.10 A marathon was conducted in a large city on September 3, 1989. Based on the entry applications, the following data were obtained.

Age Group	N	Mean Number of Marathons Completed ($\bar{X}$)	Standard Deviation σ_x
$\leqslant 30$	2300	1.9	0.6
30–49	1478	2.3	0.8
50 +	978	3.1	0.7

It is desired to take a sample of approximately 500 persons from this list for purposes of estimating the average number of miles run per week in preparation for this marathon. If it is assumed that this might be proportional to the number of marathons completed, is there much to be gained by using a stratified random sample with proportional allocation over a simple random sample?

6.11 This exercise relates to the illustrative example on screening for twins discussed in Section 6.5. White female–female pairs were constructed as described in the illustrative example on the basis of same date of birth and SS#'s matching on the first seven digits. The number of pairs so constructed is as follows:

Quartile Based on SS# Sequence Difference	Number of Pairs Constructed from Medicare Files
First Quartile	10,024
Middle Two Quartiles	20,031
Fourth Quartile	10,024

Suppose that you guess that the overall prevalence of twins among these pairs is 20%, and that the prevalence of twins in the first quartile is twice that in the second quartile, while it is 3 times that in the third quartile. If you are planning to take a stratified random sample of 300 pairs from this file for the purposes of estimating the prevalence of twins in this file, what would be the optimal allocation in each of the three quartiles?

Suppose that instead of a stratified random sample of 300 pairs, it is decided to take a simple random sample of 300 pairs and the following data are obtained:

Quartile Based on SS# Sequence Difference	Number of Pairs Sampled	Number of Twins
First quartile	90	40
Middle two quartiles	110	10
Fourth quartile	100	1

a. What is the estimated prevalence of twins and its standard error?

b. Find the poststratified estimate of the prevalence of twins and its standard error.

BIBLIOGRAPHY

The following articles present sample surveys in which stratification is used.

1. Hemphill, F. M., A sample survey of home injuries, *Public Health Reports*, 67: 1026, 1952.

2. Horvitz, D. G., Sampling and field procedures of the Pittsburgh morbidity survey, *Public Health Repors*, 67: 1003, 1952.

3. Goldberg, J., Levy, P. S., Mullner, R., Gelfand, H., Iverson, N., Lemeshow, S., and Rothrock, J., Factors affecting trauma center utilization in Illinois, *Medical Care*, 19: 547, 1981.

4. Goldberg, J., Miles, T. P., Furner, S., Meyer, J., Hinds, A., Ramakrishnan, V., Lauderdale, D., and Levy, P. S., Identification of a biracial cohort of male and female twins age 65 and above in the United States, *American Journal of Epidemiology*, 145: 175–183, 1997.

5. Barner, B. M., and Levy, P. S., State-wide shoulder belt usage by type of roadway and posted speed limit: A three year comparison, *37th Annual Proceedings*

Association for the Advancement of Automotive Medicine, Association for the Advancement of Automotive Medicine, Des Plaines, Ill., 1994.

The following are recent reviews of stratification in sample surveys.

6. Parsons, V., Stratified sampling. In *Encyclopedia of Biostatistics*, Armitage, P. and Colton, T., Eds., Wiley, Chichester, U.K., 1998.

7. Malec, D., Allocation in stratified sampling. In *Encyclopedia of Biostatistics*, Armitage, P., and Colton, T. Eds, Wiley, Chichester, U.K., 1998.

8. Brewer, K. R. W., Stratified designs. In *Encyclopedia of Statistical Sciences*, Johnson, N., and Kotz, S. Eds., Wiley, New York, 1984.

The following books provide an overview of methodology used in the construction of strata as well as a thorough overview of stratification.

9. Cochran, W. G., *Sampling Techniques*, 3rd ed., Wiley, New York, 1977.

10. Hansen, M. H., Hurwitz, W. N., and Madow, W. G., *Sample Survey Methods and Theory*, Vols. 1 and 2, Wiley, New York, 1953.

11. Kish, L., *Survey Sampling*, Wiley, New York, 1965.

The following are "classic" articles that present methodology for construction of strata.

12. Dalenius, T., *Sampling in Sweden. Contributions to the Methods and Theories of Sample Survey Practice*, Almqvist and Wicksell, Stockholm, 1957.

13. Dalenius, T., and Hodges, J. L., Jr., Minimum variance stratification, *Journal of the American Statistical Association*, 54: 88–101, 1959.

CHAPTER 7

Ratio Estimation

In this chapter we introduce the concept of a ratio $\bar{x}/\bar{y}$ of two sample means $\bar{x}$ and $\bar{y}$. This ratio serves as an estimate of the ratio $\bar{X}/\bar{Y}$ of the means of two variables $\mathcal{X}$ and $\mathcal{Y}$ in a population. But, more importantly, it also serves as a device for obtaining a more accurate estimate of a population total X than can be obtained from the estimate x' determined by simple inflation of a sample total x by N/n, the inverse of the sampling fraction. This method is called *ratio estimation*, and the resulting estimates are called *ratio estimates*.

To begin, let us look at an example of ratio estimation.

Illustrative Example. Let us consider a community having eight community areas. Suppose that we wish to estimate the ratio R of total pharmaceutical expenses X to total medical expenses Y among all persons in the community. To do this, a simple random sample of two community areas is to be taken and every household in each sample community area is to be interviewed.

With this sampling design the elements are community areas and the ratio X/Y of total pharmaceutical to total medical expenses can be estimated by r, where $r = x/y$, the ratio obtained from the sample. Let us suppose that the data for the community areas are as given in Table 7.1.

Now suppose, for example, that community areas 2 and 5 are selected in the sample. Then we have

$$x = 50{,}000 + 150{,}000 = 200{,}000$$
$$y = 200{,}000 + 450{,}000 = 650{,}000$$

and

$$r = \frac{x}{y} = \frac{200{,}000}{650{,}000} = .308$$

Thus, the ratio of total pharmaceutical expenses to total medical expenses is equal to .308. □

Table 7.1 Pharmaceutical Expenses and Total Medical Expenses Among All Residents of Eight Community Areas

Community Area	Total Pharmaceutical Expenses, X ($)	Total Medical Expenses, Y ($)
1	100,000	300,000
2	50,000	200,000
3	75,000	300,000
4	200,000	600,000
5	150,000	450,000
6	175,000	520,000
7	170,000	680,000
8	150,000	450,000
Total	1,070,000	3,500,000

7.1 RATIO ESTIMATION UNDER SIMPLE RANDOM SAMPLING

The example above can be generalized as follows. Suppose that we have a simple random sample of n elements from a population of N elements, and that we wish to estimate the *ratio R* of two population totals X and Y. Clearly R is given by

$$R = \frac{X}{Y}$$

or, equivalently, by

$$R = \frac{\bar{X}}{\bar{Y}}$$

The ratio R can be estimated by r, as given by

$$r = \frac{x'}{y'}$$

or by the two algebraically equivalent forms

$$r = \frac{x}{y} \quad \text{and} \quad r = \frac{\bar{x}}{\bar{y}}$$

The estimate r is called a ratio estimate because both the numerator $\bar{x}$ and the denominator $\bar{y}$ are subject to sampling variation.

Now, let us return to the example presented in the introduction to this chapter to see whether an estimated ratio is an unbiased estimate.

Illustrative Example. In the example given above there are $\binom{8}{2} = 28$ possible simple random samples of two elements from the population of 8 elements. These possible samples are listed in Table 7.2 along with the values of x, y, and r obtained from each sample.

The sampling distribution of the estimated ratio r has a mean $E(r)$ and a standard error $SE(r)$ given by (see Box 2.3)

$$E(r) = \left(\frac{1}{28}\right) \times (.300 + .292 + \cdots + .283) = .3054$$

$$SE(r) = \left(\frac{1}{\sqrt{28}}\right) \times [(.300 - .3054)^2 + (.292 - .3054)^2$$
$$+ \cdots + (.283 - .3054)^2]^{1/2} = .0268$$

The true value of R from Table 7.1 is

$$R = \frac{1,070,000}{3,500,000} = .3057$$

The difference between the mean $E(r)$ of the sampling distribution of the estimated ratio r and the true population ratio R is not due to rounding error. Thus we see that an estimated ratio r is not necessarily an unbiased estimate of a population ratio R. However, in most situations the bias in an estimated ratio r is small, and estimates of this form are widely used. □

Note that in order to calculate $SE(r)$ in the example above, it was necessary to generate all possible samples and compute the standard error of the sampling distribution. Of course, in actual practice we do not generate the entire sampling distribution. However, unlike other estimates (such as means, totals, and proportions) that we have considered so far in this text, the estimated ratio r has both numerator and denominator subject to sampling variability; thus an exact expression for its standard error cannot be derived. However, it has been suggested by Hansen et al. [1] that if the coefficient of variation $V(\bar{y})$ of the denominator $\bar{y}$ or r (using the form $r = \bar{x}/\bar{y}$) is less than or equal to .05, then the standard error $SE(r)$ of r can be approximated by the following expression.

$$SE(r) \approx \left(\frac{R}{\sqrt{n}}\right) \times (V_x^2 + V_y^2 - 2\rho_{xy} V_x V_y)^{1/2} \times \sqrt{\frac{N-n}{N-1}} \qquad (7.1)$$

where ρ_{xy} is the *correlation coefficient* between x and y and is defined by

$$\rho_{xy} = \frac{\sum_{i=1}^{N}(X_i - \bar{X})(Y_i - \bar{Y})/N}{\sigma_x \sigma_y} \qquad (7.2)$$

Table 7.2 Possible Samples of Two Elements from the Population of Eight Elements (Table 7.1)

Community Areas in Sample	x	y	r
1,2	150,000	500,000	.300
1,3	175,000	600,000	.292
1,4	300,000	900,000	.333
1,5	250,000	750,000	.333
1,6	275,000	820,000	.335
1,7	270,000	980,000	.276
1,8	250,000	750,000	.333
2,3	125,000	500,000	.250
2,4	250,000	800,000	.313
2,5	200,000	650,000	.308
2,6	225,000	720,000	.313
2,7	220,000	880,000	.250
2,8	200,000	650,000	.308
3,4	275,000	900,000	.306
3,5	225,000	750,000	.300
3,6	250,000	820,000	.305
3,7	245,000	980,000	.250
3,8	225,000	750,000	.300
4,5	350,000	1,050,000	.333
4,6	375,000	1,120,000	.335
4.7	370,000	1,280,000	.289
4,8	350,000	1,050,000	.333
5,6	325,000	970,000	.335
5,7	320,000	1,130,000	.283
5,8	300,000	900,000	.333
6,7	345,000	1,200,000	.288
6,8	325,000	970,000	.335
7,8	320,000	1,130,000	.283

Let us do some calculations for the example we have been working with.

Illustrative Example.   For the data given in Table 7.1 we have the following population parameters [refer to the expressions in Box 2.1 and to Equations (2.7) and (7.2)]:

$$\sigma_x = 49{,}418.5 \qquad \bar{X} = 133{,}750 \qquad R = .3057$$
$$\sigma_y = 152{,}704.8 \qquad \bar{Y} = 437{,}500 \qquad V_x = .3695$$
$$N = 8 \qquad\qquad \rho_{xy} = .9272 \qquad V_y = .3490$$

For the data of Table 7.2, the coefficient of variation of the denominator $\bar{y}$ of r is

$$V(\bar{y}) = \left(\frac{1}{\bar{Y}}\right) \times \left(\frac{\sigma_y}{\sqrt{n}}\right) \times \sqrt{\frac{N-n}{N-1}} = \left(\frac{1}{437,500}\right) \times \left(\frac{152,704.8}{\sqrt{2}}\right)$$

$$\times \sqrt{\frac{8-2}{8-1}} = .2285$$

Calculation with Equation (7.1) gives

$$\text{SE}(r) \approx \left(\frac{.3057}{\sqrt{2}}\right) \times [(.3695)^2 + (.3490)^2 - 2(.9272)(.3695)(.3490)]^{1/2}$$

$$\times \sqrt{\frac{8-2}{8-1}} = .0277$$

compared to the exact value of .0268. Since the coefficient of variation of $\bar{y}$ is greater than .05, the approximation given by Equation (7.1) should not normally be used for SE(r). However, in this instance it seems to work reasonably well.

Now consider selecting samples of size $n = 7$ from the given population. The exact distribution of r for samples of $n = 7$ elements is shown in Table 7.3.

The exact standard error SE(r) of r obtained by enumerating all possible samples is used to .0063. Calculations show that

$$V(\bar{y}) = \left(\frac{1}{437,500}\right) \times \left(\frac{152,704.8}{\sqrt{7}}\right) \times \sqrt{\frac{8-7}{8-1}} = .0499$$

Therefore, since $V(\bar{y}) = .0499 \leqslant .05$, we expect the approximation of Equation (7.1) to provide a good approximation to the true value of SE(r). This calculation is as follows:

Table 7.3 Samples of Seven Elements from the Population of Table 7.1

Sample	x	y	r
1,2,3,4,5,6,7	920,000	3,050,000	.3016
1,2,3,4,5,6,8	900,000	2,820,000	.3191
1,2,3,4,5,7,8	895,000	2,980,000	.3003
1,2,3,4,6,7,8	920,000	3,050,000	.3016
1,2,3,5,6,7,8	870,000	2,900,000	.3000
1,2,4,5,6,7,8	995,000	3,200,000	.3109
1,3,4,5,6,7,8	1,020,000	3,300,000	.3091
2,3,4,5,6,7,8	970,000	3,200,000	.3031

$$\text{SE}(r) \approx \left(\frac{.3057}{\sqrt{7}}\right) \times [(.3695)^2 + (.3490)^2 - 2(.9272)(.3695)(.3490)]^{1/2}$$

$$\times \sqrt{\frac{8-7}{8-1}} = .0061$$

Thus we see that the approximation (7.1) agrees very closely in this example with the exact standard error of r. □

The standard error of an estimated ratio can be estimated from the data by replacing $\hat{\sigma}_x^2$ for σ_x^2, $\hat{\sigma}_y^2$ for σ_y^2, $\hat{\rho}_{xy}$ for ρ_{xy}, $\bar{x}$ for $\bar{X}$, $\bar{y}$ for $\bar{Y}$, and r for R in relation (7.1). The resulting estimate, $\widehat{\text{SE}}(r)$, is given by

$$\widehat{\text{SE}}(r) = \left(\frac{r}{\sqrt{n}}\right) \times (\hat{V}_x^2 + \hat{V}_y^2 - 2\hat{\rho}_{xy}\hat{V}_x\hat{V}_y)^{1/2} \times \sqrt{\frac{N-n}{N-1}} \qquad (7.3)$$

where

$$\hat{V}_x^2 = \left(\frac{N-1}{N}\right)\left(\frac{s_x^2}{\bar{x}^2}\right)$$

$$\hat{V}_y^2 = \left(\frac{N-1}{N}\right)\left(\frac{s_y^2}{\bar{y}^2}\right)$$

$$\hat{\rho}_{xy} = \frac{\sum_{i=1}^{n}(x_i - \bar{x})(y_i - \bar{y})}{(n-1)s_x s_y}$$

Generally this approximation will be used only when the following inequality is satisfied:

$$\frac{s_y}{\sqrt{n} \times \bar{y}} \times \sqrt{\frac{N-n}{N}} \leqslant .05$$

For convenience, formulas that can be used for ratio estimation are summarized in Box 7.1.

Illustrative Example. Suppose we take the sample consisting of community areas 1, 2, 3, 4, 5, 6, 8 from Table 7.1. We calculate $s_y = 141,033.6$, $\bar{y} = 402,857.1$, and $s_y/\sqrt{n}\bar{y} \times \sqrt{(N-n)/N} = .0468$, which is less than .05. Thus we expect approximation (7.3) to provide a good estimate of the standard error of the estimated ratio r. For this example we have

BOX 7.1   FORMULAS FOR RATIO ESTIMATION UNDER SIMPLE RANDOM SAMPLING

Population Parameters

$$R = \frac{X}{Y} = \frac{\bar{X}}{\bar{Y}}$$

$$\text{SE}(r) \approx \left(\frac{R}{\sqrt{n}}\right) \times (V_x^2 + V_y^2 - 2\rho_{xy}V_xV_y)^{1/2} \times \sqrt{\frac{N-n}{N-1}}$$

Sample Estimates

$$r = \frac{x'}{y'} = \frac{x}{y} = \frac{\bar{x}}{\bar{y}}$$

$$\widehat{\text{SE}}(r) = \left(\frac{r}{\sqrt{n}}\right) \times (\hat{V}_x^2 + \hat{V}_y^2 - 2\hat{\rho}_{xy}\hat{V}_x\hat{V}_y)^{1/2} \times \sqrt{\frac{N-n}{N-1}}$$

A $100(1 - \alpha)\%$ confidence interval may be constructed as

$$r - z_{1-(\alpha/2)}\widehat{\text{SE}}(r) \leqslant R \leqslant r + z_{1-(\alpha/2)}\widehat{\text{SE}}(r)$$

V_x and V_y are defined in Equation (2.7); X, $\bar{X}$, σ_x, Y, $\bar{Y}$, and σ_y are as defined in Box 2.1. ρ_{xy} is as defined in Equation (7.2); x, $\bar{x}$, x', y, $\bar{y}$, y', s_x^2, and s_y^2 are as defined in Box 2.2. Then

$$\hat{V}_x^2 = \left(\frac{N-1}{N}\right)\left(\frac{s_x^2}{\bar{x}^2}\right)$$

$$\hat{V}_y^2 = \left(\frac{N-1}{N}\right)\left(\frac{s_y^2}{\bar{y}^2}\right)$$

$$\hat{\rho}_{xy} = \sum_{i=1}^{n} \frac{(x_i - \bar{x})(y_i - \bar{y})}{(n-1)s_xs_y}$$

$$r = .3191 \qquad \hat{\rho}_{xy} = .9900$$
$$s_x = 54{,}826.6 \qquad s_y = 141{,}033.6$$
$$\bar{x} = 128{,}571.4 \qquad \bar{y} = 402{,}857.1$$
$$\hat{V}_x^2 = .1591 \qquad \hat{V}_y^2 = .1072$$

Then we obtain

$$\widehat{SE}(r) = \left(\frac{.3191}{\sqrt{7}}\right) \times [.1591 + .1072 - 2(.9900)\sqrt{.1591} \times \sqrt{.1072}]^{1/2} \times \left(\frac{8-7}{8-1}\right)^{1/2}$$
$$= .0040$$

as compared to the true population value of SE(r), which is .0063. This discrepancy is not surprising since estimated variances are known to be highly variable.   □

The estimated ratio r is, in general, a biased estimate of R. However, when sample sizes are reasonably large, the bias is generally small, and approximate confidence intervals for the unknown population ratio R can be constructed by use of the estimated standard error, $\widehat{SE}(r)$, of r.

Estimates of ratios are important in sample surveys, especially when the enumeration units are not the same as the elementary units. For example, if a simple random sample is taken for purposes of estimating the mean number of days lost from work per person because of acute illness, a ratio estimate having the form discussed above could be used, with the numerator being number of days lost from work per household, and the denominator being number of persons per household. Both the numerator and denominator would be subject to sampling variability.

In Section 3.5, we discussed the estimation of population means for subgroups of a population under simple random sampling. The estimate appropriate for this situation is a special case of an estimated ratio, where the denominator is the number of members of the subgroup in the sample. If the sampling plan is that of a simple random sample of elements, this form of ratio estimate is an unbiased estimate of the appropriate subgroup mean.

Estimation of ratios and their standard errors can be performed in SUDAAN by use of the *PROC RATIO* module in that software package. The following illustrates the set of commands that would be used for the previous illustrative example.

```
1  PROC RATIO DATA=TAB7PT1 FILETYPE=SAS DESIGN=STRWOR;
2  TOTCNT TOTCNT;
3  WEIGHT WT1;
4  NEST _ONE_;
5  NUMER PHARMEXP;
6  DENOM TOTMEDEX;
```

7 SETENV COLWIDTH = 1;
8 SETENV DECWIDTH = 4

The first statement indicates that the procedure, *PROC RATIO*, is to be used and that the sample data are in the SAS data file, *TAB7PT1.SSD*. This file has the following appearance:

AREA	PHARMEXP	TOTMEDEX	TOTCNT	WT1
1	100000	300000	8	1.1428571
2	50000	200000	8	1.1428571
3	75000	300000	8	1.1428571
4	200000	600000	8	1.1428571
5	150000	450000	8	1.1428571
6	175000	520000	8	1.1428571
8	150000	450000	8	1.1428571

The above data file consists of 7 records, one for each sample community area. Each record has the following five variables:

area = the community area identification number.

pharmexp = the total pharmaceutical expenses associated with each community area.

totmedex = the total medical expenses associated with each community area.

totcnt = the total number, N, of community areas in the population.

wt1 = the sampling weight, N/n.

The phrase, DESIGN = STRWOR, along with the fourth statement, NEST = _ONE_, indicates that the sampling design is simple random sampling without replacement. The second statement specifies that the population size, N, is on each record as the variable, TOTCNT, and is equal to 8 in this example. The third statement specifies that the sampling weight $(8/7 = 1.1429)$ appears as the variable, *WT1*, on each sample record. Finally, the fifth and sixth statements specify the numerator and denominator variables for the ratio, and the seventh statement specifies the column width and number of decimal places in the resulting output.

The output generated by the above commands is shown below. Note that the estimated standard error is exactly equal to that obtained from the formula shown in Box 7.1. This is not surprising since SUDAAN uses the exact same formula.

Variable		One 1
PHARMEXP/TOTMEDEX	Sample Size	7.0000
	Weighted Size	8.0000
	Weighted X-Sum	3222978.0000
	Weighted Y-Sum	1028610.0000
	Ratio Est.	0.3191
	SE Ratio	0.0040

Estimation using STATA can be performed on the STATA data file *tab7pt1.dta* with the following commands:

```
. use a:tab7pt1
. svyset fpc totcnt
. svyset pweight wt1
. svyratio pharmexp/totmedex
```

The file *tab7pt1.dta* has the same structure as the file *tab7pt1.ssd* used in the SUDAAN analysis.

These commands would generate the output shown below:

Survey ratio estimation

pweight: wt1	Number of obs =	7
Strata: < one >	Number of strata =	1
PSU: < observations >	Number of PSUs =	7
FPC: totcnt	Population size =	8

Ratio	Estimate	Std. Err.	[95% Conf. Interval]		Deff
pharmexp/totmedex	.3191489	.0040067	.309345	.3289529	1

Finite population correction (FPC) assumes simple random sampling without replacement of PSUs within each stratum with no subsampling within PSUs.

7.2 ESTIMATION OF RATIOS FOR SUBDOMAINS UNDER SIMPLE RANDOM SAMPLING

In Section 3.6 we discussed, in a relatively informal way, estimation of means for subdomains under simple random sampling. We noted that the mean for a subdomain is, in reality, a ratio estimate with numerator equal to the sample aggregate of the variable being estimated over all sample elements belonging to the subdomain, and denominator equal to the number of sample elements belonging to the subdomain. In this section, we will generalize estimation of ratios for subdomains to situations where the denominator of the ratio is not necessarily a count of subdomain elements in the sample.

Let us suppose we take a simple random sample of n elements from a population containing N elements, and wish to estimate the ratio $R_{(k)}$, which is defined as follows:

$$R_{(k)} = \frac{X_{(k)}}{Y_{(k)}}$$

where $X_{(k)}$ and $Y_{(k)}$ are totals of variables X and Y over all elements in a defined subdomain, k. By use of a transformation of the numerator and denominator variables, we can use the estimation procedures developed in Section 7.1 and the formulas shown in Box 7.1. This is shown below. Let

$$\delta_{ik} = \begin{cases} 1 & \text{if element } i \text{ is in subdomain } k \\ 0 & \text{if otherwise} \end{cases}$$

and

$$r_{(k)} = \frac{x_{(k)}}{y_{(k)}}$$

The standard error of the estimated subdomain ratio, $r_{(k)}$, can be estimated by the formula shown in Box 7.1. This is illustrated by the following example.

Illustrative Example. Suppose we take a sample of 56 hospitals from an area containing 101 hospitals and, for each sample hospital, review the records of all babies born at the hospital during the previous calendar year for purposes of determining whether the mother's status with respect to hepatitis B surface antigen (HBsAG) was recorded on the newborn's patient medical record. The presence of this information on the infant's record is considered important, because if the mother is positive for the antigen, the newborn should receive immune globulin to prevent occurrence of hepatitis B.

The hospitals are classified according to the level of their obstetrics and gynecological services (1 = "basic"; 2 = "intermediate"; 3 = "tertiary"), and it is desired to estimate for intermediate level hospitals the proportion of newborns whose mothers' HBsAG status was recorded on their newborn medical records. Data relevant to this illustrative example are in the file *BHRATIO.DAT*. For purposes of illustration, relevant variables from the first 10 records on that data file are shown in the table.

Sample Hospital	Number of Records having Mother's Antigen Recorded (x_i)	Number of Births (y_i)	Obstetrics Level of Hospital	Indicator Variable for Subdomain (δ_i)	Transformed Numerator Variable (x_i)	Transformed Denominator Variable (y_i)
1	2898	2898	2	1	2898	2898
2	1095	1304	2	1	1095	1304
3	1860	2022	2	1	1860	2022
4	1227	1395	2	1	1227	1395
5	618	773	2	1	618	773
6	1499	1630	2	1	1499	1630
7	1321	1436	2	1	1321	1436
8	0	2525	2	1	0	2525
9	3595	4674	3	0	0	0
10	1732	2279	2	1	1732	2279

Among the first 10 sample records shown in the table, only one record (that for sample hospital 9) is affected by the transformation, since it is from the only hospital among the first 10 that is not in the subdomain of interest. Among the entire sample of 56 hospitals, 13 are not obstetrics level "2" hospitals and would be affected by the transformation; the other 43 are obstetrics level "2" hospitals. Summary statistics for the sample of 56 hospitals are shown below:

$$N = 101 \qquad n = 56$$

$$x_{(k)} = \sum_{i=1}^{56} x_i \delta_{ik} = 43{,}910 \qquad y_{(k)} = \sum_{i=1}^{56} y_i \delta_{ik} = 58{,}082$$

$$r_{(k)} = \frac{x_{(k)}}{y_{(k)}} = 0.7560$$

$$s_{x_{(k)}}^2 = 547{,}393.079 \qquad s_{y_{(k)}}^2 = 639{,}484.913$$

$$\bar{x}_{(k)} = \frac{x_{(k)}}{56} = 784.107 \qquad \bar{y}_{(k)} = \frac{y_{(k)}}{56} = 1037.179$$

$$\hat{V}_{x_{(k)}} = \sqrt{\frac{100}{101}} \frac{s_{x_{(k)}}}{\bar{x}_{(k)}} = .9389$$

$$\hat{V}_{y_{(k)}} = .7672 \quad \hat{\rho}_{x_{(k)},y_{(k)}} = 0.825$$

Then from the formula in Box 7.1

$$\widehat{SE}(r_{(k)}) = .0360$$

Thus, it is estimated that, among obstetric level "2" hospitals, 75.6% of all newborns have his/her mother's hepatitis B surface antigen status recorded on the newborn medical record, and that the standard error of that estimate is 0.0360.

$\square$

7.3 POSTSTRATIFIED RATIO ESTIMATES UNDER SIMPLE RANDOM SAMPLING

The technique of *poststratification*, as generally used in sampling methodology, is an estimation technique that uses known population information for subgroups or subdomains to produce estimates that can have much improved precision. In Chapter 6, Section 6.6, we discussed poststratified estimates of population means under simple random sampling. The discussion in that section is equally applicable to other linear estimates such as totals and proportions. In this section, we will discuss the use of poststratification in ratio estimation under simple random sampling.

Let us suppose that we have a simple random sample of n elements from a population of N elements and that we wish to estimate the ratio:

$$R = X/Y$$

The ratio estimate, r, specified in Section 7.1, can be put in the form

$$r = \frac{x'}{y'} = \frac{\sum\limits_{i=1}^{n} w_i x_i}{\sum\limits_{i=1}^{n} w_i y_i}$$

where

$$w_i = \frac{N}{n}$$

If there are K mutually exclusive and exhaustive subdomains or subgroups, then the following is true for x':

$$x' = \sum_{k=1}^{K} \sum_{i=1}^{n} w_i \delta_{ik} x_i = \frac{N}{n} \sum_{k=1}^{K} x_{(k)}$$

where

$$x_{(k)} = \sum_{i=1}^{n} \delta_{ik} x_i$$

and

$$\delta_{ik} = \begin{cases} 1 & \text{if element } i \text{ is in subdomain } k \\ 0 & \text{if otherwise} \end{cases}$$

The entity, $x_{(k)}$, is simply the sample total of the variable X for all sample elements that are in the subdomain k. Likewise, the entity, $n_{(k)} = \sum_{i=1}^{n} \delta_{ik}$ is the number of sample elements that are in subdomain k. The ratio $x_{(k)}/n_{(k)}$ estimates from the sample the level of X per element in domain k, and if the total number, N_k, of elements in the domain k population were known, then the ratio $(N_k/n_{(k)})x_{(k)}$, is a more "specific" estimate of the total X in domain k. Finally, using this "correction" for each domain and for the Y variable as well, we obtain the poststratified ratio estimate, r_{pstr}, shown below:

$$r_{\text{pstr}} = \frac{\displaystyle\sum_{k=1}^{K} \frac{N_k}{n_{(k)}} x_{(k)}}{\displaystyle\sum_{k=1}^{K} \frac{N_k}{n_{(k)}} y_{(k)}}$$

where

$$x_{(k)} = \sum_{i=1}^{n} \delta_{ik} x_i$$

$$y_{(k)} = \sum_{i=1}^{n} \delta_{ik} y_i$$

and

$$n_{(k)} = \sum_{i=1}^{n} \delta_{ik}$$

Since the entities $x_{(k)}$, $y_{(k)}$, and $n_{(k)}$ are all subject to sampling variability, it follows that the poststratified ratio estimate, r_{pstr}, is really the ratio of the sum of K ratio estimates involving $x_{(k)}$ and $n_{(k)}$ divided by the sum of K ratio estimates involving $y_{(k)}$ and $n_{(k)}$. The standard error of r_{pstr} does not have a simple form and will not be given here but can be estimated by Taylor series linearization (see Chapter 12), and is available in SUDAAN.

Illustrative Example. Let us consider the sample of 56 hospitals discussed in Section 7.2 (the data from this sample are in the ASCII file, BHRATIO.DAT). A straightforward use of the ratio estimation formulas in Box 7.1 would yield an estimate of .756 with estimated standard error .036 for the proportion of all newborns who have their mother's hepatitis B surface antigen status recorded on their newborn medical record.

It is known, moreover, that 29 (51.8%) of the 56 sample hospitals have written policies stating that the newborn should not be discharged until the mother's status with respect to Hepatitis B surface antigen is documented on the newborn's record. It is also known that 66 (65.4%) of the 101 hospitals in the corresponding population from which this sample was drawn have this written policy. Since it is logical that hospitals having this policy should have a higher proportion of newborns with their mother's HBsAG status documented on their records, and since the population distribution of hospitals having and not having this policy is known, it is a situation where one might reasonably use a poststratified ratio estimate. Letting subdomain 1 be the subdomain having written policy requiring newborns to have information about mother's HBsAG status on the medical record before discharge, and subdomain 2 be the subdomain of hospitals not having this policy, we obtain the following summary statistics.

$n_{(1)} = 29 =$ the number of hospitals in the sample belonging to subdomain 1
$n_{(2)} = 27 =$ the number of sample hospitals in subdomain 2
$x_{(1)} = 42,749 =$ the total number of newborns in the subdomain 1 sample hospitals having their mother's HBsAG status on the medical record
$x_{(2)} = 22,560 =$ the total number of newborns in the subdomain 2 sample hospitals having their mother's HBsAG status on the medical record
$y_{(1)} = 47,850 =$ the total number of newborns in the sample of subdomain 1 hospitals
$y_{(2)} = 38,929 =$ the total number of newborns in the sample of subdomain 2 hospitals
$N_1 = 66 =$ the known population number of subdomain 1 hospitals
$N_2 = 35 =$ the known population number of subdomain 2 hospitals

From these summary statistics, we construct the poststratified ratio estimate as shown below:

$$r_{pstr} = \frac{\frac{66}{29} 42,749 + \frac{35}{27} 22,560}{\frac{66}{29} 47,850 + \frac{35}{27} 38,929} = .794$$

The following compares the poststratified ratio estimate with the usual ratio estimate for this example:

| | | **Estimated** |
Estimate	**Estimated Ratio**	**Standard Error**
Ordinary	$r = .756$	$SE(r) = .036$
Poststratified	$r_{pstr} = .794$	$SE(r_{pstr}) = .022$

Clearly, in this example, the poststratified ratio estimate is different from the ordinary ratio estimate and its standard error is much lower. The reason for this is that the subdomain ratios differ considerably and the sample has a higher proportion of subdomain 2 hospitals than is represented in the population.   □

7.4 RATIO ESTIMATION OF TOTALS UNDER SIMPLE RANDOM SAMPLING

The estimates of totals or aggregates discussed so far have been obtained from simple inflation of a sample total by the ratio N/n. We have discussed the fact that estimates x' of this type are unbiased estimates, and we have developed an expression for the standard error of such estimates and the methodology for constructing approximate confidence intervals for the unknown total X under simple random sampling. Sometimes, however, we are in a position to use additional information available to us for purposes of constructing a different estimator of a population total, one which is based on an estimated ratio, so that the resulting estimator has a smaller mean square error than the simple inflation estimator x'.

Let us investigate this idea by looking at an example.

Illustrative Example. Let us suppose that a village comprises six census tracts having the 1990 population given in Table 7.4. The school enrollment (considered unknown in advance of the survey) is also given in Table 7.4.

Let us suppose that we wish to estimate the total present school enrollment by taking a simple random sample of two census tracts and ascertaining the school enrollment in each sample tract by surveying each school within the tract, counting heads, and inflating the sample totals by N/n as discussed in Chapter 3. The $\binom{6}{2} = 15$ possible samples are listed in Table 7.5 along with the values of x', the estimated total.

From our results on simple random sampling, we know that the estimated total x' is an unbiased estimate of the population total. The standard error of x' (computed by enumeration of all the samples listed below) is, according to Box 2.3,

$$SE(x') = 1568.4577$$

Table 7.4 Population (1990 Census) and Present School Enrollment by Census Tract

Census Tract	1990 Population	Present School Enrollment*
1	6,657	2269
2	4,057	1324
3	3,642	952
4	5,320	1558
5	4,480	1352
6	5,880	1796
Total	30,036	9251

*Unknown until the schools are surveyed.

Table 7.5 Possible Samples of Two Schools Taken from Data of Table 7.4

Schools in Sample	Estimated School Enrollment	Schools in Sample	Estimated School Enrollment
1, 2	10,779	2, 6	9,360
1, 3	9,663	3, 4	7,530
1, 4	11,481	3, 5	6,912
1, 5	10,863	3, 6	8,244
1, 6	12,195	4, 5	8,730
2, 3	6,828	4, 6	10,062
2, 4	8,646	5, 6	9,444
2, 5	8,028		

Instead of using the estimate x' as we did in the example above, we can estimate the total school enrollment X by using the data on the 1990 population that is available for each census tract. Each sample of census tracts enables us not only to estimate school enrollment from the sample but also to estimate total population from the sample. Suppose we use the following notation:

Y = the total number of persons in the population

Y_i = the number of persons in census tract i

y_i = the number of persons in sample tract i

$y = \sum_{i=1}^{n} y_i$ = the total number of persons in the sample census tracts

Then the estimated population total y' is given by

$$y' = \left(\frac{N}{n}\right) \times y$$

where

$N =$ the total number of tracts in the population
$n =$ the total number of tracts in the sample

Each sample gives us an estimate x' of X and y' of Y. But since the true value of Y is known to us from census data, then it might make sense, if school enrollment and population size are strongly correlated, to assume that the estimator x' of X might differ from X in the same proportion that the estimator y' differs from Y. That is, $X/x' = Y/y'$. This motivates the use of an estimator x'' of X given by

$$x'' = \left(\frac{x'}{y'}\right) \times Y \tag{7.4}$$

or its algebraic equivalent

$$x'' = r \times Y \tag{7.5}$$

where r is an estimated ratio.

Further insight into this estimator is evident if one writes it as follows:

$$x'' = \left(\frac{Y}{y'}\right) \times x'$$

If the estimated population size y' is less than the known true total Y, then y' underestimates Y. We would expect also that the estimate x' obtained from the same sample underestimates to a similar extent the true unknown total X since $\mathscr{X}$ and $\mathscr{Y}$ are correlated. But note that the ratio Y/y' would be greater than unity in this case, and x'' would be greater than the simple inflation estimate x'. The opposite occurs when y' is greater than Y. Thus we see that even for particularly bad samples (i.e., those that yield values of x' that differ greatly from X in absolute value), the ratio Y/y' would adjust for this, and the estimator x'' would not differ from X by as much as x' does.

Let us examine all of these ideas in some examples.　　　　　□

Illustrative Example. For samples of $n = 2$ census tracts taken from the population shown in Table 7.4, let us investigate the sample values of x' and x''. These values are listed in Table 7.6.

We see from the sampling distribution shown in Table 7.6 that the mean $E(x'')$, the standard error $SE(x'')$, and the mean square error $MSE(x'')$ are (refer to Box 2.3)

$$E(x'') = \frac{10{,}073 + 9394 + \cdots + 9127}{15} = 9211.07$$

$$SE(x'') = \left[\frac{(10{,}073 - 9211.07)^2 + (9394 - 9211.07)^2 + \cdots + (9127 - 9211.07)^2}{15}\right]^{1/2}$$

$$= 466.38$$

$$MSE(x'') = Var(x'') + B^2(x'') = 217{,}512.33 + (9211.07 - 9251)^2$$
$$= 219{,}106.73$$

Since the simple inflation estimate x' is an unbiased estimate of X, its MSE is equal to its variance:

$$MSE(x') = Var(x') = (1568.4577)^2 = 2{,}460{,}059.56$$

Thus, even though x'' is a biased estimate of X, its mean square error in this example is much less than that of x'. ☐

Illustrative Example. The data from Table 5.1 can also be used to illustrate estimation of a total by a ratio. If we wish to estimate the total number X of truck miles driven from a simple random sample of $n = 3$ segments, we can

Table 7.6 Values of x' and x'' for Samples in Table 7.5

Sample	x'	x''
1, 2	10,779	10,073
1, 3	9,663	9,394
1, 4	11,481	9,597
1, 5	10,863	9,766
1, 6	12,195	9,739
2, 3	6,828	8,879
2, 4	8,646	9,231
2, 5	8,028	9,415
2, 6	9,360	9,431
3, 4	7,530	8,412
3, 5	6,912	8,520
3, 6	8,244	8,668
4, 5	8,730	8,919
4, 6	10,062	8,995
5, 6	9,444	9,127

estimate the ratio r of truck miles to accidents involving trucks from the sample. If the total number Y of accidents involving trucks is known for the entire road, the estimate x'' can be constructed. For example, if segments 1, 3, and 4 are sampled, we have the following calculations (refer to Boxes 3.1 and 7.1):

$$x' = \left(\frac{8}{3}\right) \times (6327 + 8691 + 7834) = 60{,}938.67$$

   = simple inflation estimate of truck miles driven

$$y' = \left(\frac{8}{3}\right) \times (8 + 9 + 9) = 69.33$$

   = simple inflation estimate of number of accidents involving trucks

$$r = \frac{x'}{y'} = 878.9230$$

   = estimated ratio of truck miles to accidents involving trucks

The total number Y of accidents involving trucks is known; specifically,

$$Y = 50$$

Hence,

$$x'' = \left(\frac{x'}{y'}\right) \times Y = 878.9230 \times 50 = 43{,}946.15 \text{ truck miles}$$

which is closer to the true total $(X = 34{,}054)$ than is the simple inflation estimate x'.   □

The estimate x'' is of the form rY where r is an estimated ratio and Y is a known population total. Hence it follows that its *standard error* $SE(x'')$ is equal to $Y \times SE(r)$, which can be approximated by the following expression provided that $V(\bar{y})$, the coefficient of variation of $\bar{y}$, is less than .05:

$$SE(x'') = \left(\frac{YR}{\sqrt{n}}\right) \times (V_x^2 + V_y^2 - 2\rho_{xy}V_xV_y)^{1/2} \times \sqrt{\frac{N-n}{N-1}} \qquad (7.6)$$

Likewise, an estimate $\widehat{SE}(x'')$ of $SE(x'')$ can be obtained from data by substituting $\widehat{SE}(r)$ [relation (7.3)] for $SE(r)$ in expression (7.6) as given below:

$$\widehat{SE}(x'') = \left(\frac{Yr}{\sqrt{n}}\right) \times (\hat{V}_x^2 + \hat{V}_y^2 - 2\hat{\rho}_{xy}\hat{V}_x\hat{V}_y)^{1/2} \times \sqrt{\frac{N-n}{N-1}} \qquad (7.7)$$

Expression (7.7) can be used to obtain approximate confidence intervals for an unknown total X provided that $\hat{V}(\bar{y})$, the estimated coefficient of variation of $\bar{y}$, is less than .05.

Let us look at another example.

Illustrative Example. If segments 1, 3, and 4 are sampled in the data from Table 5.1, we have the sample data given in Table 7.7. We than have the following summary statistics:

$$
\begin{array}{llll}
n = 3 & \bar{x} = 7617.33 & s_x = 1196.80 & \hat{V}_x^2 = .0216 \\
N = 8 & \bar{y} = 8.67 & s_y = .5774 & \hat{V}_y^2 = .003883 \\
\hat{\rho}_{xy} = .9337 & Y = 50 & r = 878.9231 & x'' = 43{,}946.15
\end{array}
$$

The estimated coefficient of variation $\hat{V}(\bar{y})$ is*

$$
\hat{V}(\bar{y}) = \left(\frac{s_y}{\bar{y}\sqrt{n}}\right) \times \sqrt{\frac{N-n}{N}} = \left[\frac{.5774}{8.67\sqrt{3}}\right] \times \sqrt{\frac{8-3}{8}} = .0304
$$

Since $\hat{V}(\bar{y}) < .05$, expression (7.7) can be used to estimate the standard error of x'' as follows:

$$
\widehat{SE}(x'') = \left[\frac{50 \times 878.5848}{\sqrt{3}}\right] \times [.0245 + .003883 - 2 \times .9337
$$

$$
\times \sqrt{.0216} \times \sqrt{.003883}]^{1/2} \times \sqrt{\frac{8-3}{8-1}}
$$

$$
= 1963.04
$$

Table 7.7 Sample Data from Table 5.1

Segments in Sample	No. of Truck Miles (x_i)	No. of Accidents Involving Trucks (y_i)
1	6,327	8
3	8,691	9
4	7,834	9

*The formula for $V(\bar{y})$ is given in Equation (3.7). Substituting $(\hat{V}_y^2)^{1/2}$ as given in Box 7.1 into formula (3.7), we obtain

$$
\hat{V}(\bar{y}) = \left(\frac{\hat{V}_y}{\sqrt{n}}\right) \times \sqrt{\frac{N-n}{N-1}} = \left[\sqrt{\frac{N-1}{N}} \times \left(\frac{s_y^2}{\bar{y}^2}\right)^{1/2} \times \frac{1}{\sqrt{n}}\right] \times \sqrt{\frac{N-n}{N-1}}
$$

$$
= \left(\frac{s_y}{\bar{y}\sqrt{n}}\right) \times \sqrt{\frac{N-n}{N}}
$$

We then have the following 95% confidence interval for the estimated total number of truck miles driven:

$$x'' - 1.96 \times \widehat{SE}(x'') \leqslant X \leqslant x'' + 1.96 \times \widehat{SE}(x'')$$
$$43{,}946.15 - 1.96 \times 1963.04 \leqslant X \leqslant 43{,}946.15 + 196 \times 1963.04$$
$$40{,}098 \leqslant X \leqslant 47{,}793.71$$

Note that for this particular sample the 95% confidence interval does not cover the true population total. $\square$

7.5 COMPARISON OF RATIO ESTIMATE WITH SIMPLE INFLATION ESTIMATE

Let us assume that the approximation to the standard error of the ratio estimate of a total under simple random sampling, given by relation (7.6), is valid and that the bias in the ratio estimate can be ignored. Then we can evaluate whether a ratio estimate x'' is likely to result in an improved estimate of a total over a simple inflation estimate by examining the ratio of the variance of x'' to that of x' as follows:

$$\frac{\text{Var}(x'')}{\text{Var}(x')} = \frac{V_x^2 + V_y^2 - 2\rho_{xy}V_xV_y}{V_x^2}$$

Since

$$\text{Var}(x'') = Y^2 \times \text{Var}(r)$$
$$= Y^2 \times \left(\frac{R^2}{n}\right) \times (V_x^2 + V_y^2 - 2\rho_{xy}V_xV_y) \times \left(\frac{N-n}{N-1}\right)$$

and

$$\text{Var}(x') = \left(\frac{N^2}{n}\right) \times \sigma_x^2 \times \left(\frac{N-n}{N-1}\right)$$
$$= \left(\frac{N^2}{n}\right) \times (\bar{X}^2 V_x^2) \times \left(\frac{N-n}{N-1}\right) = \left(\frac{X^2}{n}\right) \times V_x^2 \times \left(\frac{N-n}{N-1}\right)$$

it follows that x'' will have smaller variance than x' whenever

$$V_x^2 + V_y^2 - 2\rho_{xy}V_xV_y < V_x^2$$

or equivalently, whenever

$$\frac{V_y}{V_x} < 2\rho_{xy} \tag{7.8}$$

Thus for fixed values of coefficients of variation of $\mathscr{X}$ and $\mathscr{Y}$ in the population, the greater the correlation between $\mathscr{X}$ and $\mathscr{Y}$, the more likely it is that a total estimated by x'' will have lower variance than when estimated by x', the simple inflation estimate.

7.6 APPROXIMATION TO THE STANDARD ERROR OF THE RATIO ESTIMATED TOTAL

A special situation of interest occurs when the relationship between $\mathscr{X}$ and $\mathscr{Y}$ can be represented reasonably closely by a straight line through the origin. In other words, suppose that the relationship between $\mathscr{X}$ and $\mathscr{Y}$ can be expressed by the *regression model*

$$X_i = \beta Y_i + \varepsilon_i \tag{7.9}$$

where β is the *slope* of the regression line of $\mathscr{X}$ on $\mathscr{Y}$ and

$$\sum_{i=1}^{N} \varepsilon_i = 0$$

Then the expression for ρ_{xy} becomes

$$\rho_{xy} = \frac{\sum_{i=1}^{N}(\beta Y_i + \varepsilon_i - \beta \bar{Y})(Y_i - \bar{Y})/N}{\sigma_x \sigma_y}$$

$$= \frac{\beta \sum_{i=1}^{N}(Y_i - \bar{Y})^2 + \sum_{i=1}^{N}\varepsilon_i(Y_i - \bar{Y})}{N\sigma_x \sigma_y}$$

If the expression $\sum_{i=1}^{N}\varepsilon_i(Y_i - \bar{Y})$ is close to zero (which it will be if the model represented above fits the data well), then ρ_{xy} is approximately equal to the expression

$$\rho_{xy} \approx \frac{\beta \sum_{i=1}^{N}(Y_i - \bar{Y})^2}{N\sigma_x \sigma_y}.$$

Since it follows from expression (7.9) that $\beta = \bar{X}/\bar{Y}$, and since

$$\sum_{i=1}^{N}(Y_i - \bar{Y})^2 = N\sigma_y^2,$$

we have

$$\rho_{xy} \approx \frac{\bar{X}\sigma_y}{\bar{Y}\sigma_x} = \frac{V_y}{V_x}. \tag{7.10}$$

This gives us, from relation (7.6), the following *approximation to the standard error* of x'', the total estimated from a ratio:

$$\text{SE}(x'') \approx \left(\frac{YR}{\sqrt{n}}\right) \times (V_x^2 - V_y^2)^{1/2}\sqrt{\frac{N-n}{N-1}} \tag{7.11}$$

which can be *estimated* from the data by the expression

$$\widehat{\text{SE}}(x'') \approx \left(\frac{Yr}{\sqrt{n}}\right) \times (\hat{V}_x^2 - \hat{V}_y^2)^{1/2}\sqrt{\frac{N-n}{N-1}}. \tag{7.12}$$

The expressions above are especially useful since they do not involve the correlation coefficient in explicit form.

For the example given earlier in which three segments were sampled, under the assumption that the regression is linear and passes through the origin, the estimated standard error, $\widehat{\text{SE}}(x'')$, as given by approximation (7.12) is

$$\widehat{\text{SE}}(x'') = \left[\frac{50 \times 878.5848}{\sqrt{3}}\right](.0245 - .004435)^{1/2}\sqrt{\frac{8-3}{8-1}} = 3036.33$$

which is larger than the standard error obtained from relation (7.7).

7.7 DETERMINATION OF SAMPLE SIZE

In order to be $100 \times (1 - \alpha)\%$ confident that the estimated ratio r or a ratio estimated total x'' is within $100 \times \varepsilon\%$ of the true value of R (or X), the approximate *sample size* needed is given by

$$n = \frac{z_{1-(\alpha/2)}^2 \times N \times (V_x^2 + V_y^2 - 2\rho_{xy}V_xV_y)}{z_{1-(\alpha/2)}^2 \times (V_x^2 + V_y^2 - 2\rho_{xy}V_xV_y) + (N-1)\varepsilon^2} \tag{7.13}$$

If the parameters in expression (7.13) can either be guessed or estimated from preliminary data, a sample size can be determined.

7.8 REGRESSION ESTIMATION OF TOTALS

The estimate x'' of a total X based on a ratio r is a special case of a *regression estimate* of a total. The *regression estimate* x''' has the form given by

$$x''' = x' + b(Y - y') \tag{7.14}$$

where b is an estimated slope, and x' and y' are simple inflation estimates. The estimated slope has the form

$$b = \hat{\rho}'_{xy} \frac{\widehat{SE}(x')}{\widehat{SE}(y')} \tag{7.15}$$

where $\hat{\rho}'_{xy}$ is the estimated correlation coefficient between the estimated totals x' and y'. For simple random sampling, this reduces to

$$b = \frac{\sum_{i=1}^{n}(x_i - \bar{x})(y_i - \bar{y})}{\sum_{i=1}^{n}(y_i - \bar{y})^2}. \tag{7.16}$$

An estimate of the variance of the regression estimate x''' valid for large sample sizes under simple random sampling is given by

$$\widehat{Var}(x''') = \widehat{Var}(x') \times (1 - \hat{\rho}^2_{xy}) \tag{7.17}$$

Under certain conditions, this estimate will have lower variance than the ratio estimate. The following example will illustrate the use of this estimate.

Illustrative Example. A city consists of four geographically defined community areas. In 1985, a survey of health care providers including hospitals and long term care facilities was performed in order to obtain an estimate of the number of persons diagnosed as having hepatitis related to intravenous drug use during that year. It was desired to obtain a similar estimate for 1990 for the city as a whole, but funds were available to examine this only for a sample of two of the four community areas. Let us assume that the true (unknown) population data are as follows:

Number of Persons Having Drug-Related Hepatitis

Community Area	1990 (X_i)	1985 (Y_i)
1	40	30
2	103	60
3	115	70
4	23	21
Total	281	181

If community areas 2 and 3 were chosen, the regression estimate x''' would be obtained as follows:

$$x' = 2 \times (103 + 115) = 436$$
$$y' = 2 \times (60 + 70) = 260$$
$$\bar{x} = (103 + 115)/2 = 109$$
$$\bar{y} = (60 + 70)/2 = 65$$
$$b = \frac{(103 - 109)(60 - 65) + (115 - 109)(70 - 65)}{(60 - 65)^2 + (70 - 65)^2} = 1.20$$
$$Y = 181$$

and

$$x''' = x' + b(Y - y') = 436 + 1.20(181 - 260) = 341.2.$$

The ratio estimate x'' is given by

$$x'' = (x'/y') \times Y = (436/260) \times 181 = 303.5.$$

The distributions of the regression estimate x''', the ratio estimate x'', and the simple inflation estimate x' over the six possible samples are shown below:

Sample	Simple Inflation Estimate x'	Ratio Estimate x''	Regression Estimate x'''
1, 2	286	287.59	288.10
1, 3	310	280.55	274.38
1, 4	126	223.59	275.22
2, 3	436	303.52	341.20
2, 4	252	281.56	290.97
3, 4	276	274.48	274.12

From the distributions shown above, the variances, biases, and mean square errors (MSEs) of the three estimates are:

Estimate	Variance	(Bias)^2	MSE
x'	8297	0	82.97
x''	619.83	33.47	648.30
x'''	556.33	93.43	649.76

One can see that in this example, both the regression estimate x''' and the ratio estimate x'' have mean square errors that are considerably lower than the MSE for the simple inflation estimate x'. In this instance, the regression estimated total x''', despite having the highest bias has an MSE approximately the same as that of the ratio estimated total. ☐

Both the ratio estimated total x'' and the regression estimated total x''' use the relationship between the variable of interest $\mathscr{X}$ and an ancillary variable $\mathscr{Y}$ to obtain a more accurate estimate of the true total X. The regression estimated total is, in fact, a generalization of the ratio estimated total and reduces to it when the regression coefficient b is equal to x'/y'.

7.9 RATIO ESTIMATION IN STRATIFIED RANDOM SAMPLING

There are two methods for estimating ratios that are generally used when the sampling design is stratified random sampling, namely the *combined ratio estimate*, r_{strc}, and the *separate ratio estimate*, r_{strs}. These are given below.

COMBINED RATIO ESTIMATE, r_{strc}

$$r_{\text{strc}} = \frac{\bar{x}_{\text{str}}}{\bar{y}_{\text{str}}} \qquad (7.18)$$

where $\bar{x}_{\text{str}}$ and $\bar{y}_{\text{str}}$ are estimated means appropriate for stratified random sampling as given in Chapter 6. Its variance is approximated by

$$\text{Var}(r_{\text{strc}}) \approx \left(\frac{1}{N^2 \bar{Y}^2}\right) \sum_{h=1}^{L} \frac{N_h^2(N_h - n_h)}{n_h(N_h - 1)} \sigma_{hz}^2 \qquad (7.19)$$

where

$$\sigma_{hz}^2 = \sigma_{hx}^2 + R^2 \sigma_{hy}^2 - 2R\rho_{hxy}\sigma_{hx}\sigma_{hy}$$

and σ_{hx}^2, σ_{hy}^2 are within stratum variances of $\mathcal{X}$ and $\mathcal{Y}$, and ρ_{hxy} is the correlation coefficient between $\mathcal{X}$ and $\mathcal{Y}$.

SEPARATE RATIO ESTIMATE, r_{strs}

$$r_{strs} = \frac{\sum_{h=1}^{L} x_h''}{Y} \tag{7.20}$$

where

$$x_h'' = Y_h \times \frac{\bar{x}_h}{\bar{y}_h}$$

$\bar{x}_h$ and $\bar{y}_h$; $h = 1, \ldots, L$, are estimated stratum specific means,

Y_h; $h = 1, \ldots, L$, are known stratum specific totals for $\mathcal{Y}$

and

$$Y = \sum_{h=1}^{L} Y_h$$

Its approximate variance is

$$\text{Var}(r_{strs}) \approx \left(\frac{1}{Y^2}\right) \sum_{h=1}^{L} \text{Var}(x_h'') \tag{7.21}$$

where $\text{Var}(x_h'')$ for $h = 1, \ldots, L$ is the variance of the ratio estimated total within stratum h as discussed in Section 7.2.

The separate ratio estimate, r_{strs} requires knowledge of the stratum totals Y_h in order to be used. Conditions where one of these is preferable to the other are complex and are discussed in some detail by Hansen et al. [1] and by Cochran [2]. In general, when the within-stratum ratios, R_h, are not too diverse, little is gained by using the separate ratio estimate. Estimates of the variances of both the combined and separate ratio estimates can be constructed by substituting the appropriate sample statistics for the parameters shown in relations (7.19) and (7.21).

Illustrative Example. A large university gives employees the choice of joining one of two health maintenance organizations (HMOs) as part of their employee benefit plan. In order to determine the cost to the university per patient encounter, a stratified random sample was taken of 200 persons within each of the two HMOs and the following data were obtained:

HMO	N_h	n_h	$\bar{x}_h$	$\hat{\sigma}_{hx}$	$\bar{y}_h$	$\hat{\sigma}_{hy}$	$\hat{\rho}_{hxy}$	Y_h
1	1295	200	$1,346	$564	3.2	0.9	0.69	690
2	2310	200	$785	$345	2.5	0.6	0.65	472

where

N_h = number of employees subscribing to HMO h ($h = 1, 2$)
n_h = number of employees sampled in HMO h ($h = 1, 2$)
$\bar{x}_h$ = estimated mean annual cost per person in HMO h ($h = 1, 2$)
$\hat{\sigma}_{hx}$ = estimated standard deviation of the distribution of mean annual cost per person in HMO h ($h = 1, 2$)
$\bar{y}_h$ = estimated annual number of visits per person in HMO h ($h = 1, 2$)
$\hat{\sigma}_{hy}$ = estimated standard deviation of the distribution of annual number of visits per person in HMO h ($h = 1, 2$)
$\hat{\rho}_{hxy}$ = estimated correlation between annual costs per person and annual visits per person in HMO h ($h = 1, 2$)
Y_h = total annual visits among all persons in HMO h ($h = 1, 2$)

The separate ratio estimate r_{strs} is calculated as follows:

$$r_{strs} = \left(\frac{1}{1162}\right)\left(\frac{1346}{3.2} \times 690 + \frac{785}{2.5} \times 472\right) = 377.31.$$

From relations (7.12) and (7.21), its standard error is estimated by

$$\widehat{SE}(r_{strs}) = 5.72$$

The combined ratio estimate r_{strc} is given by

$$r_{strc} = \frac{\bar{x}_{str}}{\bar{y}_{str}} = \frac{986.5243}{2.751456} = 358.55$$

and from relation (7.19), its standard error is estimated by

$$\widehat{SE}(r_{strc}) = 14.92.$$

In this particular example, since the individual stratum ratios are diverse ($r_1 = 420.62$ and $r_2 = 314.00$), the separate ratio estimate is preferable to the combined ratio estimate, and this is reflected in the estimated standard errors of the two estimates. $\square$

7.10 SUMMARY

In this chapter we developed the basic concepts of ratio estimation, a technique often used to estimate population ratios as well as population totals. Ratio estimation can be used with any sampling plan, and when used to estimate population totals, it often produces estimates that have lower mean square errors than those produced by simple inflation estimates. Particular emphasis was given in this chapter to ratio estimation under simple random sampling. For this type of sampling, we discussed the sampling distributions of ratio estimates and presented methods for estimating standard errors, for determining sample sizes, and for constructing confidence intervals. Finally, we discussed the regression estimated total, which is similar to the ratio estimated total in that it uses ancillary information to produce a more accurate estimate of the population total.

EXERCISES

7.1 A sample survey is being planned in which it is desired to estimate the average ratio of medical expenses to family income in a large city containing 234,785 families. Based on data in the table accompanying Exercise 7.2, how many families would have to be sampled if it is desired to estimate with 95% certainty this parameter to within 5% of its true value?

7.2 The accompanying table, based on a simple random sample of 33 families from a community of 600 families, gives the family size, weekly net family income, and weekly cost of medical expenditures including pharmaceuticals. The community contains 2700 persons.

    a. Estimate and give a 95% confidence interval for the average weekly medical expenditure per family.

    b. Estimate and give a 95% confidence interval for the average weekly medical expenditure per person. Justify your method of estimation.

    c. Estimate and give a 95% confidence interval for the average proportion of family income spent on medical expenses.

    d. Estimate and give a 95% confidence interval for the total weekly medical expenses paid by the community.

    e. Estimate and give a 95% confidence interval for the average proportion of family income spent on medical expenses for families whose weekly net income is less than $400. Do the same for those whose weekly net income is greater than $400.

Family Number	Family Size	Weekly Net Income ($)	Weekly Medical Expenses ($)
1	2	372	28.60
2	3	372	41.60
3	3	522	45.40
4	5	390	61.00
5	4	348	82.40
6	7	552	56.40
7	2	528	48.40
8	4	574	60.00
9	2	498	48.40
10	5	372	88.80
11	3	378	26.80
12	6	372	39.60
13	4	360	58.80
14	4	450	54.20
15	2	540	44.20
16	5	450	75.40
17	3	414	45.20
18	4	498	72.00
19	2	510	21.20
20	4	438	55.40
21	2	396	51.90
22	5	348	46.60
23	3	462	79.60
24	4	414	33.60
25	7	390	75.60
26	3	462	69.60
27	3	414	57.40
28	6	570	126.00
29	2	462	39.10
30	2	414	43.20
31	6	414	36.40
32	4	402	40.20
33	2	378	41.40

7.3 For the city cited in Exercise 7.2, it is also desired to estimate with virtual certainty the total moneys spent on medical expenses to within 10% of its true value. How many families would have to be sampled if these specifications were to be met?

7.4 For the data in the table accompanying Exercise 7.2, obtain a regression estimate of the total weekly medical expenditures paid by the community. Give 95% confidence intervals for the true value of this parameter based on this regression estimate.

7.5 It is desired to estimate the total X of nurse practitioner hours spent in direct patient care in a large HMO during a given year. This is to be done by taking a simple random sample of patients, and determining for each visit during the year, the number of nurse practitioner hours spent during the visit. It is known that there are 3524 members of the HMO and that 8950 visits took place during that year. A small pilot sample of 10 patients yielded the following data:

Patient	Visits	Nurse Practitioner Hours
1	0	0
2	5	3
3	1	0
4	2	6
5	3	3
6	7	0
7	1	0
8	1	2
9	0	0
10	4	3

Based on these pilot data, would you recommend a simple inflation estimate or a ratio estimate as the estimation method for the sample survey? Document the reasons for your recommendation.

7.6 Based on the data in Exercise 7.5, how many patients would have to be sampled if a simple inflation estimate were to be used?

7.7 Based on the data in Exercise 7.5, how many patients would have to be sampled if a ratio estimate were to be used?

7.8 A sample survey is to be conducted in which it is desired to estimate the proportion of persons over 70 years of age who have evidence of a cognitive impairment. This is to be done by taking a sample of households and giving a simple test of cognitive functioning to all members of the household over 70 years of age. A pilot study of 25 households yielded an average of 1.2 persons over 70 years of age per household with standard deviation equal to .8 and an average of .24 persons over 70 years of age per household showing evidence of cognitive impairment with standard deviation equal to .76. It is known that there are 3058 households in the community and 2949 persons over 70 years of age. How many households should be sampled if it is desired to estimate with 95% confidence the proportion of persons over 70 who show evidence of cognitive impairment within 20% of its true value?

7.9 Show that for simple random sampling the correlation ρ'_{xy} between estimated totals x' and y' of characteristics $\mathcal{X}$ and $\mathcal{Y}$ is equal to ρ_{xy}, the correlation between $\mathcal{X}$ and $\mathcal{Y}$.

7.10 The following exercise was suggested by an article appearing in *Public Health Reports* [3]. A survey was taken to determine the incidence of HIV seroconversion among first-time blood donors at a blood center located in a large city. During a particular month, 180 first-time donors gave blood at the center. Of these, 175 were seronegative. A sample of 60 from the seronegative first-time donors was selected and given appointments to give blood again over the next 6 months. The following data were obtained from these persons.

Months Since First Blood Donation	No. of Persons	HIV Status	
		Positive	Negative
3	18	2	16
4	10	2	8
5	8	1	7
6	7	0	7
7	6	2	4
8	5	0	5
9	4	1	3
10	2	1	1

From these data, estimate the annual incidence of HIV seroconversion among first-time blood donors at this center. Give 95% confidence intervals for this incidence rate.

7.11 A large plant has 1000 workers. A simple random sample of 25 workers is taken to find the ratio of work-loss days to total days employed during the previous calendar year. The following data were obtained from the survey:

Total work-loss days among the 25 individuals sampled: 250
Total days employed among the 25 individuals sampled: 4375

   a. What is the estimated ratio of work-loss days to total days employed among workers in this plant?
   b. What further information would you need to estimate the standard error of this estimate?

    c. From the information given above, estimate the total work-loss days among the 1000 workers in the cohort.

    d. It so happens that the 1000 workers in the plant in aggregate had 140,000 employment days during the previous calendar year. Based on this information, what would you infer about the estimate of total work-loss days computed in part (c)? Give reasons for your response.

7.12 For the illustrative example in Section 7.3, suppose that the known number of hospitals in subdomain 1 is 50, and in subdomain 2 is 51.

    a. Determine the poststratified ratio estimate of the proportion of newborns discharged with the mother's hepatitis B surface antigen status documented on the newborn's record.

    b. Give reasons why this estimate is closer to the ordinary rate estimate than the poststratified estimate that was obtained in the illustrative example.

BIBLIOGRAPHY

The following texts contain more detailed discussions of ratio and regression estimation.

1. Hansen, M. H., Hurwitz, W. N., and Madow, W. G. *Sample Survey Methods and Theory*, Vols. 1 and 2, Wiley, New York, 1953.

2. Cochran, W. G., *Sampling Techniques*, 2nd ed, Wiley, New York, 1962.

The following article gives an example of the use of a ratio estimate in an HIV seroconversion survey.

3. Petersen, L. R., Dodd, R., and Dondero, T. J., Jr., Methodological approaches to surveillance of HIV infection among blood donors, *Public Health Reports* 105: 153, 1990.

The following three review articles present an overview of ratio and regression estimators along with a long list of references including "classic" articles.

4. Rao, P. S. R. S., Ratio and regression estimators. In *Handbook of Statistics*, Krishnaian, P. R. and Rao, C. R., Eds., Vol. 6, *Sampling*, Chap. 18, pp 449–468, Elsevier, Amsterdam and New York, 1988.

5. Rao, J. N. K., Ratio estimators. In *Encyclopedia of Statistical Sciences*, Kotz, S., and Johnson, N. L., Eds., Vol. 7, pp. 639–646, New York, Wiley, 1986.

6. Cumberland, W. G., Ratio and regression estimators. In *Encyclopedia of Biostatistics*, Armitage, P. and T., Colton, Ed., Wiley, Chichester, U.K., 1998.

CHAPTER 8

Cluster Sampling:
Introduction and Overview

The sampling techniques discussed in previous chapters all require sampling frames that list the individual enumeration units (or listing units). Sometimes, however, especially in sample surveys of human populations, it is not feasible—and perhaps not even possible—to compile sampling frames that list all enumeration units for the entire population. On the other hand, sampling frames can often be constructed that identify groups or *clusters* of enumeration units without listing explicitly the individual enumeration units. One can perform sampling from such frames by taking a sample of the clusters, obtaining a list of enumeration units only for those clusters that have been selected in the sample, and then selecting a sample of the enumeration units. These sample designs are known as *cluster samples* and are widely used in practice. In this chapter we introduce some basic concepts of cluster sampling, and in the following three chapters we will discuss some specific techniques of cluster sampling that are widely used.

To illustrate the process of cluster sampling and to contrast it with designs based on direct sampling of enumeration units, let us consider a simple example.

Illustrative Example. Suppose that we wish to select a sample of households in a medium-size city for purposes of investigating utilization of health services among residents of the city. If an up-to-date city directory that lists all households in the city is available, it can serve as a sampling frame from which the sample can be selected. However, if such a directory or some other list of households is not available, it would be very expensive in terms of person-hours to construct such a sampling frame.

It might be relatively easy, however, to construct a list of city blocks. For many cities, maps that identify and label each city block are available from the U.S. Bureau of the Census. This list of city blocks can serve as a sampling frame. Each city block can be considered as a cluster of households, and every household in the city would be associated with a particular block. The sample of households can be taken by first taking a sample of blocks and then, within each of the blocks selected in the sample, listing each household. From this resulting list of households the final sample of households can be drawn. Note that it is necessary to list only those households that are on the blocks selected in the sample of blocks.   □

8.1 WHAT IS CLUSTER SAMPLING?

The term *cluster*, when used in sample survey methodology, can be defined as any sampling unit with which one or more listing units can be associated. The unit can be geographic, temporal, or spatial in nature. Some examples of clusters that might occur in practice are shown in Table 8.1.

For purposes of further illustration let us consider the second example of a cluster shown in the table. If we wish to estimate the proportion of all hospitalized patients discharged dead in a particular state during a particular year, we might first list all counties in the state and take a sample of counties from this list. For each of the counties selected in the sample we might then list all hospitals in the county and select a sample of individual hospitals. Finally, for each hospital selected in the sample, we would obtain the total number of persons admitted during the year and the total discharged dead. From these data the proportion discharged dead can be estimated for the entire state.

For the last example of a cluster shown in Table 8.1, a list consisting of 52 calendar weeks can be compiled and a sample of weeks can be selected from this list. For each of the weeks selected in the sample, a sample of days can be selected, and on each sample day ozone measurements can be made.

The relationship between clusters and listing units is very similar to that between listing units and elementary units. A cluster has listing units associated with it in the same way that a listing unit has elementary units associated with it. As we shall see later, cluster sampling is a hierarchical kind of sampling in which the elementary units are often at least two steps removed from the original sampling of clusters.

Now that we have introduced the concept of clusters, we can define *cluster sampling* broadly as any sampling plan that uses a frame consisting of clusters of listing units. The above definition is broader than that used in some other texts in that it includes sampling that is done in more than one stage (i.e., *multistage sampling*). Some investigators confine the term *cluster sampling* to those sampling designs in which clusters are selected by some sampling plan and each enumeration unit within each cluster is then sampled. In this text, we refer to such designs as *single-stage cluster sampling*.

With this broader definition of cluster sampling in mind, we list below some important features of cluster sampling.

Table 8.1 Some Practical Examples of Clusters

Cluster	Listing Unit	Elementary Unit	Application
City block	Household	Person	Estimation of total persons in city having hypertension
County	Hospital	Patient	Estimation of the proportion discharged dead in a particular state
School	Classroom	Student	Estimation of mean scholastic achievement among students in a school district
Batch of syringes	Individual syringe	Individual syringe	Estimation of the proportion of all syringes having defects
File drawer	Individual file folder	Account	Estimation of accounts that are overdue
Page of text	Line of text	Word	Estimation of total number of words in a book
Week	Day	Day	Estimation of all days having maximum ozone level above some specified level

1. The process by which a sample of listing units is selected might be step-wise. For example, if city blocks are clusters and households are listing units, there might be two steps involved in selecting the sample of households. The first step might entail selecting a sample of blocks, and the second step might entail selecting a sample of households within each of the blocks selected at the first step. In sampling terminology these steps are called *stages*, and sampling plans are often characterized in terms of the number of stages involved. For example, a *single-stage cluster sample* is one in which the sampling is done in

only one step. That is, once the sample of clusters is selected, every listing unit within each of the selected clusters is included in the sample.

In many surveys covering large geographical areas, several stages of sampling are often involved. For example, an immunization survey of school children in a state might entail five stages. First, we take a sample of counties within the state. Second, we take a sample of townships or other minor civil divisions within each of the counties that were selected at the first stage. Third, we take a sample of school districts within each of the townships selected at the second stage. Fourth, we take a sample of schools within each of the school districts selected at the third stage. Fifth, we take a sample of classrooms within each of the schools selected at the fourth stage. And finally, we take every child within the classrooms selected at the fifth stage. In this example, the children are the elementary units and the classrooms are the listing units. There are five stages of sampling involving four types of clusters: counties, townships, school districts, and schools. In sample designs involving two or more stages, the clusters used at the first stage of sampling are generally referred to as *primary sampling units*, or in abbreviated form, as PSUs.

2. Clusters can be selected by a variety of sampling techniques. For example, we can select a sample of clusters by simple random sampling or by systematic sampling. We can group the clusters into strata and take a stratified random sample of clusters.

When clusters are selected by simple random sampling, the term *simple cluster sampling* is generally used to describe the sampling design. More specifically, the term *simple one-stage cluster sampling* is used to categorize sample designs in which there is one stage of sampling and the clusters are selected by simple random sampling. Similarly, *simple two-stage cluster sampling* is used to describe sampling designs in which the clusters are selected at the first stage by simple random sampling; the listing units are selected at the second stage independently within each sample cluster, also by simple random sampling; and the fraction of listing units chosen at the second stage is the same for each sample cluster. Simple one-stage cluster sampling is discussed in Chapter 9, and simple two-stage cluster sampling is discussed in Chapter 10.

Another type of cluster sampling often used in practice is called *sampling with probability proportional to size*, or PPS sampling. This type of sampling, which is discussed in Chapter 11, is one in which the clusters are not selected by simple random sampling.

3. More than one sampling frame might be involved in the process. To illustrate this situation, we refer back to the example above in which an immunization survey is taken by a five-step procedure. The sampling frame at the first stage is a list of all counties in the state. The sampling frame at the second stage is a list of townships or other minor civil divisions within each of the counties selected at the first stage. The sampling frame at the third stage is a list of all school districts located within those townships or minor civil divisions selected at the second stage. At the fourth stage of sampling the sampling frame is a list of schools within each of the school districts at the third stage. Finally, the sampling frame used at the fifth stage is a list of classrooms within each of the schools sampled at the fourth stage.

4. After the first stage of sampling, the sampling frame is compiled from only those clusters chosen in the sample. Once the sample clusters are selected at the first stage, the listing of second-stage sampling units is compiled only for the sample clusters. Likewise, if there are more than two stages of sampling, sampling units at any later stage are listed only for those sampling units selected at the previous stage. Since the listing of clusters or of listing units is often an expensive field operation, listing costs are often much lower for cluster sampling designs than for other designs.

8.2 WHY IS CLUSTER SAMPLING WIDELY USED?

The two most important reasons cluster sampling is so widely used in practice, especially in sample surveys of human populations and in sample surveys covering large geographic areas, are *feasibility* and *economy*.

Cluster sampling is often the only feasible method of sampling because the only sampling frames readily available for the target populations are lists of clusters. This is especially true for surveys of human populations for which the household serves as the listing unit. It is almost never feasible in terms of time and resources to compile a list of households for any sizeable population (e.g., the United States, a state, or even a city) for the sole purpose of conducting a survey. However, lists of blocks or other geographical units can be compiled relatively easily, and these can serve as the sampling frame.

Cluster sampling is often the most economical form of sampling. Not only are listing costs almost always lowest for cluster sampling, but also traveling costs are often lowest. For example, if a cluster is a geographical unit such as a census tract, then once households are selected within census tracts, the costs of traveling within the sample tracts from household to household are relatively low. Thus a cluster sample of households within a few sample census tracts involves considerably less travel than a simple random sample of the same number of households spread over many more census tracts.

Cluster sampling may be advantageous in surveys of institutions such as hospitals. It is often very expensive and time-consuming to enlist an institution into a study. For example, to obtain permission from a hospital administrator to take a sample of patient records from the hospital may entail a great deal of effort, some public relations expertise, and sometimes even a great deal of influence. Therefore, once access is gained into hospital records, it is often worthwhile to sample many records rather than just a few.

To illustrate further how cluster sampling can lower the costs of a sample survey, let us consider the following example.

Illustrative Example. Suppose that scattered throughout a particular county there are five housing developments for senior citizens, and each of these developments contains 20 apartments. Suppose that a sample of 10 apartments is to be selected for purposes of estimating the total number of senior citizens in these developments that have need for the services of a visiting nurse. Further, let us suppose that the households are the listing units and that the major field costs of the survey involve listing and interviewing tasks.

In order to list all the apartments in a housing development, let us suppose that a member of the field staff would have to travel to the development and jot down the names of families from mailboxes. Assume that it would take 0.5 h to travel to the development and 3 min to list each household, or $3 \times 20 = 60$ min to list all households in the development. We then assume that it would take 1.5 person-hours to list an entire development (1 h of listing plus 0.5 h of travel) and 7.5 h (1.5 h per development times 5 developments) to list all five developments.

Suppose that it takes 15 min (0.25 h) to interview each household selected in the sample. Then the interviewing costs in person-hours at a particular development is equal to 0.25 times the number of households selected in the development plus the cost of traveling to the development (0.5 person-hours per trip).

Let us now compare two sampling designs with respect to the interviewing and listing costs for a sample of 10 households. The first design is simple random sampling, and let us assume that households from four of the developments are chosen in the sample. The second design is a simple two-stage cluster sample of ten households, five households from each of two developments. The listing and interviewing costs for each design are shown in Table 8.2.

From the calculations in Table 8.2 we see that even for this small sample, the field costs involved in cluster sampling can be very much lower than the field

Table 8.2 Comparison of Costs for Two Sampling Designs

	Design	
Costs	Simple Random Sampling	Simple Two-Stage Cluster Sampling
Listing costs	1.5 per development × 5 developments = 7.5	1.5 per development × 2 developments = 3.0
Interviewing costs in person-hours	Travel to 4 developments + interviewing 10 households: $4 \times 0.5 + 10 \times 0.25 = 4.5$	Travel to 2 developments + interviewing 10 households: $2 \times 0.5 + 10 \times 0.25 = 3.5$
Total field costs in person-hours	12.0	6.5

costs of simple random sampling. The particular savings are in the listing and traveling costs.   □

8.3 A DISADVANTAGE OF CLUSTER SAMPLING: HIGH STANDARD ERRORS

Now that we have shown how economical cluster sampling can be and how feasible it often is, we must point out that the standard errors of estimates obtained from cluster sampling designs are often high compared with those obtained from samples of the same number of listing units chosen by other sampling designs. The reason for this situation is that listing units within the same cluster are often homogeneous with respect to many characteristics. For example, households on the same block are often quite similar with respect to socioeconomic status, ethnicity, and other variables. Because of homogeneity among listing units within the same cluster, selection of more than one household within the same cluster, as is done in cluster sampling, is in a sense redundant. The effect of this redundancy becomes evident in the high standard errors of estimates that are so often seen in cluster sampling.

If we were to choose between cluster sampling and some alternative design solely on the basis of cost or feasibility, cluster sampling would inevitably be the sampling design of choice. On the other hand, if we were to choose a design solely on the basis of reliability of estimates, then cluster sampling would never be the design of choice. However, because it is possible to take a larger sample for a fixed cost with cluster sampling, greater precision may be attained than is possible with other methods. Generally, in choosing between cluster sampling and alternatives, we use criteria that incorporate both reliability and cost. In fact, we generally choose the sampling design that gives the lowest possible standard error at a specified cost—or, conversely, the sampling design that yields, at the lowest cost, estimates having specified standard errors.

8.4 HOW CLUSTER SAMPLING IS TREATED IN THIS BOOK

Following the overview of cluster sampling given in this chapter, we develop specific cluster sampling designs in the next three chapters by going from very simple to very complex sampling designs. The simplest type of cluster sampling is *single-stage cluster sampling* where clusters are selected by simple random sampling, and this type of cluster sampling is discussed in the next chapter (Chapter 9). The following two chapters (Chapters 10 and 11) both deal with two-stage cluster sampling. In two-stage cluster sampling, estimates of population characteristics and estimates of the standard errors of those statistics that serve to estimate population characteristics are relatively easy to obtain if each cluster in the population has the same number of listing units. Two-stage cluster sampling in this situation is treated in Chapter 10. Two-stage cluster sampling at its most complex occurs when each cluster in the population does not have the same number of listing units. Unfortunately, this happens in many practical situations, and we feel that it should be covered in this book in spite of the fact that it entails the use of formulas that are more cumbersome than those that appear in the rest of this book. We develop this type of cluster sampling in Chapter 11. Over the past 25 years, considerable advances have been made in development of statistical methodology and software for estimating the standard errors of estimates from even very complex cluster sampling designs. As has been done in previous chapters, we will show how two currently available software packages, SUDAAN and STATA, can be used to estimate standard errors of estimated population characteristics under complex cluster sampling designs. In Chapter 12, we discuss more fully some of the more widely used statistical methods for obtaining estimates of these standard errors. Our treatment of cluster sampling is very similar to our treatment of other sampling designs. In particular, we devote discussion to how samples are taken, how estimates are obtained, the nature of the sampling distributions of these estimates, and the methods of estimating the standard errors of these estimates.

8.5   SUMMARY

In this chapter we presented an overview of cluster sampling. We introduced the concept of a cluster of enumeration or listing units, and we defined cluster sampling as any sampling design that uses a sampling frame consisting of clusters of listing units. Some examples of clusters were given and some characteristics of cluster sampling were discussed, such as its sequential stepwise nature and the fact that the listing units need to be listed only from sample clusters rather than from all clusters. We pointed out the advantages of cluster sampling (namely feasibility and economy) as well as its major disadvantage (namely the high standard errors of estimates). However, because of the potential for taking more observations for the same budget than is possible with other designs, it is often possible to reduce the standard errors to the point where cluster sampling is the method of choice.

EXERCISES

8.1   Given a sample of 100 elements, which of the following designs is likely to yield estimates having the highest standard errors?
   a. Systematic sampling
   b. Cluster sampling
   c. Simple random sampling
   d. Stratified random sampling

8.2 If one wished to sample this page for misspelled words, what would be a logical cluster?

8.3 If one wished to sample this entire book for misspelled words according to a three-stage cluster sampling design, what could serve as primary sampling units, as secondary sampling units, as listing units, and as elementary units?

BIBLIOGRAPHY

Cluster sampling is discussed in all of the texts on sampling referenced in previous chapters. References to specific methods and applications of cluster sampling are given in Chapters 9, 10, 11, and 14.

CHAPTER 9

Simple One-Stage Cluster Sampling

We begin our development of some of the most commonly used cluster sampling designs with a discussion of simple one-stage cluster sampling. As we mentioned in Chapter 8, *simple one-stage cluster sampling* is a sampling plan in which clusters are chosen by simple random sampling and, within each sample cluster, all listing units are selected.

Simple one-stage cluster sampling is frequently used in situations in which the cost of obtaining every listing unit within a cluster is no higher, or only slightly higher, than the cost of obtaining a sample of listing units. Let us consider, for example, a sample survey in which hospitals are clusters and patients hospitalized with a certain diagnosis are listing units. If the information needed for the survey can be obtained from computer printouts that summarize the experience of each patient, and if these are either already available or can be furnished readily by the hospital record librarian, it might be cheaper and more convenient to select every patient having the specified diagnosis than to select a sample of these patients. On the other hand, if the data needed from each patient must be extracted from information on the original hospital medical record for that patient (which is often a costly and time-consuming process), then it might be more economical to select a sample of these patients rather than to take all of them.

As we shall see later in this chapter, the estimation procedures associated with simple one-stage cluster sampling are virtually identical to those associated with simple random sampling if we consider the cluster itself to be the effective listing unit. We shall elaborate on this concept later on in this chapter. A disadvantage of this type of sampling, however, is that the sampling errors associated with estimates obtained from simple one-stage cluster sampling are generally much higher than those obtained from a simple random sample of the same number of listing units, especially when listing units within clusters are homogeneous with respect to the variable being measured. Suppose, for example, that we are attempting to estimate the proportion of all families below the poverty level in a community from a simple one-stage cluster sample in which city blocks are the clusters and households are the listing units. Since the households within any city block are likely to contain families of very similar income, the inclusion in the sample of every household on a selected block is a wasteful way of allocating the sample listing units and is likely to yield estimates having high sampling errors.

9.1 HOW TO TAKE A SIMPLE ONE-STAGE CLUSTER SAMPLE

We take a one-stage cluster sample by first listing all clusters in the population and then taking, in the usual manner, a simple random sample of clusters. Within each of the clusters selected in the sample, we then include all listing units.

For example, let us suppose that the total number of persons over 65 and the number of persons over 65 requiring the services of a visiting nurse are as given in Table 9.1 for the five housing developments discussed in Chapter 8. We will use these data to illustrate how cluster sampling is performed.

Suppose that we wish to take a simple one-stage cluster sample of two housing developments from the housing developments in Table 9.1. We would choose two random numbers between 1 and 5 and then interview every household in the two housing developments chosen in the sample. Suppose that the random numbers chosen were 2 and 5. Then all households in developments 2 and 5 would be interviewed and the relevant data would be collected.

9.2 ESTIMATION OF POPULATION CHARACTERISTICS

Once the sample of clusters is selected, the required data are collected from every listing unit within the chosen clusters. The forms used to collect these data would, of course, depend on the type of information needed and the manner in which the data are to be collected (e.g., mail, personal interview, telephone, extraction from records, etc.). Then the estimates of population characteristics are calculated from the data that have been collected.

Let us investigate the estimation procedures by considering an example.

Illustrative Example. Suppose that from the sample of two housing units discussed above, we wish to estimate the following population characteristics:

1. The total number of persons over 65 years of age in the five housing developments;
2. The total number of persons over 65 years of age requiring the services of a visiting nurse; and
3. The proportion of all persons over 65 years of age requiring the services of a visiting nurse;

Table 9.1 Number of Persons over 65 Years of Age and Number over 65 Years Needing Services of a Visiting Nurse for Five Housing Developments

House-hold	Development 1 No. of Persons over 65	Development 1 No. over 65 Needing Nurse	Development 2 No. of Persons over 65	Development 2 No. over 65 Needing Nurse	Development 3 No. of Persons over 65	Development 3 No. over 65 Needing Nurse	Development 4 No. of Persons over 65	Development 4 No. over 65 Needing Nurse	Development 5 No. of Persons over 65	Development 5 No. over 65 Needing Nurse
1	3	1	2	1	3	0	3	0	1	1
2	1	0	1	0	2	1	1	0	1	0
3	1	1	2	0	2	1	3	0	1	1
4	1	1	1	1	3	1	1	0	3	1
5	1	1	1	0	2	1	2	0	2	0
6	1	1	1	0	2	1	2	0	1	1
7	1	1	2	1	1	0	1	0	3	0
8	1	0	1	1	1	0	1	0	1	0
9	3	1	3	1	3	0	3	1	1	0
10	3	2	1	1	3	1	1	1	3	2
11	3	2	1	0	2	0	1	0	2	1
12	1	1	2	1	3	1	1	0	3	0
13	1	0	1	0	1	1	3	1	1	1
14	1	1	3	1	1	1	3	0	1	0
15	1	0	1	0	2	2	1	0	2	1
16	3	1	3	2	1	0	1	0	2	1
17	1	1	1	0	1	1	1	0	1	0
18	3	2	2	0	3	0	1	1	2	0
19	1	1	1	1	1	0	1	0	2	0
20	1	1	3	0	2	2	1	0	1	1
Total	32	19	33	11	39	14	32	4	34	12

237

4. The mean number of persons over 65 years of age per housing development

5. The proportion of all households having at least one individual over 65 years of age who requires the services of a visiting nurse

To obtain these estimates, the form shown in Figure 9.1 might be suitable for collecting the data by personal interview.

If housing developments 2 and 5 are those selected in the sample, then the form shown in Figure 9.1 illustrates data that may have been collected from household 10 in development 5 (sample development 2). Note that there are three individuals over 65 years of age in this household and that two of them require the services of a visiting nurse. There would be 20 such forms collected from this housing development and also from housing development 2 (sample development 1).

From these household forms summary information for each sample development is tabulated in a format similar to that shown in Table 9.2. We then obtain the desired estimates as follows from the summary data shown in the table.

To find the estimated total number of persons over 65 years of age, we first compute the average number of persons over 65 per sample cluster. Then the estimated total number of persons over 65 years of age in the population is obtained by multiplying this cluster average by the total number of clusters in the population. That is,

———

Housing Development: *Kingswood Manor Apartments*
Sample Development No.: 2
Household Number: 10
Name of Household Head: *Jones, John*
List All Persons in Household Beginning With the Respondent:
  Does this person require the services of a visiting nurse? (Answer yes or no only for patients over 65 years of age)

Person	Age	Yes	No
1. Lydia Jones	67		×
2. John Jones	68	×	
3. Samantha Jones	75	×	
4. Edgar Jones	60		
5.			
6.			
7.			

Figure 9.1 Form for collecting the data from sample households in housing developments.

$$\text{Cluster average} = \frac{67}{2} = 33.5$$

Estimated population total of persons over 65 = $5 \times 33.5 = 167.5$

Alternately, the sample total may be inflated by the ratio of total clusters in the population to total sample clusters (i.e., 5/2). Then the estimated population total of persons over 65 is $(5/2) \times 67 = 167.5$.

To find the estimated total number of persons over 65 years needing the services of a visiting nurse, we inflate the sample total by 5/2, as we did above:

Estimated total over 65 needing nurse = $(5/2) \times 23 = 57.5$

To find the proportion of all persons over 65 years of age requiring the services of a visiting nurse, we take the ratio of the appropriate sample totals:

$$\begin{array}{c}\text{Estimated proportion of all} \\ \text{persons over 65 needing nurse}\end{array} = 23/67 = .3433$$

To find the estimated mean number of persons over 65 years of age per housing development, we divide the total number of persons over 65 years in the sample by the total number of housing developments in the sample:

Estimated mean number over 65 per development = $67/2 = 33.5$

To find the estimated proportion of all households having at least one individual over 65 years who requires the services of a visiting nurse, we divide the total number of households in the sample having at least one individual over 65 who requires the services of a visiting nurse by the number of households in the sample:

Table 9.2 Summary Data for the Two Clusters Selected in the Sample

Sample Development	No. of Households	No. of Persons over 65	No. of Households with at least One Person over 65 Needing Nurse	No. over 65 Needing Nurse
1. Housing development 2	20	33	10	11
2. Housing development 5	20	34	11	12
Total	40	67	21	23

Estimated proportion of households with 1 or
more over 65 needing nurse $= 21/40 = .525$

The estimates shown above include estimated population totals, ratios, and means.   □

In cluster sampling the mean level of a characteristic $\mathscr{X}$ per cluster is generally denoted by $\bar{X}$, as opposed to $\bar{\bar{X}}$, which is used to denote the mean level of $\mathscr{X}$ per listing unit. To generalize, let us use the notation shown in Box 9.1.

Using the notation of Box 9.1, we list in Box 9.2 the formulas used to compute estimated population characteristics and estimated standard errors of these estimated population characteristics. Note that the subscript "clu" is used to indicate that the estimate is obtained by cluster sampling. For example, x'_{clu} indicates an estimated population total obtained by cluster sampling.

Examining the expressions for estimates given in Box 9.2, we see their close resemblance to the expressions for equivalent estimates under simple random sampling developed in Chapter 3. Since in simple one-stage cluster sampling every listing unit within every sample cluster is selected in the sample, the sampling variability among listing units within clusters is not a factor in determining the sampling variability of estimates under this sampling plan. Effectively, then, cluster totals are the building blocks on which the estimation formulas in Box 9.2 are built. Use of these formulas for the data in Table 9.2 is illustrated next.

Illustrative Example.   Let us consider the data in Table 9.2. Then we have

$m = 2$ housing developments in sample

$M = 5$ housing developments in population

$N = 100$ households in population

$N_1 = N_2 = 20$ households per development $= \bar{N}$

First we consider the estimation of the mean number of persons over 65 years of age per housing development requiring the services of a visiting nurse. The computations for $\bar{x}_{\text{clu}}$ are

$$x_1 = 11 \qquad x_2 = 12 \qquad x = 23$$
$$\bar{x}_{\text{clu}} = \frac{23}{2} = 11.5$$

BOX 9.1   NOTATION USED IN SIMPLE ONE-STAGE CLUSTER SAMPLING

General Notation

$M =$ number clusters in the population

$m =$ number of clusters in the sample

$x_{ij} =$ level of characteristic $\mathcal{X}$ for sample listing unit j in sample cluster i

$y_{ij} =$ level of characteristic $\mathcal{Y}$ for sample listing unit j in sample cluster i

$N_i =$ number of listing units in sample cluster i

$x_i = \sum_{j=1}^{N_i} x_{ij} =$ aggregate of characteristic $\mathcal{X}$ for the ith sample cluster

$y_i = \sum_{j=1}^{N_i} y_{ij} =$ aggregate of characteristic $\mathcal{Y}$ for the ith sample cluster

$x = \sum_{i=1}^{m} x_i =$ sample total for characteristic $\mathcal{X}$

$y = \sum_{i=1}^{m} y_i =$ sample total for characteristic $\mathcal{Y}$

$N =$ total number of listing units in population

$\bar{N} = N/M =$ average number of listing units per cluster in the population

Population Characteristics

$X_{ij} =$ level of characteristic $\mathcal{X}$ for population listing unit j in population cluster i

$Y_{ij} =$ level of characteristic $\mathcal{Y}$ for population listing unit j in population cluster i

$X_i = \sum_{j=1}^{N_i} X_{ij} =$ aggregate of characteristic $\mathcal{X}$ for ith population cluster

$Y_i = \sum_{j=1}^{N_i} Y_{ij} =$ aggregate of characteristic $\mathcal{Y}$ for ith population cluster

$X = \sum_{i=1}^{M} \sum_{j=1}^{N_i} X_{ij} =$ population total for characteristic $\mathcal{X}$

$\bar{X} = X/M =$ mean level of $\mathcal{X}$ per cluster

$Y = \sum_{i=1}^{M} \sum_{j=1}^{N_1} Y_{ij} =$ population total for characteristic $\mathcal{Y}$

$\bar{Y} = Y/M =$ mean level of $\mathcal{Y}$ per cluster

$\bar{\bar{X}} = X/N =$ mean level of $\mathcal{X}$ per listing unit

$\bar{\bar{Y}} = Y/N =$ mean level of $\mathcal{Y}$ per listing unit

$\sigma_{1x}^2 = \sum_{i=1}^{M}(X_i - \bar{X})^2/M =$ variance of distribution of $\mathcal{X}$ over all clusters

$\sigma_{1y}^2 = \sum_{i=1}^{M}(Y_i - \bar{Y})^2/M =$ variance of distribution of $\mathcal{Y}$ over all clusters

$\sigma_{1xy} = \sum_{i=1}^{M}(X_i - \bar{X})(Y_i - \bar{Y})/M =$ covariance of cluster totals X_i and Y_i over all clusters

BOX 9.2   ESTIMATED POPULATION CHARACTERISTICS AND ESTIMATED STANDARD ERRORS FOR SIMPLE ONE-STAGE CLUSTER SAMPLING

Total, X

$$x'_{clu} = \left(\frac{M}{m}\right)x \qquad \widehat{SE}(x'_{clu}) = \left(\frac{M}{\sqrt{m}}\right)\hat{\sigma}_{1x}\sqrt{\frac{M-m}{M-1}}$$

Mean Per Cluster, $\bar{X}$

$$\bar{x}_{clu} = \frac{x}{m} \qquad \widehat{SE}(\bar{x}_{clu}) = \left(\frac{1}{\sqrt{m}}\right)\hat{\sigma}_{1x}\sqrt{\frac{M-m}{M-1}}$$

Mean Per Listing Unit, $\bar{\bar{X}}$

$$\bar{\bar{x}}_{clu} = \frac{x}{m\bar{N}} \qquad \widehat{SE}(\bar{\bar{x}}_{clu}) = \left(\frac{1}{\sqrt{m}\bar{N}}\right)\hat{\sigma}_{1x}\sqrt{\frac{M-m}{M-1}}$$

Ratio, $R = X/Y$

$$r_{clu} = \frac{x}{y}$$

$$\widehat{SE}(r_{clu}) = r_{clu}\left\{\frac{[\widehat{SE}(\bar{x}_{clu})]^2}{\bar{x}_{clu}^2} + \frac{[\widehat{SE}(\bar{y}_{clu})]^2}{\bar{y}_{clu}^2} - \frac{2}{m} \times \left(\frac{M-m}{M}\right) \times \left(\frac{1}{\bar{x}_{clu}\bar{y}_{clu}}\right)\right.$$

$$\left. \times \left[\frac{\sum_{i=1}^{m}(x_i - \bar{x}_{clu})(y_i - \bar{y}_{clu})}{m-1}\right]\right\}^{1/2}$$

where $\hat{\sigma}_{1x}$ is defined as

$$\hat{\sigma}_{1x} = \left[\frac{\sum_{i=1}^{m}(x_i - \bar{x}_{clu})^2}{m-1}\right]^{1/2}\sqrt{\frac{M-1}{M}}$$

and $\hat{\sigma}_{1y}$ is defined in a similar fashion. All other notation is defined in Box 9.1.

The computations for $\widehat{SE}(\bar{x}_{clu})$ are

$$\frac{\sum_{i=1}^{m}(x_i - \bar{x}_{clu})^2}{m-1} = \frac{(11 - 11.5)^2 + (12 - 11.5)^2}{(2-1)} = .5$$

$$\hat{\sigma}_{1x} = \left[\frac{\sum_{i=1}^{m}(x_i - \bar{x}_{clu})^2}{m-1}\right]^{1/2}\sqrt{\frac{M-1}{M}}$$

$$= (.5)^{1/2}\left(\frac{5-1}{5}\right)^{1/2} = .6325$$

$$\widehat{SE}(\bar{x}_{clu}) = \left(\frac{1}{\sqrt{m}}\right)\hat{\sigma}_{1x}\sqrt{\frac{M-m}{M-1}}$$

$$= \left(\frac{1}{\sqrt{2}}\right) \times .6325\sqrt{\frac{5-2}{5-1}} = .3873$$

A 95% confidence interval for $\bar{X}$ is

$$\bar{x}_{clu} - 1.96 \times \widehat{SE}(\bar{x}_{clu}) \leqslant \bar{X} \leqslant \bar{x}_{clu} + 1.96 \times \widehat{SE}(\bar{x}_{clu})$$
$$11.5 - 1.96 \times .3873 \leqslant \bar{X} \leqslant 11.5 + 1.96 \times .3873$$
$$10.74 \leqslant \bar{X} \leqslant 12.26$$

Now we consider the estimation of the total number of persons over 65 years of age requiring the services of a visiting nurse. The computation of x'_{clu} is

$$x'_{clu} = \left(\frac{M}{m}\right)x = \left(\frac{5}{2}\right) \times 23 = 57.5$$

The computation of $\widehat{SE}(x'_{clu})$ is

$$\widehat{SE}(x'_{clu}) = \left(\frac{M}{\sqrt{m}}\right)\hat{\sigma}_{1x}\sqrt{\frac{M-m}{M-1}} = \left(\frac{5}{\sqrt{2}}\right) \times .6325\sqrt{\frac{5-2}{5-1}} = 1.94$$

A 95% confidence interval for X is

$$x'_{clu} - 1.96 \times \widehat{SE}(x'_{clu}) \leqslant X \leqslant x'_{clu} + 1.96 \times \widehat{SE}(x'_{clu})$$
$$57.5 - 1.96 \times 1.94 \leqslant X \leqslant 57.5 + 1.96 \times 1.94$$
$$53.7 \leqslant X \leqslant 61.3$$

Now we consider the estimation of the mean number of persons over 65 years of age requiring the services of a visiting nurse per household. The computation of $\bar{\bar{x}}_{clu}$ is

$$\bar{\bar{x}}_{\text{clu}} = \frac{x}{m\bar{N}} = \frac{23}{2 \times 20} = .5750$$

The computation of $\widehat{\text{SE}}(\bar{\bar{x}}_{\text{clu}})$ is

$$\widehat{\text{SE}}(\bar{\bar{x}}_{\text{clu}}) = \left(\frac{1}{\sqrt{m\bar{N}}}\right)\hat{\sigma}_{1x}\sqrt{\frac{M-m}{M-1}}$$

$$= \left(\frac{1}{\sqrt{2(20)}}\right) \times .6325 \times \sqrt{\frac{5-2}{5-1}} = .0194$$

A 95% confidence interval for $\bar{\bar{X}}$ is

$$\bar{\bar{x}}_{\text{clu}} - 1.96 \times \widehat{\text{SE}}(\bar{\bar{x}}_{\text{clu}}) \leqslant \bar{\bar{X}} \leqslant \bar{\bar{x}}_{\text{clu}} + 1.96 \times \widehat{\text{SE}}(\bar{\bar{x}}_{\text{clu}})$$

$$.5750 - 1.96 \times .0194 \leqslant \bar{\bar{X}} \leqslant .5750 + 1.96 \times .0194$$

$$.5370 \leqslant \bar{\bar{X}} \leqslant .6130$$

Now we consider the estimation of the mean number of persons over 65 years of age per housing development. The computations for $\bar{y}_{\text{clu}}$ are

$$y_1 = 33 \qquad y_2 = 34 \qquad y = 67$$

$$\bar{y}_{\text{clu}} = \frac{y}{m} = \frac{67}{2} = 33.5$$

The computations for $\widehat{\text{SE}}(\bar{y}_{\text{clu}})$ are

$$\frac{\sum_{i=1}^{m}(y_i - \bar{y}_{\text{clu}})^2}{m-1} = \frac{(33 - 33.5)^2 + (34 - 33.5)^2}{2-1} = .5$$

$$\hat{\sigma}_{1y} = \left(\frac{\sum_{i=1}^{m}(y_i - \bar{y}_{\text{clu}})^2}{m-1}\right)^{1/2} \times \sqrt{\frac{M-1}{M}}$$

$$= (.5)^{1/2} \times \sqrt{\frac{5-1}{5}} = .6325$$

$$\widehat{\text{SE}}(\bar{y}_{\text{clu}}) = \frac{\hat{\sigma}_{1y}}{\sqrt{m}} \times \sqrt{\frac{M-m}{M-1}} = \frac{.6325}{\sqrt{2}} \times \sqrt{\frac{5-2}{5-1}} = .3873$$

A 95% confidence interval for $\bar{Y}$ is

$$\bar{y}_{\text{clu}} - 1.96 \times \widehat{\text{SE}}(\bar{y}_{\text{clu}}) \leqslant \bar{Y} \leqslant \bar{y}_{\text{clu}} + 1.96 \times \widehat{\text{SE}}(\bar{y}_{\text{clu}})$$

$$33.5 - 1.96 \times .3873 \leqslant \bar{Y} \leqslant 33.5 + 1.96 \times .3873$$

$$32.7 \leqslant \bar{Y} \leqslant 34.3$$

Finally, we consider the estimation of the proportion of persons over 65 years of age requiring the services of a visiting nurse. The computation of r_{clu} is

$$r_{clu} = \frac{x}{y} = \frac{23}{67} = .3433$$

The computations for $\widehat{SE}(r_{clu})$ are

$$\frac{\sum_{i=1}^{m}(x_i - \bar{x}_{clu})(y_i - \bar{y}_{clu})}{m-1} = \frac{(11 - 11.5)(33 - 33.5) + (12 - 11.5)(34 - 33.5)}{2-1} = .5$$

$$\widehat{SE}(r_{clu}) = r_{clu} \times \left\{ \frac{[\widehat{SE}(\bar{x}_{clu})]^2}{\bar{x}_{clu}^2} + \frac{[\widehat{SE}(\bar{y}_{clu})]^2}{\bar{y}_{clu}^2} \right.$$

$$- \frac{2}{m} \times \left(\frac{M-m}{M}\right) \times \left(\frac{1}{\bar{x}_{clu}\bar{y}_{clu}}\right)$$

$$\times \left. \left[\frac{\sum_{i=1}^{m}(x_i - \bar{x}_{clu})(y_i - \bar{y}_{clu})}{m-1}\right]\right\}^{1/2}$$

$$= .3433 \times \left\{ \frac{.3873^2}{11.5^2} + \frac{.3873^2}{33.5^2} - \frac{2}{2} \times \frac{5-2}{5} \right.$$

$$\left. \times \frac{1}{11.5 \times 33.5} \times .5 \right\}^{1/2}$$

$$= .0076$$

A 95% confidence interval for R is

$$r_{clu} - 1.96 \times \widehat{SE}(r_{clu}) \leqslant R \leqslant r_{clu} + 1.96 \times \widehat{SE}(r_{clu})$$
$$.3433 - 1.96 \times .0076 \leqslant R \leqslant .3433 + 1.96 \times .0076$$
$$.3284 \leqslant R \leqslant .3582 \qquad \qquad \square$$

USE OF STATISTICAL SOFTWARE FOR ESTIMATION. We will illustrate how estimation can be performed for the previous illustrative example by use of both STATA and SUDAAN, and will first illustrate use of STATA. The STATA data file, TAB9_1A.DTA, consists of 40 records (20 households in each of 2 housing developments) as shown below:

devlpmnt	hh	wt1	M	Nhh	nge65	nvstnrs	hhneedvn	nge65dv
2	1	2.5	5	20	2	1	1	40
2	2	2.5	5	20	1	0	0	20
2	3	2.5	5	20	2	0	0	40
2	4	2.5	5	20	1	1	1	20
2	5	2.5	5	20	1	0	0	20
2	6	2.5	5	20	1	0	0	20
2	7	2.5	5	20	2	1	1	40
2	8	2.5	5	20	1	1	1	20
2	9	2.5	5	20	3	1	1	60
2	10	2.5	5	20	1	1	1	20
2	11	2.5	5	20	1	0	0	20
2	12	2.5	5	20	2	1	1	40
2	13	2.5	5	20	1	0	0	20
2	14	2.5	5	20	3	1	1	60
2	15	2.5	5	20	1	0	0	20
2	16	2.5	5	20	3	2	1	60
2	17	2.5	5	20	1	0	0	20
2	18	2.5	5	20	2	0	0	40
2	19	2.5	5	20	1	1	1	20
2	20	2.5	5	20	3	0	0	60
5	1	2.5	5	20	1	1	1	20
5	2	2.5	5	20	1	0	0	20
5	3	2.5	5	20	1	1	1	20
5	4	2.5	5	20	3	1	1	60
5	5	2.5	5	20	2	0	0	40
5	6	2.5	5	20	1	1	1	20
5	7	2.5	5	20	3	0	0	60
5	8	2.5	5	20	1	0	0	20
5	9	2.5	5	20	1	0	0	20
5	10	2.5	5	20	3	2	1	60
5	11	2.5	5	20	2	1	1	40
5	12	2.5	5	20	3	0	0	60
5	13	2.5	5	20	1	1	1	20
5	14	2.5	5	20	1	0	0	20
5	15	2.5	5	20	2	1	1	40
5	16	2.5	5	20	2	1	1	40
5	17	2.5	5	20	1	0	0	20
5	18	2.5	5	20	2	0	0	40
5	19	2.5	5	20	2	1	1	40
5	20	2.5	5	20	1	1	1	20

Note that each record corresponds to a particular sample household, and that the housing development in which the household resides is indicated on each record, as is the sampling weight.

Each record contains the following variables:

1. *devlpmnt*—the housing development (2 selected from the 5 in the population)
2. *hh*—the household number within the development
3. *wt1*—the sampling weight ($= M/m = 5/2 = 2.5$ for all households)
4. *M*—the number of housing developments in the population ($= 5$)
5. *Nhh*—the number of households within each housing development ($= 20$)
6. *nge65*—the number of persons over 65 in each household
7. *nvstnrs*—the number of persons over 65 in each household who require the services of a visiting nurse
8. *hhneedvn*—dummy variable set equal to "1" if the household has at least 1 person over 65 years of age who requires the services of a visiting nurse; "0" if otherwise
9. *nge65dv*—This equals *nge65**20, which is a transformed variable used to estimate the mean number of persons 65 years old or older per development

The following set of STATA commands can be used to perform the required estimation.

```
use "a:\tab9_la.dta",clear
.svyset pweight wt1
.svyset fpc M
.svyset psu devlpmnt
.svytotal nvstnrs nge65
.svymean nvstnrs hhneedvn
.svyratio nvstnrs nge65
.svymean nge65dv
```

These commands generate the following output (which we annotate as regular text).

```
use "a:\tab9_1a.dta", clear
. svyset pweight wt1
. svyset fpc M
. svyset psu devlpmnt
```

The above three commands set the required sample design parameters. The sampling weight is denoted by the variable, *wt1*, and is equal to 2.5 for each household. The finite population correction (fpc) is computed on the basis of the number of clusters ($M = 5$) in the population. The primary sampling units (or clusters) are identified in the variable *devlpmnt*.

```
svytotal nvstnrs nge65
```

The above command estimates the total number of persons 65 years of age or older in the 5 developments and the total needing the services of a visiting nurse. The output for this is shown immediately below.

Survey total estimation

pweight:	wt1		Number of obs	=	40
Strata:	< one >		Number of strata	=	1
PSU:	devlpmnt		Number of PSUs	=	2
FPC:	M		Population size	=	100

Total	Estimate	Std. Err.	[95% Conf.	Interval]	Deff
nvstnrs	57.5	1.936492	32.89454	82.10546	.0707804
nge65	167.5	1.936492	142.8945	192.1055	.0393542

Finite population correction (FPC) assumes simple random sampling without replacement of PSUs within each stratum with no subsampling within PSUs.

Note that for the above estimation and all others, the estimates and standard errors are identical to those derived from the appropriate formulas shown in the body of the text. The confidence intervals, however, are wider than those shown in the text because those in STATA are based on Student's t-distribution, whereas those in the text are based on the normal distribution. Since, in this illustrative example, there are only 2 sample clusters and hence 1 degree of freedom, the differences with respect to the width of the confidence interval are dramatic.

```
svymean nvstnrs hhneedvn
```

The above command results in estimation of the total number of persons 65 years or older in the 5 developments who require the services of a visiting nurse; also the total number of households in the 5 developments having 1 or more persons 65 years of age or older who require the services of a visiting nurse. The resulting output is shown below:

Survey mean estimation

pweight:	wt1			Number of obts	=	40
Strata:	< one >			Number of strata	=	1
PSU:	devlpmnt			Number of PSUs	=	2
FPC:	M			Population size	=	100

Mean	Estimate	Std. Err.	[95% Conf.	Interval]	Deff
nvstnrs	.575	.0193649	.3289454	.8210546	.0707804
hhneedvn	.525	.0193649	.2789454	.7710546	.0977444

Finite population correction (FPC) assumes simple random sampling without replacement of PSUs within each stratum with no subsampling within PSUs

svyratio nvstnrs nge65

The above command results in computation of a ratio estimator which estimates the proportion of persons 65 years of age or older who require the services of a visiting nurse. Output is shown below:

Survey ratio estimation

pweight:	wt1			Number of obts	=	40
Strata:	< one >			Number of strata	=	1
PSU:	devlpmnt			Number of PSUs	=	2
FPC:	M			Population size	=	100

Ratio	Estimate	Std. Err.	[95% Conf.	Interval]	Deff
nvstnrs/nge65	.3432836	.0075924	.2468131	.4397541	.0325067

Finite population correction (FPC) assumes simple random sampling without replacement of PSUs within each stratum with no subsampling within PSUs

svymean nge65dv

The above command results in estimation of the mean number of individuals 65 years of age or older per housing development. Output is below:

Survey mean estimation

pweight:	wt1			Number of obts	=	40
Strata:	< one >			Number of strata	=	1
PSU:	devlpmnt			Number of PSUs	=	2
FPC:	M			Population size	=	100

Mean	Estimate	Std. Err.	[95% Conf.	Interval]	Deff
nge65dv	33.5	.3872983	28.57891	38.42109	.0393542

Finite population correction (FPC) assumes simple random sampling without replacement of PSUs within each stratum with no subsampling within PSUs.
.exit, clear

We will now show how SUDAAN can provide estimates for the SAS data set, *tab9_lc.SSd*, which has the same data and variables as the STATA data set *tab9_1c.dta* used in the above demonstration.

The following set of commands will provide estimates from SUDAAN for the total number of persons 65 years of age and older, the total number of persons 65 and older requiring the services of a visiting nurse, the total number of households having one or more persons requiring the services of a visiting nurse, and the proportion of all persons 65 and older requiring the services of a visiting nurse.

```
proc descript data = tab9_lc filetype = sas design = WOR means totals;
nest _one_ devlpmnt;
totcnt M _zero_;
weight wt1;
var nge65 nvstnrs hhneedvn;
setenv colwidth = 13 decwidth = 5;
proc ratio data = tab9_lc filetype = sas design = WOR;
nest _one_ devlpmnt;
totcnt M _zero_;
weight wt1
numer nvstnrs;
denom nge65;
setenv colwidth = 13 decwidth = 5;
```

These commands will produce the output shown overleaf.

Illustrative Example. The following example is introduced here as another example of ratio estimation under simple one-stage cluster sampling. It will also be used to illustrate other concepts in later sections of this chapter. We will perform computations using the ratio estimation procedure in SUDAAN.

A particular region contains 26 district courts, and it is desired to conduct a sample survey of these courts for purposes of determining certain information on individuals placed on probation with recommendation that they receive treatment for substance abuse. A single-stage cluster sample is taken of 10 of these district courts and, within each selected court, records were identified of all cases heard during the previous year that resulted in probation with recommendation of substance abuse treatment. For every case identified, information is obtained on whether the individual actually received substance abuse treatment. The most important objective is to estimate the proportion of those individuals who actually received the recommended treatment.

Prior to the survey, there were no lists available which identified those individuals eligible for the study. Thus, for each district court sampled, eligible cases had to be identified by screening the records of all court cases resulting in probation during the study period. The following data were obtained from the sample of 10 district courts.

```
1  PROC DESCRIPT DATA = TAB9_1C FILETYPE = SAS DESIGN = WOR MEANS
   TOTALS;
2  NEST _ONE_ DEVLPMNT;
3  TOTCNT M _ZERO_;
4  WEIGHT WT1;
5  VAR NGE65 NVSTNRS HHNEEDVN;
6  SETENV COLWIDTH = 13 DECWIDTH = 5;
```

Number of observations read   :   40   Weighted count :   100
Number of observations skipped :   0
(WEIGHT variable nonpositive)
Denominator degrees of freedom :   1

Table : 1

by: Variable, One.

Variable		One 1
NGE65	Sample Size Weighted Size Total SE Total Mean SE Mean	40.00000 100.00000 167.50000 1.93649 1.67500 0.01936
NVSTNRS	Sample Size Weighted Size Total SE Total Mean SE Mean	40.00000 100.00000 57.50000 1.93649 0.57500 0.01936
HHNEEDVN	Sample Size Weighted Size Total SE Total Mean SE Mean	40.00000 100.00000 52.50000 1.93649 0.52500 0.01936

```
7  PROC RATIO DATA = TAB9_1C FILETYPE = SAS DESIGN = WOR;
8  NEST _ONE_ DEVLPMNT;
9  TOTCNT M _ZERO_;
10 WEIGHT WT1;
11 NUMER NVSTNRS;
12 DENOM NGE65;
13 SETENV COLWIDTH = 13 DECWIDTH = 5;
```

Number of observations read :	40	Weighted count : 100
Number of observations skipped :	0	
(WEIGHT variable nonpositive)		
Denominator degrees of freedom :	1	

by: Variable, One.

Variable		One 1
NVSTNRS/NGE65	Sample Size	40.00000
	Weighted Size	100.00000
	Weighted X-Sum	167.50000
	Weighted Y-Sum	57.50000
	Ratio Est.	0.34328
	SE Ratio	0.00759

Data from 10 District Courts

District Court	Number of Eligible Persons	Number Receiving Substance Abuse Treatment
6	486	79
10	240	94
14	428	17
15	343	57
17	1130	63
19	983	10
20	333	58
21	13	0
22	1506	101
25	1755	411
Total	7217	890

Since the number of eligible individuals in the sample is subject to sampling variability, the resulting estimate of the proportion receiving substance abuse treatment is a ratio estimate as shown in Box 9.2. Using that notation, we have the following summary statistics and estimates:

$$M = 26 \qquad m = 10$$

$$\bar{x}_{clu} = 89 \qquad s_x = 118.303 \qquad \widehat{SE}(\bar{x}_{clu}) = 29.3473$$

$$\bar{y}_{clu} = 721.700 \qquad s_y = 585.797 \qquad \widehat{SE}(\bar{y}_{clu}) = 145.3185$$

$$\frac{\sum_{i=1}^{m}(x_i - \bar{x}_{clu})(y_i - \bar{y}_{clu})}{m-1} = 46{,}579.222$$

$$r_{clu} = \frac{89}{721.700} = .1233$$

$$\widehat{SE}(r_{clu}) = .0302$$

Thus, one would estimate that $12.33\% \pm 3.02\%$ of eligible individuals received substance abuse treatment.

One can analyze these data using SUDAAN from a file in which the basic record is the cluster as shown below:

Record	District	Eligible	Treated	W	N
1	6	486	79	2.6	26
2	10	240	94	2.6	26
3	14	428	17	2.6	26
4	15	343	57	2.6	26
5	17	1130	63	2.6	26
6	19	983	10	2.6	26
7	20	333	58	2.6	26
8	21	13	0	2.6	26
9	22	1506	101	2.6	26
10	25	1755	411	2.6	26

The command file for obtaining the ratio estimate, r_{clu}, and its estimated standard error is shown below:

```
PROC RATIO DATA = PROBBKSM FILETYPE = SAS DESIGN = STRWOR;
NEST _ONE_;
TOTCNT N;
WEIGHT W;
NUMER TREATED;
DENOM ELIGIBLE;
SETENV COLWIDTH = 13;
SETENV DECWIDTH = 3;
```

The first line calls for a ratio estimate, identifies the name of the data file, indicates that it is a SAS file, and specifies the SUDAAN design, STRWOR. The second statement, NEST _ONE_, indicates that there is only one stratum. The net effect of the design statement in combination with the nest statement is that there is one stage of sampling, one stratum, and that the sampling is without replacement. The third line indicates that the total number of records in the population is given by the variable, N. In this instance, it is 26. The fourth line specifies that the sampling weight is given by the variable, W. In this instance, it is 2.6 (26/10). The last three statements specify the numerator and denominator variables and the appearance of the output. Note that this command file is exactly the same as would be used for a simple random sample without replacement. In this instance, however, the variables being processed are cluster aggregates rather than values for individual elements.

Note that the data file could have been constructed using the enumeration units (which in this example are the eligible cases) as the basic records, as was done in the previous illustrative example. This would have entailed, however, working with a data set containing 7217 records, which would have been somewhat cumbersome. The SUDAAN output for this example is shown below:

Variable		One 1
TREATED/ELIGIBLE	Sample Size	10.000
	Weighted Size	26.000
	Weighted X-Sum	18764.199
	Weighted Y-Sum	2314.000
	Ratio Est.	0.123
	SE Ratio	0.030

Note that the estimated ratio and its standard error agree with those obtained by use of the formulas in Box 9.2.   □

9.3 SAMPLING DISTRIBUTIONS OF ESTIMATES

In cluster sampling, the clusters themselves are often constructs used to provide an efficient sampling plan, and it is often not of primary importance to estimate characteristics on a per-cluster basis. In order to obtain estimates on a per-element basis from a cluster sample, ratio estimates must be used. For example, in order to estimate the proportion of all persons requiring the services of a visiting nurse, a ratio estimate is necessary since the number of persons in the sample, and hence the estimated number of persons in the universe, is a random variable subject to sampling variability. Thus, ratio estimates are very important in cluster sampling.

Let us first look at an example of the sampling distributions of estimates.

Illustrative Example.   In the earlier example in which a simple one-stage cluster sample of two housing developments is selected from a population of five housing developments, there are 10 possible samples, each having the same chance of being selected. The sampling distributions of three estimates—the total number of persons over 65 years of age requiring the services of a visiting nurse (x'_{clu}), the total number of persons over 65 years of age (y'_{clu}), and the proportion of persons over 65 years of age requiring the services of a visiting nurse (r_{clu})—are shown in Table 9.3.

The means and standard errors of x'_{clu}, y'_{clu}, and r_{clu} obtained by enumeration over all samples are shown in Table 9.4 along with the true population values (X, Y, and R).

Note that in this example $E(x'_{clu}) = X$ and $E(y'_{clu}) = Y$, and this is true in general about totals estimated from simple one-stage cluster sampling. Note also that while the ratio estimate r_{clu} is not an unbiased estimator of the population ratio R, the magnitude of this bias is small. □

Expressions for the theoretical standard errors of estimated totals, means, and ratios are shown in Box 9.3 for simple one-stage cluster sampling in terms of the population parameters. The expressions X_i and $\bar{X}$ appearing in Box 9.3 were defined in Box 9.1 and are as follows:

$$X_i = \sum_{j=1}^{N_i} X_{ij}$$

where X_{ij} is the level of characteristic $\mathcal{X}$ for the jth listing unit in cluster i

$$\bar{X} = \frac{\sum_{i=1}^{M} X_i}{M}$$

In other words, the X_i are cluster totals and $\bar{X}$ is the mean level of $\mathcal{X}$ per cluster. As in earlier chapters, these entities are capitalized when we are discussing population characteristics, and are lower case when we are discussing sample characteristics.

Table 9.3 Sampling Distribution of Three Estimates

Clusters in Sample	x'_{clu}	y'_{clu}	r_{clu}
1, 2	75.0	162.5	.462
1, 3	82.5	177.5	.465
1, 4	57.6	160.0	.359
1, 5	77.5	165.0	.470
2, 3	62.5	180.0	.347
2, 4	37.5	162.5	.231
2, 5	57.5	167.5	.343
3, 4	45.0	177.5	.254
3, 5	65.0	182.5	.356
4, 5	40.0	165.0	.242

Table 9.4   Means and Standard Errors of Estimates

Estimate	Mean of Estimate	Standard Error of Estimate	Population Value
x'_{clu}	60	14.87	$X = 60$
y'_{clu}	170	7.98	$Y = 170$
r_{clu}	.35287	.087	$R = .35294$

The use of these formulas for the population of five housing developments given in Table 9.1 is illustrated next.

Illustrative Example.   For the population given in Table 9.1, we have

$$M = 5 \quad Y_1 = 32 \quad Y_2 = 33 \quad Y_3 = 39 \quad Y_4 = 32 \quad Y_5 = 34$$

$$\bar{Y} = 34 \quad \sigma_{1y}^2 = \frac{\sum_{i=1}^{M}(Y_i - \bar{Y})^2}{M} = 6.8$$

$$X_1 = 19 \quad X_2 = 11 \quad X_3 = 14 \quad X_4 = 4 \quad X_5 = 12$$

$$\bar{X} = 12 \quad \sigma_{1x}^2 = \frac{\sum_{i=1}^{M}(X_i - \bar{X})^2}{M} = 23.6$$

$$\sigma_{1xy} = \frac{\sum_{i=1}^{M}(X_i - \bar{X})(Y_i - \bar{Y})}{M} = 2.6 \quad R = \frac{12}{34} = .353$$

Then for samples of $m = 2$ clusters, we have

$$SE(y'_{clu}) = \left(\frac{5}{\sqrt{2}}\right) \times \sqrt{6.8} \times \sqrt{\frac{5-2}{5-1}} = 7.98$$

$$SE(x'_{clu}) = \left(\frac{5}{\sqrt{2}}\right) \times \sqrt{23.6} \times \sqrt{\frac{5-2}{5-1}} = 14.87$$

$$SE(\bar{x}_{clu}) = \left(\frac{1}{\sqrt{2}}\right) \times \sqrt{23.6} \times \sqrt{\frac{5-2}{5-1}} = 2.97$$

$$SE(\bar{\bar{x}}_{clu}) = \left(\frac{1}{20\sqrt{2}}\right) \times \sqrt{23.6} \times \sqrt{\frac{5-2}{5-1}} = .149$$

$$SE(r_{clu}) = \left(\frac{.353}{\sqrt{2}}\right) \times \sqrt{\frac{5-2}{5-1}} \times \sqrt{\frac{23.6}{(12)^2} + \frac{6.8}{(34)^2} - \frac{2 \times 2.6}{12 \times 34}} = .0857 \quad \square$$

Note that in the example $SE(x'_{clu})$ and $SE(y'_{clu})$ as computed from the formulas given in Box 9.3 are exactly what was obtained earlier by complete enumeration of all samples (Table 9.4). This is true in general for estimated totals and means obtained from simple cluster sampling. The formula for the standard error of r_{clu}, however, is only an approximation.

BOX 9.3 THEORETICAL STANDARD ERRORS FOR ESTIMATES UNDER SIMPLE ONE-STAGE CLUSTER SAMPLING

Total, x'_{clu}

$$\text{SE}(x'_{clu}) = \frac{M}{\sqrt{m}} \times \left[\frac{\sum_{i=1}^{M}(X_i - \bar{X})^2}{M}\right]^{1/2} \left(\frac{M-m}{M-1}\right)^{1/2}$$

Mean Per Cluster, $\bar{x}_{clu}$

$$\text{SE}(\bar{x}_{clu}) = \frac{1}{\sqrt{m}} \times \left[\frac{\sum_{i=1}^{M}(X_i - \bar{X})^2}{M}\right]^{1/2} \left(\frac{M-m}{M-1}\right)^{1/2}$$

Mean Per Enumeration Unit, $\bar{\bar{x}}_{clu}$

$$\text{SE}(\bar{\bar{x}}_{clu}) = \frac{1}{\bar{N}\sqrt{m}} \times \left[\frac{\sum_{i=1}^{M}(X_i - \bar{X})^2}{M}\right]^{1/2} \left(\frac{M-m}{M-1}\right)^{1/2}$$

Ratio, r_{clu}

$$\text{SE}(r_{clu}) \approx \left(\frac{R}{\sqrt{m}}\right) \times \left(\frac{M-m}{M-1}\right)^{1/2} \times \left[\frac{\sum_{i=1}^{M}(X_i - \bar{X})^2}{M\bar{X}^2} + \frac{\sum_{i=1}^{M}(Y_i - \bar{Y})^2}{M\bar{Y}^2}\right.$$
$$\left. - \frac{2\sum_{i=1}^{M}(X_i - \bar{X})(Y_i - \bar{Y})}{M\bar{X}\bar{Y}}\right]^{1/2}$$

The notation used here is defined in Box 9.1. The population estimates are defined in Box 9.2.

The expression $\sum_{i=1}^{M}(X_i - \bar{X})^2/M$ that appears in the formulas in Box 9.3 is really the variance of the distribution of the cluster totals X_i. This expression, denoted by σ_{1x}^2, is often referred to as a *first-stage variance* and is descriptive of the variation among clusters with respect to the distribution of total levels of characteristic $\mathscr{X}$. In other words, for any characteristic $\mathscr{X}$,

$$\sigma_{1x}^2 = \frac{\sum_{i=1}^{M}(X_i - \bar{X})^2}{M}. \tag{9.1}$$

If we examine the formulas in Box 9.3, substituting relation (9.1) in the appropriate places, we see that these expressions are exactly the same as the expressions for the standard errors of the analogous estimates in simple random sampling with the exception that m replaces n, M replaces N, and σ_{1x}^2 replaces σ_x^2. This result is not surprising since simple one-stage cluster sampling is exactly the same as simple random sampling with the aggregate of all listing units in the cluster serving as an effective enumeration unit.

The estimated standard errors of estimated means, totals, and ratios shown in Box 9.2 are obtained from the theoretical standard errors of these estimates shown in Box 9.3 by substitution of $\hat{\sigma}_{1x}^2$ for σ_{1x}^2 in the appropriate places, where $\hat{\sigma}_{1x}^2$ is an estimate from the data of σ_{1x}^2, given by

$$\hat{\sigma}_{1x}^2 = \left[\frac{\sum_{i=1}^{m}(x_i - \bar{x}_{\text{clu}})^2}{m - 1} \right] \times \left(\frac{M - 1}{M} \right)$$

as defined in Box 9.2.

9.4   HOW LARGE A SAMPLE IS NEEDED?

Suppose that we intend to use a simple one-stage cluster sample design and wish to be virtually certain of obtaining estimates that differ in relative terms from the true values of the unknown parameters by no more than ε (where ε is as defined in Chapter 3). Then the required number of sample clusters is as given in Box 9.4. Let us look at a calculation that uses one of these formulas.

Illustrative Example.   In the example based on the data in Table 9.1, suppose that we wish to be virtually certain (i.e., $z = 3$) of estimating the total number Y of persons over 65 years of age residing in the five housing developments to within 10% of the true value. With $\sigma_{1y}^2 = 6.8$, $M = 5$, $\varepsilon = .10$, and $Y = 34$, we have

$$V_{1y}^2 = \frac{\sigma_{1y}^2}{\bar{Y}^2} = \frac{6.8}{34^2} = .0059$$

BOX 9.4 EXACT AND APPROXIMATE SAMPLE SIZES REQUIRED UNDER SIMPLE ONE-STAGE CLUSTER SAMPLING

Exact	**Approximate**

Total

$$m = \frac{z^2_{1-(\alpha/2)} M V^2_{1x}}{z^2_{1-(\alpha/2)} V^2_{1x} + (M-1)\varepsilon^2} \qquad\qquad m \approx \frac{z^2_{1-(\alpha/2)} V^2_{1x}}{\varepsilon^2}$$

Mean per Cluster

$$m = \frac{z^2_{1-(\alpha/2)} M V^2_{1x}}{z^2_{1-(\alpha/2)} V^2_{1x} + (M-1)\varepsilon^2} \qquad\qquad m \approx \frac{z^2_{1-(\alpha/2)} V^2_{1x}}{\varepsilon^2}$$

Mean per Listing Unit

$$m = \frac{z^2_{1-(\alpha/2)} M V^2_{1x}}{z^2_{1-(\alpha/2)} V^2_{1x} + (M-1)\varepsilon^2} \qquad\qquad m \approx \frac{z^2_{1-(\alpha/2)} V^2_{1x}}{\varepsilon^2}$$

Ratio

$$m = \frac{z^2_{1-(\alpha/2)} M V^2_{1R}}{z^2_{1-(\alpha/2)} V^2_{1R} + (M-1)\varepsilon^2} \qquad\qquad m \approx \frac{z^2_{1-(\alpha/2)} V^2_{1R}}{\varepsilon^2}$$

where

$$V^2_{1x} = \frac{\sigma^2_{1x}}{\bar{X}^2} \qquad V^2_{1R} = \left[\frac{\sigma^2_{1x}}{\bar{X}^2} + \frac{\sigma^2_{1y}}{\bar{Y}^2} - 2 \times \frac{\sigma_{1xy}}{\bar{X}\bar{Y}} \right]$$

$$\sigma_{1xy} = \frac{\sum_{i=1}^{M}(X_i - \bar{X})(Y_i - \bar{Y})}{M}$$

M is the number of clusters in the population; $z^2_{1-(\alpha/2)}$ is the reliability coefficient for $100[1 - (\alpha/2)]$ confidence; and ε represents the specifications set on our estimate in terms of the maximum relative difference allowed between it and the unknown population parameter.

and from Box 9.4

$$m = \frac{z_{1-(\alpha/2)}^2 M V_{1y}^2}{z_{1-(\alpha/2)}^2 V_{1y}^2 + (M-1)\varepsilon^2} = \frac{9 \times 5 \times .0059}{9 \times .0059 + 4 \times (.10)^2} = 2.85$$

Rounding up, we have $m = 3$. Thus, we would need a simple one-stage cluster sample of three clusters to meet these specifications.   □

In order to determine the sample size that meets the specifications required for the reliability of the estimate, it is necessary to know the value of V_{1x}^2, which is the ratio of σ_{1x}^2, the variance of the distribution of cluster totals, to $\bar{X}^2$, the square of the mean level of characteristic $\mathscr{X}$ per cluster. These quantities are population parameters that in general would be unknown and would have to be either estimated from preliminary studies or else guessed by means of intuition or past experience.

9.5 RELIABILITY OF ESTIMATES AND COSTS INVOLVED

One of the major advantages of simple one-stage cluster sampling is that the cost of obtaining a sample of listing units by this method is often lower than that of obtaining a sample of the same number of listing units by other methods. This was shown in the illustrative example in Chapter 8 involving comparison of the costs of taking a simple one-stage cluster sample of 10 households against that of taking a simple random sample of 10 households. In this section, we use an illustrative example to show that use of single-stage cluster sampling can reduce costs, but often at the price of resulting in estimates that have high standard errors.

Illustrative Example.   Let us consider the sample survey of district courts described earlier in this chapter. We now suppose that this sample is selected from the following underlying population of 26 district courts shown in Table 9.5 (the sampled courts are shown in italics).

If approximately 15% of all persons given probation in these district courts were recommended for substance abuse treatment, then the 15,364 eligible persons were screened from approximately 102,427 total individuals or an average of 3939 individuals per court. If the costs in personnel time of screening these individuals is approximately 20 minutes per person (this entails review of the court record for determination of eligibility), then the expected cost of screening for a sample survey of 10 district courts is approximately 13,130 person-hours (3939 × 10 ×20/60). The expected number of eligible persons identified by this screening in a sample survey of 10 courts would be approximately 5909 (3939 × 10 × 0.15).

Table 9.5 Number of Eligible Persons and Number Receiving Substance Abuse Treatment Among Individuals Sentenced to Probation in 26 District Courts

District Court	Number of Eligible Persons	Number Receiving Substance Abuse Treatment
1	514	253
2	205	78
3	329	21
4	508	145
5	224	17
6	*486*	*79*
7	275	0
8	224	18
9	83	14
10	*240*	*94*
11	305	30
12	82	22
13	74	8
14	*428*	*17*
15	*343*	*57*
16	232	11
17	1,130	63
18	1,000	165
19	*983*	*10*
20	*333*	*58*
21	*13*	*0*
22	*1,506*	*101*
23	1,181	228
24	1,398	12
25	*1,755*	*411*
26	.1,513	532
Total	15,364	2,444

For each individual identified as eligible, the probation officer for that individual is contacted and asked to verify, from his/her records, whether the person actually received substance abuse treatment. It is estimated that the cost of this verification along with the cost of abstracting and preparing the data is approximately 45 minutes per eligible person. Thus, the expected cost for the sample survey would be approximately 4432 person-hours (5909 × 45/60). The estimated total field costs for this sample survey are summarized below in person-hours (p.h.):

Cost associated with identifying eligible persons: 13,130 p.h.

Cost associated with obtaining information from eligible persons: 4432 p.h.

Total cost: 17,561 p.h.

If, instead of a single-stage cluster sample, one were to take a simple random sample of the same number (i.e., 5909) of eligible individuals, one would have to screen for eligibility all of the probation cases in all 26 courts (instead of only those in the 10 sample courts). This would require screening approximately 102,427 persons at a cost of 34,142 person-hours ($102,427 \times 20/60$). It would yield approximately 15,364 eligible individuals ($102,427 \times 0.15$). Obtaining information from the 5909 sample individuals would take (as with single one-stage cluster sampling) approximately 4432 person-hours.

The estimated field costs for a simple random sample of 5909 eligible individuals are summarized below in person-hours:

Cost associated with identifying eligible persons: 34,142 p.h.

Cost associated with obtaining information from eligible persons: 4432 p.h.

Total cost: 38,574 p.h.

From the above, we see that the total field costs for the sample survey having the simple random sample design (38,574 person-hours) is considerably higher than that for the survey having the single-stage cluster sampling design (17,561 person-hours).

Let us suppose further that the most important objective of the sample survey is to estimate the total number of eligible individuals who received substance abuse treatment. We now compare the standard errors of this variable for the two sample designs. For the single-stage cluster sample the standard error of the estimate, x'_{clu}, as given by the formula in Box 9.3, with $M = 26$, $m = 10$, and $\sigma_{1x} = 128.86$, is 847.60. For the simple random sample of 5909 eligible individuals, the estimated standard error of the estimated total, x', with $n = 5909$, $N = 15,364$, and $p = 2444/15,364 = .1591$, is equal to 57.36. This is much lower than the standard error of the estimated total from the single-stage cluster sample. The two designs are compared below for a sample of 5909 eligible cases.

Sample Design	Total Persons Screened	Total Persons Sampled	Total Field Costs in Person-Hours	Standard Error of Estimated Total Obtaining Substance Abuse Treatment
Simple Random Sampling	102,427	5,909	38,574	57.35
Simple One-Stage Cluster Sampling ($m = 10$)	39,390	5,909	17,561	847.60

Which of the two is the design of choice? The simple random sample is more expensive but has a much lower standard error than the single-stage cluster design having the same number of sample elements. In the next section, we discuss strategies for choosing between two sample designs on the basis of both cost and reliability. □

9.6 CHOOSING A SAMPLING DESIGN BASED ON COST AND RELIABILITY

There are essentially two widely used strategies for choosing among several possible sample designs. The first strategy consists of the four steps shown below (for simplicity, we will assume that only one estimate is to be taken into consideration in choosing the sample design).

1. Determine the relative error ε required for the estimate.
2. For each sample design under consideration, determine the sample size required to obtain, with specified confidence, an estimate that meets the specifications listed in Step 1.
3. For each sample design, estimate the field costs involved in obtaining the sample size given in Step 2.
4. Choose the sample design that yields the lowest field costs, as calculated in Step 3.

In other words, this strategy chooses from among the competing sample designs the sample design that meets the required specifications at the lowest field costs. Let us see how this strategy could be used by looking at an example.

Illustrative Example. Let us again consider the sample survey of district courts and the population data presented in Table 9.5 of the previous section. Suppose that we wish to choose between simple random sampling and single-stage cluster sampling and that we wish to be 95% certain of estimating the total number of eligible individuals who obtained treatment for substance abuse to within 33% of the true value. From the formula in Box 9.4 with $M = 26$, $z_{1-\alpha/2} = 1.96$, $\varepsilon = 0.33$, $\sigma_{1x} = 128.863$, and $\bar{x} = 94$, the required number, m, of sample clusters is 19.

A single-stage cluster sample of 19 district courts would entail screening approximately 74,841 records (3939×19) at a cost of 24,947 person-hours ($74,841 \times 20/60$). Approximately 11,226 individuals would be interviewed ($3939 \times .15 \times 19$) at a cost of 8420 person-hours ($11,226 \times 45/60$). Thus, the total field cost of the sample survey with a single-stage cluster sample is 33,367 person-hours.

In order to satsify the specifications stated above, a simple random sample would require 185 subjects (Box 3.5 with $N = 15,364$, $P = .1591$, $\varepsilon = 0.33$, and

$z_{1-\alpha/2} = 1.96$). This would entail screening all 102,427 case records at a cost of 34,142 person-hours (102,427 × 20/60). The cost of obtaining information about the 185 sample subjects would be 139 person-hours (185 × 45/60). Thus, the total field costs of the survey would be 34,281 person-hours, which is higher than the cost of 33,367 determined for the single-stage cluster sample design.

We have seen above that the single-stage cluster sample design will meet the reliability specification determined by the parameters $\varepsilon = 0.33$ and $z_{1-\alpha/2} = 1.96$ at a lower cost than the simple random sample design. A different specification, however, could lead to a different conclusion concerning the relative costs of the two designs. For example, if one requires 95% confidence that the estimate be within 15% of the true value (i.e., $\varepsilon = 0.15$, $z_{1-\alpha/2} = 1.96$), then the total field costs of the single-stage cluster sampling design will be higher than that of the simple random sampling design (43,903 vs. 34,782).

The relationship between the total field costs and ε for each design is shown in Figure 9.2 (for $z_{1-\alpha/2} = 1.96$). For the simple random sample design, the major costs are in screening for eligible cases, and these costs are independent of the required sample size. For the simple one-stage cluster sampling design, as ε decreases, more sample clusters are required, and this increases both the screening and data-collection costs.   □

A second strategy that is widely used in choosing among alternative sampling designs is to first determine the sample design that produces estimates having the lowest variance at the field costs that have been specified. This is done by first calculating the sample size that can be taken within the specified

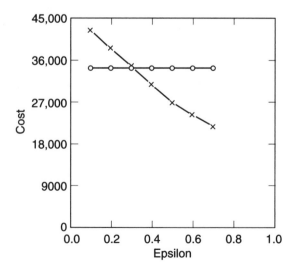

Figure 9.2 Cost: simple random sample and single-stage cluster sampling. × = Cluster; ○ = simple random sample.

field costs and then calculating the variance of the estimate for that particular sample size.

In order for this strategy to be used easily, it helps to have an equation relating sample size to field costs. Such an equation is called a *cost function* and is a very useful tool that enables an investigator to choose from among competing sample designs the one that will produce the lowest variance at a specified cost. We show below how such a simple cost function might be obtained.

Let us examine in a slightly different way the field costs involved in each of the two sample designs that we have been discussing. For the simple random sampling design, the cost of constructing the sampling frame is independent of the number of enumeration units selected in the sample, since each enumeration unit must be listed prior to the selection of the sample. The other costs, moreover, might be considered to depend on the number of enumeration units selected. Thus, a reasonable estimate of field costs for a simple random sample design might be given by the expression

$$C = C_0 + C_1 n \tag{9.2}$$

where C_0 is the cost component associated with construction of the sampling frame, plus other field costs that are not dependent on sample size, and C_1 is the data collection cost per enumeration unit. For the example given above, we have values of C_0 and C_1 given by

$$C_0 = 34{,}142 \text{ person-hours} \qquad C_1 = 0.75 \text{ person-hours}$$

As discussed earlier, the cost, C_0, is obtained by multiplying the expected number, 102,427, of total probation case records that must be screened for determination of eligibility by the estimated time, 20 minutes or 1/3 hour, that it takes to screen each case record. The cost, C_1, is the estimated time, 45 minutes or 0.75 hours, that the process of abstracting each sample record takes.

The field costs involved in simple one-stage cluster sampling have a different form. Since frame construction costs depend on the number of clusters selected, the field costs involved in a simple one-stage cluster sample can be described by the following equation:

$$C = C_1' m + C_2' m \bar{N} \tag{9.3}$$

The cost component C_1' associated with clusters includes costs of "enrolling" the cluster into the study and of constructing the sampling frame for that cluster as well as other costs that are not dependent on the number of enumeration units sampled. The cost component C_2' includes all costs that can be expressed on a per-enumeration unit basis (primarily data collection and data processing costs).

In the sample survey of district courts, the cost component, C_1', is essentially that of constructing the sampling frame for each sample court—20 minutes for each case record screened for eligibility times 3939.5 (average number of case records per district court)—and is equal to 1313.17 person-hours. The cost component, C_2', is the cost of data collection and is equal to 0.75 person-hours. Thus, we have

$$C_1' = 1313.17 \quad \text{and} \quad C_2' = 0.75$$

The cost functions discussed above are rough approximations to the true field costs and are useful in choosing between alternative sample designs. Such cost functions will be used when we discuss cost efficiency in later chapters.

Now let us examine an example of this second strategy using the same illustrative example.

Illustrative Example.   Let us suppose that we have a budget that allocates no more than 25,000 person-hours to field costs and that we wish to choose between simple one-stage cluster sampling and simple random sampling. From Equation (9.3) with $C = 25,000$, $C_1' = 1313.17$, $C_2' = 0.75$, and $\bar{N} = 590.92$, we solve for m and obtain 14.2 district courts. Thus, a simple one-stage cluster sample of $m = 14$ district courts would satisfy the cost constraint of 25,000 person-hours. If our estimate of interest is the total number, x_{clu}', of persons receiving treatment for substance abuse, then the standard error of this estimate is shown below:

$$\text{SE}(x_{\text{clu}}') = \frac{M}{\sqrt{m}}\sigma_{1x}\sqrt{\frac{M-m}{M-1}} = \frac{26}{\sqrt{14}}(128.86)\sqrt{\frac{26-14}{26-1}} = 620.37$$

Since the population total of individuals obtaining substance abuse treatment is 2444, that would give the estimate a coefficient of variation equal to 25.4% of the true value. At this cost of 25,000 person-hours, one can be 95% certain that the estimate will be within 50.8% (1.96 times the coefficient of variation of the estimate) of its true value.

In contrast, the simple random sampling design could not be implemented if field costs allocated to the sample survey were limited to 25,000 person-hours. The reason for this is that frame construction costs alone would be 34,142 person-hours. Thus, of the two sample designs, simple one-stage cluster sampling wins by default. This would not necessarily be the case if much higher field costs were allocated (e.g., 40,000 person-hours).   □

Two points should be made concerning the material in this and the previous section. The first point is that simple random sampling and single-stage cluster sampling represent two "extremes." Simple random sampling for a fixed number, n, of elements generally produces estimates having low standard errors when compared to those produced by other designs. However, costs of simple random sampling are high generally because of high frame construction costs and (for personal interview surveys) high travel costs relative to other designs.

In contrast, single-stage cluster sampling often has low costs compared to other designs for a fixed number of sample enumeration units. The reason is that frame construction costs are generally reduced because only the enumeration units in the sample cluster need to be listed. Also, the geographical clustering reduces travel costs in household surveys conducted by personal interview. When compared to other designs on a per-sample-enumeration unit basis, however, estimates produced by single-stage cluster sampling often have high standard errors. This is because similarities among members of the same cluster can result in redundancy, and the "effective" sample size becomes much less than the actual sample size. Also, if there is much variation among clusters in the total number, N_i, of enumeration units per cluster, estimates of totals under single-stage cluster sampling can have very high standard errors compared to other designs having the same number of enumeration units. In the next two chapters, we discuss other cluster sampling designs that avoid some of the problems inherent in single-stage cluster sampling.

The discussion in this section has been greatly simplified to illustrate the concepts involved in taking costs into consideration when we choose between sample designs. In our example, we made the choice on the basis of one estimate only (e.g., the total number of individuals obtaining treatment for substance abuse). In more authentic situations, many estimates would be considered important, and the design of choice would be the one that performs best in the sense discussed in this section, when all estimates are taken into consideration. Also, the cost functions developed in this section were simple linear functions of clusters or enumeration units. Although these simplified functions are often useful in practice, more complex functions are sometimes needed to describe costs in a meaningful way. Excellent discussions of cost functions are given in well-known sampling texts by Hansen et al. [2] and Jessen [3]. A more recent book by Groves [10] dealing exclusively with survey costs and survey errors provides a detailed but very readable treatment of cost components and cost functions.

9.7 SUMMARY

In this chapter we discussed the basic concepts of simple one-stage cluster sampling, a design which involves selection of a simple random sample of clusters and inclusion in the sample of every enumeration unit within each sample cluster. We developed methodology for estimating means, totals, and ratios under simple one-stage cluster sampling, and we discussed the sampling distributions of these estimates. In addition, we presented methods for estimating the standard errors of these estimates from the data in the sample.

We discussed determination of the sample size required to meet specifications set for the reliability of estimates obtained under simple one-stage cluster sampling, and the formulas developed here were found to be very similar to those developed earlier for simple random sampling, with the cluster totals serving as the effective observations. We presented strategies for choosing between alternative sample designs taking costs into consideration. Finally, we discussed the concepts of cost components and cost functions.

EXERCISES

9.1 Suppose that the elementary schools in a city are grouped into 30 school districts, with each school district containing four schools. Suppose that a simple one-stage cluster sample of three school districts is taken for purposes of estimating the number of school children in the city who are color-blind (as measured by a standard test), and that the accompanying data are obtained from this sample. Estimate and obtain a 95% confidence interval for the total number of color-blind children and the proportion of all children who are color-blind.

Sample School District	School	No. of Children	No. of Color-Blind Children
1	1	130	2
	2	150	3
	3	160	3
	4	120	5
2	1	110	2
	2	120	4
	3	100	0
	4	120	1
3	1	89	4
	2	130	2
	3	100	0
	4	150	2

9.2 A sample of patients is to be taken from the patient records of a large psychiatric outpatient clinic for purposes of estimating the total number of patients given tricyclic antidepressant drugs as part of their therapeutic regimen. The records are organized into file drawers, each containing 20 patient records, and there are 40 such file drawers.

a. Suppose that we wish to use simple random sampling of patient records. How large a sample is needed if we wish to be virtually certain of estimating the total number of persons given tricyclic anti-depressant drugs to within 10% of the true value and if we anticipate that approximately 20% of all patients were given these drugs?

b. What would be the field costs involved in taking the sample specified in part (a)? Make some assumptions about the cost components in determining these field costs.

c. What sample size is needed if the design is to be a simple one-stage cluster sample [same specifications as in part (a)]?

d. What would be the field costs for a simple one-stage cluster sample? Again, make some assumptions about the cost components in determining these field costs.

e. Which of the two alternative sample designs would you use? Why?

9.3 A simple one-stage cluster sample was taken of 10 hospitals in a midwestern state from a population of 33 hospitals that have received state and federal funds to upgrade their emergency medical services. Within each of the hospitals selected in the sample, the records of all patients hospitalized in calendar year 1988 for traumatic injuries (i.e., accidents, poisonings, violence, burns, etc.) were examined. The number of patients hospitalized for trauma conditions and the number discharged dead are shown in the accompanying table for each hospital in the sample.

Hospital	Total Number of Patients Hospitalized for Trauma Conditions	Total Number Discharged Dead Among All Patients Hospitalized with Trauma Conditions
1	560	4
2	190	4
3	260	2
4	370	4
5	190	4
6	130	0
7	170	9
8	170	2
9	60	0
10	110	1

a. For this sample, what are the clusters, what are the listing units, and what are the elementary units?

b. Estimate and give a 95% confidence interval for the total number of persons hospitalized for trauma conditions among the 33 hospitals.

   c. Estimate and give a 95% confidence interval for the total number of patients discharged dead among all persons hospitalized for trauma conditions.

   d. Estimate and give a 95% confidence interval for the proportion of patients discharged dead among those hospitalized with trauma conditions.

9.4 The number of beds in each of the ten hospitals sampled in Exercise 9.3 is shown in the accompanying table. The remaining 23 hospitals not appearing in the sample have a total of 3687 beds. Use this information to obtain improved estimates and confidence intervals for the following:

   a. The total number of persons hospitalized with trauma conditions.

   b. The total number of persons discharged dead among all persons hospitalized with trauma conditions.

Hospital	No. of Beds
1	824
2	312
3	329
4	648
5	358
6	252
7	256
8	263
9	138
10	150

9.5 A survey which used a simple one-stage cluster sampling design was conducted in a large city in China. The clusters in this instance were entities known as "neighborhood groups" (translated from the Chinese "jumin xiaozu"), which are essentially groups of contiguous households. These so-called neighborhood groups are the smallest units for which population information is available in the Peoples Republic of China (PRC). The city comprises six districts which, in this design, comprise the strata. Within each district, a simple random sample of two neighborhood groups was selected, and all individuals within each neighborhood group were interviewed concerning their overall health status. The following represents data from the survey on the number of individuals over 30 years of age who were edentulous.

District	Neighborhood Group	Number of Persons > 30 years	Number of Edentulous Persons
1	1	28	7
	2	35	9
2	1	29	12
	2	43	26
3	1	61	19
	2	48	12
4	1	15	10
	2	39	28
5	1	21	9
	2	46	15
6	1	12	0
	2	25	4

Strata 1, 2, 4 and 6 each contain 200 neighborhood groups; stratum 3 contains 175 neighborhood groups; and stratum 5 contains 150 neighborhood groups. Estimate and construct 95% confidence intervals for (1) the total number of edentulous persons 30 years of age and over, and (2) the proportion of all persons 30 years of age and older who are edentulous.

9.6 In Exercise 9.5, it was discovered during the field work that sample neighborhood group 2 in District 3 no longer existed because of redistribution of the population. With this in mind, obtain modified estimates of the parameters estimated in Exercise 9.5.

9.7 A dental HMO has 368 members and each member has 4 *quadrants* (upper left, upper right, lower left, lower right). It is desired to conduct a sample survey with the objective in mind of estimating the total number of quadrants among the membership that require some form of periodontal surgery. The sampling plan would involve taking a simple random sample of patients and evaluating, for each sample patient, the status of each of the four quadrants. A preliminary study, based on a judgmental sample of 7 patients, yielded the following data:

	Quadrant			
Patient	**1**	**2**	**3**	**4**
1	+	+	+	−
2	−	−	+	+
3	−	−	−	−
4	+	−	−	+
5	−	−	−	−
6	+	−	−	−
7	+	+	+	+

where 1 = lower left, 2 = lower right, 3 = upper left, 4 = upper right, $+$ = requires surgery, $-$ = does not require surgery.

Based on these preliminary data, how many patients are required if it is desired to estimate, with 95% certainty, the total number of quadrants among all members that require periodontal surgery to within 15% of the true value?

9.8 In the scenario described in Exercise 9.7, it is anticipated that it would take about 15 min for a dentist to examine each quadrant, and that it would take approximately 20 min of clerical time to schedule the appointment for each patient sampled and to prepare the patient for the examination. If these are the only costs involved in the survey, and if clerical time is one-third as expensive as dentist's time, what budget (expressed in dentist person-hours) would be required to meet the specifications stated in Exercise 9.7?

9.9 In many health science situations, a cluster consists of a pair of elements (e.g., in opthalmology, clusters might be patients; elements might be eyes, etc.). In this situation, derive a simplified expression for the variance of an estimated total.

9.10 In the situation described in Exercise 9.9, derive a simplified expression for the variance of an estimated ratio.

9.11 Suppose that 40,000 person-hours were allotted for field costs for the sample survey of district courts discussed in an illustrative example in this chapter. Using the cost functions and cost components developed for this example, determine which of the two sample designs—simple one-stage cluster sampling or simple random sampling—would estimate the total number of persons receiving treatment for substance abuse with the lower standard error.

9.12 For the sample survey of district courts discussed in an illustrative example in this chapter, draw a graph with the abscissa being total fixed costs and the ordinate being the coefficient of variation of the estimated total number of persons receiving treatment for substance abuse. The graph should have two lines (similar to Figure 9.2): one for a simple one-stage cluster sample design; the other for a simple random sampling design.

BIBLIOGRAPHY

The following publications contain more detailed discussions of cluster sampling.

1. Cochran, W. G., *Sampling Techniques*, 3rd ed., Wiley, New York, 1977.

2. Hansen, M. H., Hurwitz, W. N., and Madow, W. G., *Sample Survey Method and Theory*, Vol. 1, Wiley, New York, 1953.

3. Jessen, R. J., *Statistical Survey Techniques*, Wiley, New York, 1978.

4. Kish, L., *Survey Sampling*, Wiley, New York, 1965.

5. Scheaffer, R. L., Mendenhall, W., and Ott, L., *Elementary Survey Sampling*, 2nd ed., Duxbury Press, Scituate, Mass., 1979.

6. Sudman, S., *Applied Sampling*, Academic Press, New York, 1976.

The following publications report the findings of a survey which used single-stage cluster sampling.

7. Levy, P. S., Yu, E. S. H., Liu, W. T., Zhang, M. Y., Wang, Z. Y., Wong, S., and Katzman, R., A variation on single-stage cluster sampling used in a survey of elderly people in Shanghai, *International Journal of Epidemiology*, **17**: 931, 1988.

8. Levy, P. S., Yu, E. S. H., Liu, W. T., Zhang, M., Wang, Z., Wong, S., and Katzman, R. Single stage cluster sampling with a telescopic respondent rule: A variation motivated by a survey of dementia in elderly residents of Shanghai. *Statistics in Medicine*, **8**: 1225, 1989.

9. Yu, E. S. H., Liu, W. T., Levy, P. S., Zhang, M. Y., Katzman, R., Lung, C. T., Wong, S., Wang, Z. Y., and Qu, G. Y., Cognitive impairment among elderly adults in Shanghai, China. *Journal of Gerontology: Social Services*, **44**: S97, 1989.

The following book gives a very rich discussion of survey costs including determination of cost components.

10. Groves, R. M., Survey Errors and Survey Costs, Wiley, New York, 1989.

The following article gives an overview of cluster sampling using terminology very similar to that used in this chapter.

11. Levy, P. S., Cluster sampling. In *Encyclopedia of Biostatistics*. Armitage, P. A., and Colton, T. D., eds., Wiley, New York, 1998.

CHAPTER 10

Two-Stage Cluster Sampling: Clusters Sampled with Equal Probability

In the previous chapter we discussed simple one-stage cluster sampling, which involves taking a simple random sample of clusters and then sampling every enumeration or listing unit within each sample cluster. In some situations one would achieve greater efficiency if the sampling were performed in more than one stage. An obvious situation is that in which clusters are too large for all units to be sampled conveniently. Also, when the listing units within clusters are very homogeneous with respect to the variables being measured, there is a large amount of redundancy in sampling every listing unit within a sample cluster. In such situations, it is often better to take a sample of listing units within selected clusters rather than to select all of them. In other words, it is often best to draw the sample in two stages, with the first stage being a sample of clusters and the second stage being a sample of listing units within each sample cluster.

In this chapter and in the next we will discuss two-stage cluster sampling designs. The sampling designs considered in this chapter involve those commonly known as *simple two-stage cluster sampling* as defined in Chapter 8. These are designs in which clusters are selected at the first stage by simple random sampling; listing units are selected at the second stage by simple random sampling within each cluster selected at the first stage; and the sampling fraction of listing units selected at the second stage is the same (or nearly the same) for each sample cluster. The latter situation can occur when the number of listing units available for sampling is *not* the same within each cluster. For example, if one city block contains ten households and another contains six households, it would not be possible to take a 30% sample of households from each of these two blocks. However, if the general strategy is to have the second-stage sampling fractions as nearly equal as possible among the two blocks, then we would select three households from the block having ten households, and two households from the block having six households, and we would include

275

scenarios such as this under the general rubric of *simple two-stage cluster sampling*.

In this chapter, we consider only simple two-stage cluster sampling, discussing first the special situation in which all clusters in the population have the same number of enumeration units; and then discussing the more general situation in which all clusters do not have the same number of enumeration units. In Chapter 11, we treat the more complex situation in which clusters are sampled with unequal probabilities.

10.1   SITUATION IN WHICH ALL CLUSTERS HAVE THE SAME NUMBER, N_i, OF ENUMERATION UNITS

Although in most situations involving sampling of human populations, there will be differences among clusters with respect to their total number of enumeration units, there will be sampling situations in which each cluster has the same number of listing units. We begin our discussion with this special (albeit much less frequently occurring) situation because many of the estimation formulas for two-stage cluster sampling are greatly simplified, and the reader can gain considerable insight from these less complex formulas. Some examples of clusters having the same number of listing units are listed below:

- Weeks in the calendar year may serve as clusters in certain situations, with days serving as listing units. In such situations, each cluster (week) would have the same number of listing units (days).
- Health records are sometimes organized on computer tapes in reels, with each reel containing the same number of records. Hence, in a cluster sampling design which utilizes reels as clusters and individual records as listing units, each cluster (reel) would have the same number of listing units (records).
- In quality control or process control sampling, individual units of a product are often organized into batches, with each batch serving as a cluster and the individual units serving as listing units. The batches usually contain a fixed number of units.

10.1.1   How to Take a Simple Two-Stage Cluster Sample

We will use a simple example to illustrate how a simple two-stage cluster sample may be taken.

Illustrative Example.   In this example we will use the data shown in Table 10.1. Let us suppose that a local health department administers five community health centers, and that each community health center uses three nurse practitioners for primary care. Suppose further that it is desired to take a sample of

Table 10.1 Number of Patients Seen by Nurse Practitioners and Number Referred to a Physician for Five Community Health Centers

Health Center	Nurse Practitioner	Number of Patients Seen, $\mathscr{X}$	Number Referred to Physician, $\mathscr{Y}$
1	1	58	5
	2	44	6
	3	18	6
2	1	42	3
	2	53	19
	3	10	2
3	1	13	12
	2	18	6
	3	37	10
4	1	16	5
	2	32	14
	3	10	4
5	1	25	17
	2	23	9
	3	23	14

three clinics and within each clinic to take a subsample of two of the nurse practitioners employed there. Each nurse in the sample will be requested to keep a log of the patients seen during a particular week and the number of these patients referred to a physician.

To take a simple two-stage cluster sample of three community health centers and two nurse practitioners from each health center sampled, we first number the health centers from 1 to 5 and then choose three random numbers between 1 and 5 (e.g., 1, 2, and 4). Next, within each of these three sample centers we identify each nurse practitioner by a number and then we take two random numbers. The nurse practitioners corresponding to these numbers are then selected in the sample (e.g., nurse practitioners 2 and 3 from community health center 1, nurse practitioners 1 and 3 from health center 2, and nurse practitioners 1 and 2 from health center 4.   ☐

10.1.2 Estimation of Population Characteristics

Once the sample of clusters and listing units are selected, the required data are collected from every listing unit selected in the sample. The forms that are used to collect these data would, as discussed in Chapter 9, depend on the nature of the data and on the manner in which the data are collected. Then estimates of population characteristics are calculated by using the data that have been collected.

Let us investigate the estimation procedures by considering an example.

Illustrative Example. Suppose that from our sample of three community health centers and two nurse practitioners within each of the selected health centers, we wish to estimate the following population characteristics.

1. The total number of patients seen by nurse practitioners in the five community health centers
2. The total number of patients referred by nurse practitioners to physicians in the five community health centers
3. The proportion among all persons seen by nurse practitioners referred to a physician
4. The mean number of persons seen by nurse practitioners per community health center
5. The mean number of persons seen per nurse practitioner

The data might be collected by obtaining, from the records of each nurse practitioner selected in the sample, the total number of patients seen and the total number referred to physicians. Suppose that these data are as summarized in Table 10.2. We then obtain the desired estimates as follows from the summary data shown in Table 10.2.

To find the estimated total number of patients seen by nurse practitioners in the five community health centers, we first compute the total number of patients seen by all nurse practitioners in the sample. Then we divide that total by the overall sampling fraction. That is,

$$\text{Total patients seen} = 162$$

$$\text{Overall sampling fraction} = \frac{3}{5} \text{ of all centers } \times \frac{2}{3} \text{ of all nurses} = \frac{6}{15}$$

$$\text{Estimated population total of persons seen by nurses} = \frac{162}{6/15} = 405$$

Table 10.2 Summary Data for the Three Clusters Selected in the Sample

Health Center	Nurse Practitioner	Number of Patients Seen, $\mathcal{X}$	Number Referred to Physician, $\mathcal{Y}$
1	2	44	6
	3	18	6
2	1	42	3
	3	10	2
4	1	16	5
	2	32	14
Total		162	36

To find the estimated total number of patients referred by nurse practitioners to physicians in the five community health centers, we use computations similar to the previous computations:

$$\text{Total patients referred to physician} = 36$$

$$\text{Overall sampling fraction} = \frac{6}{15}$$

$$\text{Estimated total number of patients referred to physician} = \frac{36}{6/15} = 90$$

To find the estimated proportion referred to physicians among all patients seen by nurse practitioners, we compute the ratio of the two estimated totals, computed above. That is,

$$\text{Estimated proportion referred to physician} = \frac{90}{405} = .2222$$

To find the estimated mean number of patients seen by nurse practitioners per community health center, we divide the estimated total number of patients seen by nurse practitioners in all community health centers by the number of community health centers. That is,

$$\text{Estimated mean number of patients seen by nurses per center} = \frac{405}{5} = 81$$

To find the estimated mean number of patients seen per nurse practitioner, we divide the estimated total number of patients seen by nurse practitioners in all community health centers by the total number of nurse practitioners. That is,

$$\text{Estimated mean number of patients seen per nurse practitioner} = \frac{405}{15} = 27$$

The notation used in simple two-stage cluster sampling from clusters having equal numbers of listing units is very similar to the notation used for simple one-stage cluster sampling. This notation is shown in Box 10.1.   □

10.1.3 Estimation of Standard Errors

Using the notation of Box 10.1, we list in Box 10.2, the algebraic formulas used to compute estimated population characteristics and estimated standard errors of these estimated population characteristics. These estimated variances are known as *ultimate cluster variance estimates* and are discussed in the textbook by Hansen, Hurwitz, and Madow [7], who showed that this approach yields a consistent estimate of the variance so long as there are two or more clusters in

---

BOX 10.1   NOTATION USED IN SIMPLE TWO-STAGE CLUSTER SAMPLING

M = number of clusters in the population

m = number of clusters in the sample

x_{ij} = level of characteristic $\mathscr{X}$ for sample listing unit j in sample cluster i

y_{ij} = level of characteristic $\mathscr{Y}$ for sample listing unit j in sample cluster i

$\bar{n}$ = number of listing units sampled from each cluster

n = $m\bar{n}$ = total number of listing units in the sample

x_i = $\sum_{j=1}^{\bar{n}} x_{ij}$; sample total of characteristic $\mathscr{X}$ for the ith sample cluster

y_i = $\sum_{j=1}^{\bar{n}} y_{ij}$ = sample total of characteristic $\mathscr{Y}$ for the ith sample cluster

x = $\sum_{i=1}^{m} x_i$ = sample total for characteristic $\mathscr{X}$

y = $\sum_{i=1}^{m} y_i$ = sample total for characteristic $\mathscr{Y}$

$\bar{N}$ = $\dfrac{N}{M}$ = average number of listing units per cluster in the population

N = $M\bar{N}$ = total number of listing units in the population

f_1 = $\dfrac{m}{M}$ = first-stage sampling fraction

f_2 = $\dfrac{\bar{n}}{\bar{N}}$ = second-stage sampling fraction

f = $f_1 f_2$ = overall sampling fraction

$\bar{x}$ = $\dfrac{x}{m}$ = average level of characteristic $\mathscr{X}$ per cluster in the sample

$\bar{y}$ = $\dfrac{y}{m}$ = average level of characteristic $\mathscr{Y}$ per cluster in the sample

---

the sample and the second-stage sampling in one cluster does not depend on the sampling in other clusters. It should be noted that these ultimate cluster estimates are based on manipulation of the totals, x_i, over the listing units selected in each sample cluster. Also, the mean, $\bar{x}$, appearing in these formulas is not the same as $\bar{x}_{\text{clu}}$, the estimated mean per cluster. In fact, $\bar{x}_{\text{clu}} = (\bar{N}/\bar{n})\bar{x}$.

Use of these formulas with the data given in Table 10.2 is illustrated in the next example.

Illustrative Example. To use the estimation procedures shown in Box 10.2, let us consider the data shown in Table 10.2. We have the following information:

BOX 10.2 ESTIMATED POPULATION CHARACTERISTICS AND ESTIMATED STANDARD ERRORS FOR SIMPLE TWO-STAGE CLUSTER SAMPLING

Total, X

$$x'_{\text{clu}} = \frac{x}{f} \qquad \widehat{\text{SE}}(x'_{\text{clu}}) = \left(\frac{M}{\sqrt{mf_2}}\right)\left[\frac{\sum_{i=1}^{m}(x_i - \bar{x})^2}{m - 1}\right]^{1/2}\left(\frac{N - n}{N}\right)^{1/2}$$

Mean per Cluster, $\bar{X}$

$$\bar{x}_{\text{clu}} = \frac{x'_{\text{clu}}}{M} \qquad \widehat{\text{SE}}(\bar{x}_{\text{clu}}) = \left(\frac{1}{\sqrt{mf_2}}\right)\left[\frac{\sum_{i=1}^{m}(x_i - \bar{x})^2}{m - 1}\right]^{1/2}\left(\frac{N - n}{N}\right)^{1/2}$$

Mean per Listing Unit, $\bar{\bar{X}}$

$$\bar{\bar{x}}_{\text{clu}} = \frac{x'_{\text{clu}}}{N} \qquad \widehat{\text{SE}}(\bar{\bar{x}}_{\text{clu}}) = \left(\frac{1}{\bar{N}\sqrt{mf_2}}\right)\left[\frac{\sum_{i=1}^{m}(x_i - \bar{x})^2}{m - 1}\right]^{1/2}\left(\frac{N - n}{N}\right)^{1/2}$$

Ratio, R

$$r_{\text{clu}} = \frac{y}{x} \qquad \widehat{\text{SE}}(r_{\text{clu}}) = r_{\text{clu}}\sqrt{\frac{N - n}{Nm}}$$

$$\times \left(\frac{\sum_{i=1}^{m}(x_i - \bar{x})^2}{(m - 1)\bar{x}^2} + \frac{\sum_{i=1}^{m}(y_i - \bar{y})^2}{(m - 1)\bar{y}^2} - 2\frac{\sum_{i=1}^{m}(x_i - \bar{x})(y_i - \bar{y})}{(m - 1)\bar{x}\bar{y}}\right)^{1/2}$$

The notation used in these formulas is defined in Box 10.1.

$m = 3$ community health centers in the sample

$M = 5$ community health centers in the population

$\bar{n} = 2$ nurse practitioners sampled from each health center selected

$\bar{N} = 3$ nurse practitioners employed at each health center

$f_1 = \dfrac{m}{M} = \dfrac{3}{5} = .6 =$ first-stage sampling fraction

$f_2 = \dfrac{\bar{n}}{\bar{N}} = \dfrac{2}{3} = .67 =$ second-stage sampling fraction

$f = f_1 f_2 = \dfrac{3}{5} \times \dfrac{2}{3} = .4 =$ overall sampling fraction

$n = 6$ nurse practitioners in sample

$N = 15$ nurse practitioners in the population

First we consider the calculation of y'_{clu}, the total number of patients referred to a physician among those seen by the nurse practitioners in the five centers. The computations for y'_{clu} are

$$y_1 = 12 \qquad y_2 = 5 \qquad y_3 = 19 \qquad y = 36$$

$$y'_{\text{clu}} = \frac{36}{.4} = 90$$

The computations for $\widehat{\text{SE}}(y'_{\text{clu}})$ are

$$\bar{y} = \frac{12 + 5 + 19}{3} = 12$$

$$\frac{\sum_{i=1}^{m}(y_i - \bar{y})^2}{m - 1} = \frac{(12 - 12)^2 + (5 - 12)^2 + (19 - 12)^2}{3 - 1} = 49$$

$$\widehat{\text{SE}}(y'_{\text{clu}}) = \left[\frac{5}{\sqrt{3} \times .67}\right] \times \sqrt{49} \times \sqrt{\frac{15 - 6}{15}} = 23.48$$

A 95% confidence interval for Y is

$$y'_{\text{clu}} - 1.96 \times \widehat{\text{SE}}(y'_{\text{clu}}) \leqslant Y \leqslant y'_{\text{clu}} + 1.96 \times \widehat{\text{SE}}(y'_{\text{clu}})$$

$$90 - 1.96 \times 23.48 \leqslant Y \leqslant 90 + 1.96 \times 23.48$$

$$43.98 \leqslant Y \leqslant 136.02$$

Now we consider the estimation of $\bar{Y}$, the mean number of patients per health center referred to a physician by a nurse practitioner. The computation of $\bar{y}_{\text{clu}}$, the estimate of $\bar{Y}$, is

$$\bar{y}_{\text{clu}} = \frac{90}{5} = 18$$

The computation of $\widehat{SE}(\bar{y}_{clu})$ is

$$\widehat{SE}(\bar{y}_{clu}) = \left[\frac{1}{\sqrt{3} \times .67}\right] \times \sqrt{49} \times \sqrt{\frac{15-6}{15}} = 4.70$$

A 95% confidence interval for $\bar{Y}$ is

$$\bar{y}_{clu} - 1.96 \times \widehat{SE}(\bar{y}_{clu}) \leqslant \bar{Y} \leqslant \bar{y}_{clu} + 1.96 \times \widehat{SE}(\bar{y}_{clu})$$

$$18 - 1.96 \times 4.70 \leqslant \bar{Y} \leqslant 18 + 1.96 \times 4.70$$

$$8.78 \leqslant \bar{Y} \leqslant 27.21$$

Now we consider the estimation of $\bar{\bar{Y}}$, the mean number of patients referred to a physician per nurse practitoner. The computation of $\bar{\bar{y}}_{clu}$, the estimate of $\bar{\bar{Y}}$, is

$$\bar{\bar{y}}_{clu} = \frac{90}{15} = 6$$

The computation of $\widehat{SE}(\bar{\bar{y}}_{clu})$ is

$$\widehat{SE}(\bar{\bar{y}}_{clu}) = \left[\frac{1}{3\sqrt{3} \times .67}\right] \times \sqrt{49} \times \sqrt{\frac{15-6}{15}} = 1.57$$

A 95% confidence interval for $\bar{\bar{Y}}$ is

$$\bar{\bar{y}}_{clu} - 1.96 \times \widehat{SE}(\bar{\bar{y}}_{clu}) \leqslant \bar{\bar{Y}} \leqslant \bar{\bar{y}}_{clu} + 1.96 \times \widehat{SE}(\bar{\bar{y}}_{clu})$$

$$6 - 1.96 \times 1.57 \leqslant \bar{\bar{Y}} \leqslant 6 + 1.96 \times 1.57$$

$$2.92 \leqslant \bar{\bar{Y}} \leqslant 9.08$$

Finally, we consider the estimation of r_{clu}, the proportion of all patients referred to a physician among those seen by nurse practitoners. The computations for r_{clu} are

$$y = 36 \qquad x_1 = 62 \qquad x_2 = 52 \qquad x_3 = 48 \qquad x = 162$$

$$r_{clu} = \frac{36}{162} = .2222.$$

The computations for $\widehat{SE}(r_{clu})$ are

$$\bar{x} = \frac{162}{3} = 54 \qquad \bar{y} = \frac{36}{3} = 12$$

$$\frac{\sum_{i=1}^{m}(y_i - \bar{y})^2}{m-1} = \frac{(12-12)^2 + (5-12)^2 + (19-12)^2}{3-1} = 49$$

$$\frac{\sum_{i=1}^{m}(x_i - \bar{x})^2}{m-1} = \frac{(62-54)^2 + (52-54)^2 + (48-54)^2}{3-1} = 52$$

$$\frac{\sum_{i=1}^{m}(x_1 - \bar{x})(y_i - \bar{y})}{m-1} = \frac{(62-54)(12-12) + (52-54)(5-12) + (48-54)(19-12)}{3-1}$$
$$= -28$$

$$\widehat{SE}(r_{clu}) = .2222\sqrt{\frac{15-6}{(15)(3)}\left(\frac{104}{(3-1)54^2} + \frac{98}{(3-1)12^2} - 2\frac{(-28)}{(3-1)(54)(12)}\right)}^{1/2}$$
$$= .0612$$

A 95% confidence interval for R is

$$r_{clu} - 1.96 \times \widehat{SE}(r_{clu}) \leqslant R \leqslant r_{clu} + 1.96 \times \widehat{SE}(r_{clu})$$

$$.2222 - 1.96 \times .061 \leqslant R \leqslant .2222 + 1.96 \times .061$$

$$.102 \leqslant R \leqslant .342 \qquad\qquad \square$$

Estimation of the population characteristics and their standard errors can be performed using appropriate statistical software, and we illustrate this below for both STATA and SUDAAN. Either of these software packages can be used on the data file, *IL10PT1.DTA* (for STATA) and *IL10PT1.SSD* (for SUDAAN). These files consist of six records (one for each nurse sampled) and contain the following data:

CENTER	NURSE	M	NBAR	W	NPATNTS	NREFRRED
1	2	5	3	2.5	44	6
1	3	5	3	2.5	18	6
2	1	5	3	2.5	42	3
2	3	5	3	2.5	10	2
4	1	5	3	2.5	16	5
4	2	5	3	2.5	32	14

Each record contains the following variables:

CENTER: The particular community health center

NURSE: The particular nurse practitioner sampled

M: The total number of community health centers in the population

NBAR: The total number of nurse practitioners in each community health center

W: The overall sampling weight (reciprocal of the overall sampling fraction)

NPATNTS: The number of patients seen by each sampled nurse practitioner

NREFRRED: The total number of patients referred to a physician by each sampled nurse practitoner

Commands for estimation using STATA

```
Use "a:il10pt1.dta", clear
.svyset psu center
.svyset pweight w
.svytotal nrefrred
.svyratio nrefrred npatnts
```

The first command identifies the data file to be used. The next two commands indicate that the primary sampling unit is identified in the variable, CENTER, and the sampling weight is given in the variable, W. The next command calls for estimation of the total number of patients referred to a physician, and the final command calls for estimation of the proportion of all patients referred to a physician.

Commands for Estimation Using SUDAAN

```
PROC DESCRIPT DATA = IL10PT1 FILETYPE = SAS DESIGN = WOR MEANS TOTALS;
NEST _ONE_ CENTER;
WEIGHT W;
TOTCNT M NBAR;
VAR NPATNTS NREFRRED;
SETENV COLWIDTH = 13;
SETENV DECWIDTH = 3;

PROC RATIO DATA = IL10PT1 FILETYPE = SAS DESIGN = WOR;
NEST _ONE_ CENTER;
WEIGHT W;
TOTCNT M NBAR;
NUMER NREFRRED;
DENOM NPATNTS;
SETENV COLWIDTH = 13;
SETENV DECWIDTH = 3;
```

There are two sets of commands: one set generates estimates of the total number of patients referred to a physician along with the estimated standard error of this estimate, the second set of commands generates the ratio estimate of the proportion of individuals referred to a physician (and the standard error of this estimate).

The first command specifies that the SUDAAN module PROC DESCRIPT will be used, and that the file, IL10PT1.SSD is to be used; that it is a SAS data file; that means and totals are to be generated; and that the particular sample design used is called WOR (acronym for Without Replacement). This, in SUDAAN terminology, indicates that at the first stage of sampling, the clusters are sampled with equal probability without replacement, and that sampling is with equal probability with or without replacement at subsequent stages. The command also indicates that means and totals along with their estimated standard errors are to be estimated.

The second command indicates that the entire population is considered a single stratum, and that the primary sampling units are identified in the variable *CENTER*.

The third command specifies that the sampling weight for each record is in the variable, *W*.

The fourth command indicates that the total number of clusters is specified in the variable, *M*, and that the total number of enumeration units (nurse practitioners in this instance) is specified in the variable *NBAR*.

The fifth command indicates that estimates are to be obtained for the variables *NPATNTS* and *NREFRRED*.

The sixth and seventh statements indicate the form of the output.

The last 8 commands specify that a ratio estimate is to be used to estimate the proportion of patients referred to a physician by the nurse practitioner. The meaning of these commands is clear from the earlier discussion.

The SUDAAN commands shown above are appropriate for a sample design that assumes sampling is without replacement at each stage of the sampling. If one assumes that the sampling is with replacement at each stage (or that the sampling fractions are very small at each stage), then the following set of commands can be used:

```
PROC DESCRIPT DATA = IL10PTI FILETYPE = SAS DESIGN = WR MEANS TOTALS;
NEST _ONE_ CENTER;
WEIGHT W;
VAR NPATNTS NREFRRED;
SETENV COLWIDTH = 13;
SETENV DECWIDTH = 3;
```

```
PROC RATIO DATA = IL10PT1 FILETYPE = SAS DESIGN = WR;
NEST _ONE_ CENTER;
WEIGHT W;
NUMER NREFRRED;
DENOM NPATNTS;
SETENV COLWIDTH = 13;
SETENV DECWIDTH = 3;
```

All of the procedures discussed so far—formulas in Box 10.2, STATA, SUDAAN assuming sampling without replacement at each stage, and SUDAAN assuming sampling with replacement at each stage—would produce the same point estimates. However, there would be differences in the estimated standard errors of the estimates as shown below:

Estimated Standard Errors of Estimates

Estimate	Formulas in Text Box 10.2	Formulas in Text Box 10.2 Without fpc	STATA	SUDAAN Assuming WOR Design	SUDAAN Assuming WR Design
Total patients referred to physician	23.48	30.31	30.31	21.68	30.31
Proportion of patients referred to physician	0.0612	0.081	0.081	0.058	0.081

The standard errors of the estimated total patients referred to a physician not surprisingly are the same (i.e., 30.31) for SUDAAN using the WR design, for STATA, and for the ultimate cluster estimates without the finite population correction (fpc) (formulas in Box 10.2 without fpc factor $\sqrt{(N - n)/N}$. As expected, they are lower for the SUDAAN-WOR design and for the ultimate cluster estimate incorporating the fpc. The two estimates, SUDAAN-WOR and the ultimate cluster, are close to each other but not identical. This is due to the fact that for designs that assume sampling at the first stage is without replacement, SUDAAN uses an estimate based on estimated first- and second-stage components of variance rather than an ultimate cluster estimate.

For the ratio estimate, SUDAAN-WR, STATA, and the ultimate cluster estimate with the fpc not used are in agreement. The estimated variance of the ratio estimate for SUDAAN-WOR and for the ultimate cluster estimate with the fpc are expectedly lower than the others since they use an fpc. As with variance estimates for totals, SUDAAN does not use an ultimate cluster estimate of the variance of ratio estimate; hence, it does not agree with the value obtained using the formula in Box 10.2, although it is very close to that value (.058 as opposed to .0612).

10.1.4 Sampling Distribution of Estimates

Let us consider a simple two-stage cluster sample in which m clusters are chosen at the first stage from the M clusters in the population and, within each sample cluster, $\bar{n}$ listing units are selected from the $\bar{N}$ listing units in the cluster. The total number of possible samples is given by

$$\binom{M}{m}\binom{\bar{N}}{\bar{n}}^{m}$$

Let us refer to the data in Table 10.1 as an example. If we take a simple two-stage cluster sample of two health centers from the five in the population as the first-stage sample, and two nurse practitioners from the three available within each sample health center as the second-stage sample, we can select

$$\binom{5}{2}\binom{3}{2}^{2} = 10 \times 3^2 = 90 \text{ possible samples}$$

From each of these 90 samples, we can estimate population characteristics such as totals, means, and ratios.

In this section we discuss properties of the sampling distributions of the estimated population characteristics. In particular, the means, $E(x'_{\text{clu}})$, $E(\bar{x}_{\text{clu}})$, and $E(\bar{\bar{x}}_{\text{clu}})$, of the sampling distribution of estimated totals, x'_{clu}, estimated means per cluster, $\bar{x}_{\text{clu}}$, and estimated means per listing unit, $\bar{\bar{x}}_{\text{clu}}$, are equal to the corresponding population parameters, X, $\bar{X}$, and $\bar{\bar{X}}$, as defined in Box 9.1. In other words, these are unbiased estimators. Estimated ratios, r_{clu}, on the other hand, are not unbiased, but, as discussed earlier for other sample designs, their biases are generally small for reasonably large sample sizes. The theoretical standard errors of these estimates are given in Box 10.3.

Thus we see that the sampling variances of estimated means and totals from simple two-stage cluster sampling consist of two terms, one depending on the value of σ^2_{1x}, the variance among clusters of the distribution of cluster totals, X_i, and the other depending on σ^2_{2x}, a term representing the variance among listing units within the same cluster with respect to the level of characteristic $\mathcal{X}$. These terms are known as *first-stage* and *second-stage* components, respectively. If every cluster is included in the sample, or, in other words, if $m = M$, then the first-stage components in the expressions shown in Box 10.3 drop out, since the factor $(M - m)(M - 1)$ becomes zero. This makes sense intuitively, because if every cluster is included in the sample, then sampling variability due to differences among the clusters should not be a factor in the sampling distribution of estimates. The resulting estimates are then identical to those for stratified sampling. Similarly, if within each sample cluster, every listing unit is included in the sample, or, in other words, if $\bar{n} = \bar{N}$, then the second-stage components in the expressions seen in Box 10.3 drop out, since the factor $(\bar{N} - \bar{n})/(\bar{N} - 1)$ reduces to zero and the variances of the estimates become identical to those for simple one-stage cluster sampling, shown in Box 9.3. Again, this makes sense intuitively since within each sample cluster every listing unit is included. Hence, there is is no second stage of sampling and the process is, in reality, single stage cluster sampling.

If in Box 10.3 the variance components σ_{1x}^2, σ_{2x}^2, σ_{1y}^2, σ_{2y}^2, etc. are replaced by their appropriate estimators, one would obtain expressions for the estimated standard errors of x'_{clu}, $\bar{x}_{\text{clu}}$, $\bar{\bar{x}}_{\text{clu}}$, and r_{clu} that would differ from the ultimate cluster variance estimators presented in Box 10.2. The estimators based on the components would have lower bias than the ultimate cluster estimates, but could have lower stability especially when $\bar{n}$, the number of listing units sampled within clusters, is small.

Now let us illustrate, with an example, the use of the formulas of Box 10.3.

Illustrative Example. Let us consider the population shown in Table 10.1. Some preliminary calculations for this population are given in Table 10.3; for all calculations we have

$$M = 5 \qquad \bar{N} = 3 \qquad N = 15$$

Based on the information in Table 10.3 and the formulas in Box 10.3, we can make the following calculations:

$$\sigma_{1x}^2 = \frac{2837.20}{5} = 567.44 \qquad \sigma_{1y}^2 = \frac{677.2}{5} = 135.44 \qquad \sigma_{1xy} = \frac{-830.80}{5} = -166.16$$

Using the information in Table 10.4, we have the following calculations:

$$\sigma_{2x}^2 = \frac{2404.01}{15} = 160.27 \qquad \sigma_{2y}^2 = \frac{588.01}{15} = 39.20 \qquad \sigma_{2xy} = \frac{711.65}{15} = 47.44$$

Using the formula given in Box 10.3, we can calculate the theoretical standard error $\text{SE}(x'_{\text{clu}})$ of x'_{clu}, the total number of patients seen by the 15 nurse practitioners as estimated from the two-stage cluster sample of two centers and two nurses within each sample center:

$$\text{SE}(x'_{\text{clu}}) = \left[\frac{5^2}{2} \times 567.44 \times \left(\frac{5-2}{5-1} \right) + \frac{15^2}{4} \times 160.27 \times \left(\frac{3-2}{3-1} \right) \right]^{1/2} = 99.13$$

Similarly, the theoretical standard errors of $\bar{x}_{\text{clu}}$, $\bar{\bar{x}}_{\text{clu}}$, y'_{clu}, and $\bar{\bar{y}}_{\text{clu}}$ can be obtained by substituting the parameters calculated in Tables 10.3 and 10.4 into the appropriate expressions given in Box 10.3. □

BOX 10.3   STANDARD ERRORS FOR POPULATION ESTIMATES UNDER SIMPLE TWO-STAGE CLUSTER SAMPLING

Total, x'_{clu}

$$\text{SE}(x'_{clu}) = \left[\left(\frac{M^2}{m} \right) \sigma_{1x}^2 \left(\frac{M-m}{M-1} \right) + \left(\frac{N^2}{n} \right) \sigma_{2x}^2 \left(\frac{\bar{N} - \bar{n}}{\bar{N} - 1} \right) \right]^{1/2}$$

Mean Per Cluster, $\bar{x}_{clu}$

$$\text{SE}(\bar{x}_{clu}) = \left[\frac{\sigma_{1x}^2}{m} \times \left(\frac{M-m}{M-1} \right) + \left(\frac{\bar{N}^2}{n} \right) \sigma_{2x}^2 \left(\frac{\bar{N} - \bar{n}}{\bar{N} - 1} \right) \right]^{1/2}$$

Mean Per Element, $\bar{\bar{x}}_{clu}$

$$\text{SE}(\bar{\bar{x}}_{clu}) = \left[\left(\frac{1}{\bar{N}^2} \right) \times \frac{\sigma_{1x}^2}{m} \times \left(\frac{M-m}{M-1} \right) + \left(\frac{\sigma_{2x}^2}{n} \right) \left(\frac{\bar{N} - \bar{n}}{\bar{N} - 1} \right) \right]^{1/2}$$

Ratio, r_{clu}

$$\text{SE}(r_{clu}) \approx R \left[\left(\frac{\sigma_{1R}^2}{m\bar{X}^2} \right) \left(\frac{M-m}{M-1} \right) + \left(\frac{\sigma_{2R}^2}{mn\bar{\bar{x}}^2} \right) \left(\frac{\bar{N} - \bar{n}}{\bar{N} - 1} \right) \right]^{1/2}$$

The expression σ_{1x}^2 appearing in these formulas is the variance among cluster totals, defined in Chapter 9, Equation (9.1), as

$$\sigma_{1x}^2 = \frac{\sum_{i=1}^{M}(X_i - \bar{X})^2}{M}$$

BOX 10.3   **Continued**

The expression σ_{2x}^2 appearing in these expressions is given by

$$\sigma_{2x}^2 = \frac{\sum_{i=1}^{M} \sum_{j=1}^{\bar{N}} (X_{ij} - \bar{\bar{X}}_i)^2}{N} \tag{10.1}$$

where $\bar{\bar{X}}_i$ is the mean level of characteristic $\mathscr{X}$ per listing unit for those listing units in cluster i, as given by

$$\bar{\bar{X}}_i = \frac{\sum_{j=1}^{\bar{N}} X_{ij}}{\bar{N}}$$

The formula for the estimated standard error of an estimated ratio r_{clu} is an approximation that is valid whenever the coefficient of variation, $V(\bar{x}_{clu})$, of the denominator of the ratio is less than .05. The parameters σ_{1R}^2 and σ_{2R}^2 appearing in the expression for $SE(r_{clu})$ are given by

$$\sigma_{1R}^2 = \sigma_{1y}^2 + R^2\sigma_{1x}^2 - 2R\sigma_{1xy} \tag{10.2}$$
$$\sigma_{2R}^2 = \sigma_{2y}^2 + R^2\sigma_{2x}^2 - 2R\sigma_{2xy} \tag{10.3}$$

where the expressions σ_{1xy} and σ_{2xy} are first- and second-stage covariances given by

$$\sigma_{1xy} = \frac{\sum_{i=1}^{M}(X_i - \bar{X})(Y_i - \bar{Y})}{M} \tag{10.4}$$

$$\sigma_{2xy} = \frac{\sum_{i=1}^{M} \sum_{j=1}^{\bar{N}} (X_{ij} - \bar{\bar{X}}_i)(Y_{ij} - \bar{\bar{Y}}_i)}{N} \tag{10.5}$$

Other notation used in these formulas is defined in Boxes 9.1 and 101.

Table 10.3   Work Sheet for Calculations Involving Cluster Totals

Cluster	X_i	Y_i	$(X_i - \bar{X})^2$	$(Y_i - \bar{Y})^2$	$(X_i - \bar{X}) \times (Y_i - \bar{Y})$
1	120	17	1,267.36	179.56	−477.04
2	105	24	424.36	40.96	−131.84
3	68	48	268.96	309.76	−288.64
4	58	23	696.96	54.76	195.36
5	71	40	179.56	92.16	−128.64
	$X = 422$	$Y = 152$	2,837.20	677.20	−830.80
	$\bar{X} = 84.4$	$\bar{Y} = 30.4$			
	$\bar{\bar{X}} = 28.13$	$\bar{\bar{Y}} = 10.13$			

10.1.5   How Large a Sample is Needed?

In simple two-stage cluster sampling, as we shall see in a later section, the desired number $\bar{n}$ of listing units to be selected at the second stage from each cluster sampled at the first stage is determined on the basis of costs as well as on the basis of the relative sizes of the first- and second-stage variance components (e.g., σ_{1x}^2, σ_{2x}^2). Once the number $\bar{n}$ has been fixed, we might then wish to determine the total number m of clusters to be selected at the first stage of sampling in order to be $100 \times (1 - \alpha)\%$ confident of obtaining estimates that differ by no more than ε from the true value of the population characteristic being estimated. The formulas used to calculate the *number m of clusters sampled* that would satisfy these specifications are given below.

For estimated *totals* (x'_{clu}) or *means* $(\bar{x}_{clu}, \bar{\bar{x}}_{clu})$,

$$m = \frac{\left(\dfrac{\sigma_{1x}^2}{\bar{\bar{X}}^2}\right) \times \left(\dfrac{M}{M-1}\right) + \left(\dfrac{1}{\bar{n}}\right) \times \left(\dfrac{\sigma_{2x}^2}{\bar{\bar{X}}^2}\right) \times \left(\dfrac{\bar{N} - \bar{n}}{\bar{N} - 1}\right)}{\dfrac{\varepsilon^2}{z_{1-(\alpha/2)}^2} + \dfrac{\sigma_{1x}^2}{\bar{\bar{X}}^2(M-1)}}$$

(10.6)

and for estimated *ratios* $(r_{clu} = y/x)$,

$$m = \frac{\left(\dfrac{\sigma_{1R}^2}{\bar{\bar{X}}^2}\right) \times \left(\dfrac{M}{M-1}\right) + \left(\dfrac{1}{\bar{n}}\right) \times \left(\dfrac{\sigma_{2R}^2}{\bar{\bar{X}}^2}\right) \times \left(\dfrac{\bar{N} - \bar{n}}{\bar{N} - 1}\right)}{\dfrac{\varepsilon^2}{z_{1-(\alpha/2)}^2} + \dfrac{\sigma_{1R}^2}{\bar{\bar{X}}^2(M-1)}}$$

(10.7)

Illustrative Example.   Let us suppose that from the population of nurse practitioners shown in Table 10.1, we wish to take a two-stage cluster sample

Table 10.4 Work Sheet for Calculations Involving Listing Units

Cluster	j	X_{ij}	$\bar{\bar{X}}_i$	$(X_{ij} - \bar{\bar{X}}_i)^2$	Y_{ij}	$\bar{\bar{Y}}_i$	$(Y_{ij} - \bar{\bar{Y}}_i)^2$	$(X_{ij} - \bar{\bar{X}}_i)(Y_{ij} - \bar{\bar{Y}}_i)$
1	1	58		324	5		.45	−12.07
	2	44	40	16	6	5.67	.11	1.32
	3	18		484	6		.11	−7.26
2	1	42		49	3		25	−35
	2	53	35	324	19	8	121	198
	3	10		625	2		36	150
3	1	13		93.51	12		16	38.68
	2	18	22.67	21.81	6	16	100	46.70
	3	37		205.35	30		196	200.62
4	1	16		11.09	5		7.13	8.89
	2	32	19.33	160.53	14	7.67	40.07	80.20
	3	10		87.05	4		13.47	34.24
5	1	25		1.77	17		13.47	4.88
	2	23	23.67	0.45	9	13.33	18.75	2.90
	3	23		0.45	14		.45	−.45
				2404.01			588.01	711.65

with two practitioners selected at the second stage from each health center chosen in the sample at the first stage. Let us suppose that we wish to be 95% confident of obtaining an estimate x'_{clu} of the total number of patients seen by nurse practitioners that is within 30% of the true value and an estimate r_{clu} of the proportion of those patients that are referred to a physician that is also within 30% of the true value. From earler computations we have

$$\sigma^2_{1x} = 567.44 \qquad \sigma^2_{2x} = 160.27 \qquad \bar{X} = 84.4$$
$$\bar{\bar{X}} = 28.13 \qquad M = 5 \qquad \bar{N} = 3$$

Since $\bar{n} = 2$ and $\varepsilon = .3$, we have from relation (10.6)

$$m = \frac{\dfrac{567.44}{84.4^2} \times \dfrac{5}{5-1} + \dfrac{1}{2} \times \dfrac{160.27}{28.13^2} \times \left(\dfrac{3-2}{3-1}\right)}{\dfrac{.3^2}{1.96^2} + \dfrac{567.44}{84.4^2(5-1)}} = 3.47$$

That is, four clusters must be selected.

Using information determined in the previous example, we have

$$R = \frac{Y}{X} = \frac{152}{422} = .3602$$
$$\sigma^2_{1R} = \sigma^2_{1y} + R^2\sigma^2_{1x} - 2R\sigma_{1xy}$$
$$= 135.44 + .3602^2(567.44) - 2(.3602)(-166.16) = 328.76$$
$$\sigma^2_{2R} = \sigma^2_{2y} + R^2\sigma^2_{2x} - 2R\sigma_{2xy}$$
$$= 39.2 + .3602^2(160.27) - 2(.3602)(47.44) = 25.82$$

Then, from relation (10.7), we have

$$m = \frac{\dfrac{328.76}{84.4^2} \times \dfrac{5}{5-1} + \dfrac{1}{2} \times \dfrac{25.82}{28.13^2} \times \left(\dfrac{3-2}{3-1}\right)}{\dfrac{.3^2}{1.96^2} + \dfrac{328.76}{84.4^2(5-1)}} = 1.88$$

That is, two clusters must be selected.

Thus, we would need a first-stage sample of four health centers in order to be 95% confident that the estimated total number of patients seen by nurse practitioners (x'_{clu}) meets the stated specifications. However, we would need a sample of only two health centers in order to be 95% confident that the estimated proportion referred to a physician meets the stated specifications. Therefore, we would take a sample of four health centers if we wish both of these estimates to meet the given specifications.

In practice, the parameters, σ_{1x}^2, σ_{2x}^2, and so forth, which are needed for determination of the required number m of sample clusters, are rarely known and must be either estimated from available data, or guessed from experience or intuition.   □

10.1.6 Choosing the Optimal Cluster Size $\bar{n}$ Considering Costs

Suppose that we wish to choose, from among several sample designs, that design which meets, at the lowest cost, the specifications set on the reliability of the estimates, and suppose that we wish to investigate simple two-stage cluster sampling as a possible design. Simple two-stage cluster sampling, however, is a class of designs characterized by a first-stage number m of clusters and a second-stage number $\bar{n}$ of listing units. The problem then, is to investigate which combination of m and $\bar{n}$ would meet the required specifications at the lowest cost. Let us explore this problem through an example.

Illustrative Example. Let us use the population of five housing projects shown in Table 9.1. We have already discussed the cost components associated with this example for simple random sampling, stratified random sampling, and simple one-stage cluster sampling. In particular, we showed that for simple one-stage cluster sampling, the approximate field costs C are characterized by the following function [Equation (9.3)]:

$$C = C_1'm + C_2'm\bar{N}.$$

The *field costs* for a two-stage simple cluster sample can be approximated by a similar function of the form

$$C = C_1^*m + C_2^*m\bar{n} \tag{10.8}$$

where C_1^* is composed of the cost of traveling to each sample cluster for the purpose of listing the $\bar{N}$ sampling units, the cost of listing these $\bar{N}$ listing units, the cost of selecting a sample of $\bar{n}$ units from each list, and the cost of traveling back to the cluster to do the interviewing. C_2^* is the cost of interviewing each of the sampling units selected.

In the example considered in Chapter 9, it cost .5 person-hours to travel to each of the sample clusters. Suppose it costs 1 person-hour to list the 20 sampling units in the selected clusters and to then select a random sample of these sampling units, and it costs .5 person-hours to return to the cluster for the purpose of interviewing. Hence, $C_1^* = .50 + 1.00 + .50 = 2.00$. Also, as in the example of Chapter 9, the cost of interviewing each of the sampled households is .25 person-hours. Hence, $C_2^* = .25$, and the cost function (10.8) then becomes

$$C = 2.00m + .25m\bar{n}$$

Note that the expressions $m\bar{N}$ appearing in the second term of relation (9.3) is the total number of listing units included in the sample for the simple one-stage cluster sampling design. Likewise, the expression $m\bar{n}$ appearing in the second term of relation (10.8) is the number of listing units included in the sample for the simple two-stage cluster sampling design. Thus, the cost functions (9.3) and (10.8) are very similar.

Suppose that we wish to estimate the total number of persons in the five housing developments and we wish to be virtually certain that this estimate will be within 25% of the true value. Let us examine, using relation (10.6), the number of clusters m required to meet this specification for various second-stage cluster sizes $\bar{n}$. Then we will use relation (10.8) to determine the field costs for each of these designs. Those designs that satisfy the specification are listed in Table 10.5.

To illustrate how computations in Table 10.5 are made, let us consider a simple two-stage cluster sampling design with the number of households to be sampled set equal to 5 (i.e., $\bar{n} = 5$). From Table 9.1 we can calculate the following:

$$\sigma_{1y}^2 = 6.8 \qquad \bar{Y} = 34 \qquad \sigma_{2y}^2 = .693$$
$$\bar{\bar{Y}} = 1.7 \qquad M = 5 \qquad \bar{N} = 20$$

Table 10.5 Designs Satisfying Specifications on Total

Number of Listing Units Taken in Second Stage, $\bar{n}$	Number of Clusters m Needed to Meet Specification $\varepsilon = .25$	Field Cost (in person-hours) $C = 2.0m + .25m\bar{n}$
6	5	17.5
7	4	15.0
8	4	16.0
9	3	12.75
10	3	13.5
11	3	14.25
12	2	10.0
13	2	10.5
14	2	11.0
15	2	11.5
16	2	12.0
17	2	12.5
18	2	13.0
19	1	6.75
20	1	7.0

Then from relation (10.6) we have

$$m = \frac{\dfrac{6.8}{34^2} \times \dfrac{5}{5-1} + \dfrac{1}{5} \times \dfrac{.693}{1.7^2} \times \left(\dfrac{20-5}{20-1}\right)}{\dfrac{(.25)^2}{3^2} + \dfrac{6.8}{34^2(5-1)}} = 5.23$$

That is, six clusters must be selected. Thus, it would take a sample of six clusters to meet the specification. Since there are only five clusters in the population, it would be impossible for the specification to be met if $\bar{n} = 5$.

Let us now set $\bar{n} = 6$. From relation (10.6), we have

$$m = \frac{\dfrac{6.8}{34^2} \times \dfrac{5}{5-1} + \dfrac{1}{6} \times \dfrac{.693}{1.7^2} \times \left(\dfrac{20-6}{20-1}\right)}{\dfrac{(.25)^2}{3^2} + \dfrac{6.8}{34^2(5-1)}} = 4.37$$

That is, five clusters must be selected. Thus a sample of $m = 5$ clusters (i.e., every cluster in the population) would meet the specification if $\bar{n} = 6$. The field costs of such a sample design are

$$C = 2.00 \times 5 + .25 \times 5 \times 6 = 17.5 \text{ person-hours}$$

Among all the simple two-stage cluster sampling designs listed in Table 10.5 that satisfy the specifications, the design characterized by a first-stage selection of $m = 1$ cluster followed by a second-stage sample of $\bar{n} = 19$ listing units would do so at the lowest possible field costs (i.e., 6.75 person-hours) and hence would be the design of choice.

If we wished to estimate a ratio—for example, the proportion R of all persons requiring the services of a visiting nurse—we would go through the same process, except that we would use relation (10.7) rather than relation (10.6). If we set $\varepsilon = .25$ again, the two-stage cluster sampling designs listed in Table 10.6 would satisfy this specification on the estimated ratio.

From the data in Table 9.1 we can calculate the following values in order to determine the costs given in Table 10.6: $X = 60$, $Y = 170$, $R = .35294$, $\sigma_{1x}^2 = 23.6$, $\sigma_{1y}^2 = 6.8$, $\sigma_{1xy} = 2.6$, $\sigma_{2y}^2 = .693$, $\sigma_{2x}^2 = .321$, $\sigma_{2xy} = .1435$, $\sigma_{1R}^2 = 22.61$, $\sigma_{2R}^2 = .3060$.

Examining Table 10.6, we see that a two-stage cluster sample with all five housing developments sampled at the first stage and 12 households sampled from each housing development at the second stage would be the design that would satisfy, at the lowest field costs, the specification set for estimation of the proportion R of persons requiring the services of a visiting nurse. $\square$

Table 10.6   Designs Satisfying Specifications on Ratio

Number of Listing Units Taken in Second Stage, $\bar{n}$	Number of Clusters m Needed to Meet Specification $\varepsilon = .25$	Field Cost (in person-hours), $C = 2.0m + .25m\bar{n}$
12	5	25.00
13	5	26.25
14	5	27.50
15	5	28.75
16	5	30.00
17	5	31.25
18	5	32.50
19	5	33.75
20	5	35.00

10.1.7   Some Shortcut Formulas for Determining the Optimal Number $\bar{n}$

In the previous section we chose, in the following way, the values of $\bar{n}$ and m that would meet the specifications at the lowest possible field costs. We enumerated all possible combinations of m and $\bar{n}$, eliminating those combinations that would not meet the specifications [by use of relations (10.6) and (10.7)]. Then, from among those designs remaining, we chose the one that would meet the specifications at the lowest possible cost. This process can be very tedious, especially if M and $\bar{N}$ are large numbers.

There is a shortcut formula that can be used for choosing the optimal value of $\bar{n}$. It is useful if the field costs can be approximated by a function of the form $C_1^* m + C_2^* m\bar{n}$ and if the number of clusters M in the population is large in comparison with the number of clusters chosen in the sample. This formula (valid for estimating means or totals) is

$$\bar{n} = \left[\left(\frac{C_1^*}{C_2^*}\right)\left(\frac{1 - \delta_x}{\delta_x}\right)\right]^{1/2} \tag{10.9}$$

where C_1^* and C_2^* are the cost components introduced earlier, and δ_x is the *intraclass correlation coefficient* defined previously in our discussion of systematic sampling [Equation (4.5)]. It can be expressed in the form

$$\delta_x = \frac{(1/\bar{N})\sigma_{1x}^2 - \sigma_x^2}{(\bar{N} - 1)\sigma_x^2} \tag{10.10}$$

which is algebraically identical to expression (4.5) provided that the number of listing units N_i are the same for each cluster.

Once the optimal cluster size $\bar{n}$ is obtained from relation (10.9), the number m of clusters to be selected at the first stage is then obtained from relation (10.6).

For estimation of ratios, relations (10.9) and (10.10) are modified as follows:

$$\bar{n} = \left[\left(\frac{C_1^*}{C_2^*}\right)\left(\frac{1 - \delta_R}{\delta_R}\right)\right]^{1/2} \tag{10.11}$$

and

$$\delta_R = \frac{(1/\bar{N})\sigma_{1R}^2 - \sigma_R^2}{(\bar{N} - 1)\sigma_R^2} \tag{10.12}$$

To illustrate these concepts, let us consider the following example.

Illustrative Example. Suppose that a survey is to be taken in a general hospital for purposes of estimating the total amount of money billed to Medicare during a particular quarter (13 weeks). A cluster sample is to be selected by taking a simple random sample of weeks followed by a simple random sample of days within each selected week. For each day chosen in the sample, the amount billed to Medicare is obtained by a review of all items billed during that day. The data for the entire quarter (not known, of course, in advance of the survey) are shown, by days, in Table 10.7.

With weeks as clusters, days as listing units, and X as the amount billed to Medicare on a particular day, we have the following calculations:

$$\sigma_x^2 = \frac{\sum_{i=1}^{13} \sum_{j=1}^{7}(X_{ij} - \bar{\bar{X}})^2}{91} = 1304.58 \qquad \sigma_{1x}^2 = \frac{\sum_{i=1}^{13}(X_i - \bar{X})^2}{13} = 26{,}624.44$$

$$\bar{\bar{X}} = 110.45 \qquad \bar{X} = 773.15 \qquad \sigma_{2x}^2 = 761.22$$
$$M = 13 \qquad \bar{N} = 7 \qquad N = 91$$

$$\delta_x = \frac{(1/7)(26,\,624.44) - 1304.58}{(7 - 1)(1304.58)} = .3192$$

Let us now consider the field costs that might be involved in collecting the data. For each day selected in the sample it would be necessary to obtain data pertaining to the amount billed on that day to Medicare for each patient hospitalized. This could take a considerable amount of record retrieval and abstracting. Let us assume that there are an average of five patients per day in the hospital who are covered by Medicare and that for each patient 0.5 hour of time is required for retrieval and abstracting on the part of a research assistant who is paid $8.00 per hour. In addition, let us assume that for each patient it costs approximately $6.00 to code the data, prepare it for the computer, and process it. Then the total cost C_2^* per listing unit (day) selected in the sample is

Table 10.7 Amount of Money Billed to Medicare by Day and Week

Week	Sunday	Monday	Tuesday	Wednesday	Thursday	Friday	Saturday	X_i	$\sum(X_{ij} - \bar{X}_i)^2$
				Amount Billed ($\times\$10$)					
1	121	88	138	69	85	59	63	623	5418
2	152	105	179	127	145	116	165	989	4273.43
3	134	62	44	128	92	127	141	728	8882
4	94	123	81	109	110	101	34	652	5134.86
5	210	182	120	120	154	98	178	1062	9907.43
6	104	100	70	115	142	139	131	801	3929.71
7	80	43	59	50	20	69	64	385	2312
8	123	59	140	146	149	109	111	837	5847.71
9	137	168	84	120	123	87	121	840	4988
10	110	132	104	65	97	98	84	690	2619.71
11	158	114	93	147	91	125	132	860	3890.86
12	79	156	142	154	133	74	83	821	8219.43
13	97	96	110	83	89	146	142	763	3848

$C_2^* = (5 \text{ patients per day}) \times (.5 \times 8.00 + 6.00) \text{ per patient} = \$50.00 \text{ per day}$

Let us suppose that patient cost records are organized on computer tape by week and that for each week chosen in the sample the *entire week's* records must be listed by computer in order for the daily costs to be identified and that this costs \$100 in computer time and other data processing costs. Let us assume that other costs associated with the clusters (weeks) are negligible, so that the cost component C_1^* is given by

$$C_1^* = \$100 \text{ per sample week}$$

Since $\delta_x \approx .32$ for these data, we have the optimal cluster size $\bar{n}$ given by

$$\bar{n} = \sqrt{\left(\frac{100}{50}\right)\left(\frac{.68}{.32}\right)} \approx 2$$

Then from relation (10.6) with $M = 13, \bar{n} = 2, \sigma_{1x}^2 = 26{,}624.44, \sigma_{2x}^2 = 761.22$, $\bar{\bar{X}} = 110.45, \bar{X} = 773.15$, and $\bar{N} = 7$, if we wish to be virtually certain of estimating the total amount of money billed to Medicare during the quarter to within 25% of the true value (i.e., $\varepsilon = .25$) we have

$$m = \frac{\dfrac{26{,}624.44}{(773.15)^2} \times \dfrac{13}{13 - 1} + \dfrac{1}{2} \times \dfrac{761.22}{(110.45)^2} \times \left(\dfrac{7 - 2}{7 - 1}\right)}{\dfrac{(.25)^2}{3^2} + \dfrac{26{,}624.44}{(773.15)^2(13 - 1)}} = 6.97$$

Hence, seven clusters must be selected.

Thus with a two-stage cluster sample of $m = 7$ weeks and $\bar{n} = 2$ days, the specifications can be met at minimal cost in relation to other two-stage cluster sampling designs. This can be verified by examining the costs of other cluster sampling designs meeting these specifications, as shown in Table 10.8

The intraclass correlation coefficient δ_x is a parameter that is very important in sampling theory. It is useful, as shown above, in determining the optimal number of listing units that should be selected at the second stage of cluster sampling. It is also useful in relating the standard error of an estimated mean or total from a two-stage cluster sample to one that would have been obtained from a simple random sample of the same number of listing units. If the number M of clusters in the population is large in comparison to the number selected at the first stage of sampling, then the following relations are true:

Table 10.8 Designs Satisfying Specifications on Total

Number of Listing Units in Sample, $\bar{n}$	Number of Clusters, m, Needed to Meet Specification $\varepsilon = .25$	Field Costs (in dollars), $C = 100m + 50m\bar{n}$
1	10	1,500
2	7	1,400
3	7	1,750
4	6	1,800
5	6	2,100
6	6	2,400
7	6	2,700

$$\text{SE}(x'_{\text{clu}}) = \left(\frac{N\sigma_x}{\sqrt{n}}\right)\sqrt{1 + \delta_x(\bar{n} - 1)} \tag{10.13}$$

$$\text{SE}(\bar{x}_{\text{clu}}) = \left(\frac{N\sigma_x}{\sqrt{Mn}}\right)\sqrt{1 + \delta_x(\bar{n} - 1)} \tag{10.14}$$

$$\text{SE}(\bar{\bar{x}}_{\text{clu}}) = \left(\frac{\sigma_x}{\sqrt{n}}\right)\sqrt{1 + \delta_x(\bar{n} - 1)} \tag{10.15}$$

These relations are important because they show that the standard errors of estimated means and totals obtained from cluster samples are approximately $\sqrt{1 + \delta_x(\bar{n} - 1)}$ times as large as those obtained from a simple random sample of the same number n of listing units. This factor, $\sqrt{1 + \delta_x(\bar{n} - 1)}$, is known as the *design effect* and depends on the intraclass correlation coefficient δ_x as well as the number $\bar{n}$ of listing units sampled in each cluster.

It can be seen by algebraic manipulation of relation (10.10) that the intraclass correlation coefficient δ_x is a number lying between $-1/(\bar{N} - 1)$ and $+1$. It is essentially a measure of the homogeneity of listing units within clusters with respect to levels of the characteristic $\mathscr{X}$ being measured. If listing units within clusters tend to be similar in this respect, the value of δ_x will tend to be high and the design effect $\sqrt{1 + \delta_x(\bar{n} - 1)}$ would be potentially high if $\bar{n}$ were large. This makes sense intuitively because a high value of δ_x implies that taking a large number of listing units within a sample cluster would be a wasteful procedure, since the listing units within clusters are similar with respect to levels of the characteristic $\mathscr{X}$ being measured.

Knowledge of the value of δ_x for different types of clusters and different variables is extremely useful in planning surveys. More detailed discussion of this is available in other texts, [1, 2].   □

10.2 SITUATION IN WHICH NOT ALL CLUSTERS HAVE THE SAME NUMBER, N_i, OF ENUMERATION UNITS

In the previous section, we assumed the very limited scenario that all clusters used as primary sampling units have the same number of enumeration units. This situation led to relatively simple formulas for estimating population parameters and for estimating the standard errors of such estimates. In most situations involving the sampling of human populations, however, the primary sampling units do not contain the same number of enumeration units. As will be discussed in the next chapter, the strategy of sampling clusters with equal probability and having approximately equal second-stage sampling fractions within each sample cluster will often result in large sampling errors—especially in estimation of population totals. Keeping this in mind, we will nevertheless devote the remainder of this chapter to estimation of population parameters from two-stage simple cluster sampling designs when there are differences among clusters with respect to the number of enumeration units within clusters.

10.2.1 How to Take a Simple Two-Stage Cluster Sample for This Design

As before, the clusters will be selected by labeling them from 1 to M and then taking m random numbers between 1 and M. Those clusters corresponding to the random numbers selected will be in the sample. Within each sample cluster, we then take a simple random sample of n_i enumeration units, where n_i is chosen in such a way that the second-stage sampling fraction, n_i/N_i, is as close as possible to the predetermined second-stage sampling fraction, f_2, which has been set for each sample cluster.

With this in mind, we would label the listing units within the ith cluster selected at the first stage from 1 to N_i, and choose n_i different random numbers between 1 and N_i. Those listing units corresponding to the random numbers would appear in the sample.

We illustrate the procedure in the following example.

Illustrative Example. Let us consider an administrative area containing 10 hospitals, with total 1987 admissions, total 1987 admissions with life-threatening conditions, and total 1987 admissions discharged dead as given in Table 10.9.

Let us suppose that we wish to take a simple random sample of three hospitals and within each selected hospital, take a simple random sample of approximately 5% of all admission records for purposes of estimating the total number of patients discharged dead among all patients admitted to these ten hospitals with life-threatening conditions. To do this, we first choose three random numbers between 1 and 10 (e.g. 1, 2, and 8). We then identify each admission within each sample hospital with a number from 1 to N_i, and then choose by random numbers that number n_i of admissions that makes the ratio n_i/N_i closest to .05, the desired second-stage sampling fraction. For example, in

Table 10.9   Total Admissions with Life-Threatening Conditions, and Total Admissions Discharged Dead from Ten Hospitals, 1987

Hospital	Total Admissions	Total with Life-Threatening Conditions	Total Discharged Dead Among Those with Life-threatening Conditions
1	4,288	501	42
2	5,036	785	78
3	1,178	213	17
4	638	173	9
5	27,010	3404	338
6	1,122	217	17
7	2,134	424	37
8	1,824	246	18
9	4,672	778	68
10	2,154	346	27

hospital 1, $N_1 = 4288$ and $.05 \times 4288 = 214.4$. Thus we would take $n_1 = 214$ admissions from hospital 1. In a similar manner, we would decide to select $n_2 = 252$ admissions from hospital 2 and $n_3 = 91$ admissions from hospital 8.

10.2.2   Estimation of Population Characteristics

Estimated totals, means, and ratios from this type of cluster sampling, in which there are unequal numbers N_i of listing units in each sample cluster, are defined in Box 10.4.

Note that if the number N_i of listing units is the same for each cluster (i.e., $N_i = \bar{N}$) and if the second-stage sampling fraction is the same for each sample cluster (i.e., $n_i = \bar{n}$), then the formulas shown in Box 10.4 reduce to those shown in Box 10.2.   □

10.2.3   Estimation of Standard Errors of Estimates

Estimating the standard errors of estimates obtained from sampling clusters having unequal numbers of listing units is somewhat cumbersome when the clusters are chosen by simple random sampling. If, however, the second-stage sampling fractions, $f_2 = n_i/N_i$, are the same for each cluster, then the ultimate cluster estimates shown in Box 10.2 can be used. To illustrate let us look at an example.

Illustrative Example.   Let us suppose that a simple random sample of three hospitals was taken from the population of ten hospitals shown in Table 10.9

BOX 10.4 ESTIMATES OF POPULATION CHARACTERISTICS UNDER SIMPLE TWO-STAGE CLUSTER SAMPLING, UNEQUAL NUMBERS OF LISTING UNITS

Total, x'_{clu}

$$x'_{\text{clu}} = \left(\frac{M}{m}\right) \times \sum_{i=1}^{m} \left(\frac{N_i}{n_i}\right) \sum_{j=1}^{n_i} x_{ij}$$

Mean Per Cluster, $\bar{x}_{\text{clu}}$

$$\bar{x}_{\text{clu}} = \left(\frac{1}{m}\right) \times \sum_{i=1}^{m} \left(\frac{N_i}{n_i}\right) \sum_{j=1}^{n_i} x_{ij}$$

Mean Per Listing Unit, $\bar{\bar{x}}_{\text{clu}}$

$$\bar{\bar{x}}_{\text{clu}} = \frac{x'_{\text{clu}}}{N}$$

The above formula is usable when the total number N of listing units is known in advance of the sampling. When N is not known, the mean per listing unit can be estimated by use of a ratio estimate where the denominator is an estimate from the sample of the number of listing units in the population. This ratio estimate often has lower variance than the estimate $\bar{\bar{x}}_{\text{clu}}$, even when the latter can be used.

Ratio, r_{clu}

$$r_{\text{clu}} = \frac{\bar{x}_{\text{clu}}}{\bar{y}_{\text{clu}}}$$

where N_i is the number of listing units in each cluster, n_i is the number of listing units sampled from each cluster, and other notation is as defined in Box 10.1.

and that a subsample of 10% (to the nearest integer) was taken from the hospitals selected in the sample. Suppose that hospitals 1, 4, and 10 were selected and that the data shown in Table 10.10 were obtained. We will use these data and the formulas given in Boxes 10.4 and 10.2 to estimate population parameters and standard errors.

First we consider estimation of the total number of persons discharged dead among those with life-threatening conditions. The computations for x'_{clu} are as follows:

$$x_1 = 5 \qquad N_1 = 4288 \qquad n_1 = 429 \qquad \left(\frac{N_1}{n_1}\right)x_1 = 49.98$$

$$x_2 = 7 \qquad N_2 = 638 \qquad n_2 = 64 \qquad \left(\frac{N_2}{n_2}\right)x_2 = 69.78$$

$$x_3 = 3 \qquad N_3 = 2154 \qquad n_3 = 215 \qquad \left(\frac{N_3}{n_3}\right)x_3 = 30.06$$

$$M = 10 \qquad m = 3$$

$$x'_{clu} = \left(\frac{M}{m}\right) \times \sum_{i=1}^{m}\left(\frac{N_i}{n_i}\right)x_i = \left(\frac{10}{3}\right)(49.98 + 69.78 + 30.06) = 499.38$$

The computations for $\widehat{SE}(x'_{clu})$ are

$$\bar{x} = \frac{5+7+3}{3} = 5 \qquad f_2 = .10 \qquad N = 50{,}056 \qquad n = 708$$

Table 10.10 Summary Data for a Sample of Three Hospitals Selected from the Ten Hospitals in Table 10.9

Hospital	Total Admissions, N_i	Total Admissions Sampled, n_i	Total Patients with Life-Threatening Conditions, y_i	Total Patients Discharged Dead Among Those with Life-Threatening Conditions, x_i
1	4,288	429	47	5
4	638	64	17	7
10	2,154	215	24	3
Total	7,080	708	88	15

$$\frac{\sum_{i=1}^{m}(x_i - \bar{x})^2}{m-1} = \frac{(5-5)^2 + (7-5)^2 + (3-5)^2}{3-1} = 4$$

$$\widehat{SE}(x'_{\text{clu}}) = \left(\frac{10}{\sqrt{3} \times .10}\right)\sqrt{4}\sqrt{\frac{50,056 - 708}{50,056}} = 114.65$$

A 95% confidence interval for X is

$$x'_{\text{clu}} - 1.96 \times \widehat{SE}(x'_{\text{clu}}) \leqslant X \leqslant x'_{\text{clu}} + 1.96 \times \widehat{SE}(x'_{\text{clu}})$$

$$499.38 - 1.96 \times 114.65 \leqslant X \leqslant 499.38 + 1.96 \times 114.65$$

$$274.67 \leqslant X \leqslant 724.09$$

Next, we consider estimation of the mean number of persons discharged dead per hospital among those having life-threatening conditions. The computation of $\bar{x}_{\text{clu}}$ is

$$\bar{x}_{\text{clu}} = \left(\frac{1}{m}\right)\left[\sum_{i=1}^{m}\left(\frac{N_i}{n_i}\right)x_i\right] = \left(\frac{1}{3}\right)(49.98 + 69.78 + 30.06) = 49.94$$

The computation of $\widehat{SE}(\bar{x}_{\text{clu}})$ is

$$\widehat{SE}(\bar{x}_{\text{clu}}) = \left(\frac{1}{(.10)\sqrt{3}}\right)\sqrt{4}\sqrt{\frac{50,056 - 708}{50,056}} = 11.47$$

A 95% confidence interval for $\bar{X}$ is

$$\bar{x}_{\text{clu}} - 1.96 \times \widehat{SE}(\bar{x}_{\text{clu}}) \leqslant \bar{X} \leqslant \bar{x}_{\text{clu}} + 1.96 \times \widehat{SE}(\bar{x}_{\text{clu}})$$

$$49.94 - 1.96 \times 11.47 \leqslant \bar{X} \leqslant 49.94 + 1.96 \times 11.47$$

$$27.46 \leqslant \bar{X} \leqslant 72.42$$

Next we consider the mean number of persons discharged dead per person admitted to the hospital. The computation of $\bar{\bar{x}}_{\text{clu}}$ is

$$\bar{\bar{x}}_{\text{clu}} = \frac{x'_{\text{clu}}}{N} = \frac{499.38}{50,056} = .0098$$

The computation of $\widehat{SE}(\bar{\bar{x}}_{\text{clu}})$ is

$$\widehat{SE}(\bar{\bar{x}}_{\text{clu}}) = \left(\frac{10}{5005.6\sqrt{3}(.10)}\right)\sqrt{4}\sqrt{\frac{50,056 - 708}{50,056}} = .0023$$

A 95% confidence interval for $\bar{\bar{X}}$ is

$$\bar{x}_{\text{clu}} - 1.96 \times \widehat{\text{SE}}(\bar{x}_{\text{clu}}) \leqslant \bar{\bar{X}} \leqslant \bar{x}_{\text{clu}} + 1.96 \times \widehat{\text{SE}}(\bar{x}_{\text{clu}})$$

$$.0098 - 1.96 \times .0023 \leqslant \bar{\bar{X}} \leqslant .0098 + 1.96 \times .0023$$

$$.0053 \leqslant \bar{\bar{X}} \leqslant .0143$$

Finally, we consider estimation of the proportion of persons discharged dead among those having life-threatening conditions. The computations for r_{clu} are

$$\bar{y}_{\text{clu}} = \left(\frac{1}{m}\right)\left[\sum_{i=1}^{m}\left(\frac{N_i}{n_i}\right)y_i\right] = \left(\frac{1}{3}\right)\left[\left(\frac{4,288}{429}\right)(47) + \left(\frac{638}{64}\right)(17) + \left(\frac{2,154}{215}\right)(24)\right]$$

$$= 293.23$$

$$r_{\text{clu}} = \frac{\bar{x}_{\text{clu}}}{\bar{y}_{\text{clu}}} = \frac{49.94}{293.23} = .1703$$

The computations for $\widehat{\text{SE}}(r_{\text{clu}})$ are

$$\bar{x} = \frac{5+7+3}{3} = 5 \qquad \bar{y} = \frac{47+17+24}{3} = 29.33$$

$$\frac{\sum\limits_{i=1}^{m}(y_i - \bar{y})^2}{m-1} = 246.33$$

$$\frac{\sum\limits_{i=1}^{m}(x_i - \bar{x})^2}{m-1} = 4.00$$

$$\frac{\sum\limits_{i=1}^{m}(x_i - \bar{x})(y_i - \bar{y})}{m-1} = -7$$

$$\widehat{\text{SE}}(r_{\text{clu}}) = 0.1703\sqrt{\frac{50,056 - 708}{(50,056 \times 3)}\left(\frac{4}{5^2} + \frac{246.33}{29.33^2} - 2\frac{(-7)}{(5 \times 29.33)}\right)^{1/2}} = 0.0719$$

A 95% confidence interval for R is

$$r_{\text{clu}} - 1.96 \times \widehat{\text{SE}}(r_{\text{clu}}) \leqslant R \leqslant r_{\text{clu}} + 1.96 \times \widehat{\text{SE}}(r_{\text{clu}})$$

$$.1703 - 1.96 \times .0719 \leqslant R \leqslant .1703 + 1.96 \times .0719$$

$$.0294 \leqslant R \leqslant .3112$$

It should be emphasized that the expressions for the estimated standard errors of estimates are applicable only if the clusters are selected by simple random sampling and the sampling fraction of listing units taken at the second stage is the same for each cluster selected in the sample. Under this allocation every listing unit in the population has the same chance of being selected in the sample. In other words, the sample is self-weighting, as we discussed earlier in terms of stratified sampling. For sample designs that are not self-weighting, variance estimation becomes much more complicated. □

As with previous sampling designs, estimation of population parameters and their standard errors can be performed using appropriate statistical software, and we show below how this can be accomplished using STATA and SUDAAN. The data file needed for processing consists of 708 records containing information on sample patients (enumeration units) admitted to the three sample hospitals (clusters or PSU's). The format of these records and the variables used in the computations are shown below:

HOSPNO	ID	LIFETHRT	DXDEAD	M	NI	W
1	1	1	1	10	4288	33.31779
1	2	1	1	10	4288	33.31779
⋮	⋮	⋮	⋮	⋮	⋮	⋮
1	429	0	0	10	4288	33.31779
4	1	1	1	10	638	33.22916
4	2	1	1	10	638	33.22916
⋮	⋮	⋮	⋮	⋮	⋮	⋮
4	64	0	0	10	638	33.22916
10	1	1	0	10	2154	33.39535
10	2	1	0	10	2154	33.39535
⋮	⋮	⋮	⋮	⋮	⋮	⋮
10	215	0	0	10	2154	33.39535

HOSPNO is the identification number of the sample hospital to which the patient was admitted.

ID is a number identifying the particular patient.

LIFETHRT is a variable indicating whether or not the patient was admitted with a life-threatening condition.

DXDEAD is a variable indicating whether or not the patient was discharged dead.

M indicates the number of primary sampling units or clusters in the population from which the sample was selected. This is used by SUDAAN in determining a finite population correction for the first stage of sampling.

NI indicates the total number of enumeration units (e.g., patients admitted to the hospital) in the ith cluster (e.g., hospital). Note, that it is not the same for each cluster. This is used by SUDAAN in determining a finite population correction for the second stage of sampling.

W is the sampling weight (inverse of overall sampling fraction) for each record. Note that it is *not* exactly the same for each cluster since differences among clusters in total number of enumeration units make it impossible to obtain exactly the same second-stage sampling fraction.

The following STATA commands are used with the STATA data file, *il10pt2.dta*, which has a structure in the form shown above.

```
use "a:\il10pt2.dta", clear
.svyset psu hospno
.svyset pweight w
.svytotal dxdead
.svyratio dxdead lifethrt
```

The first two commands indicate the cluster and sampling weight variables, and the last two commands indicate the estimation procedures to be performed. As stated earlier, STATA does not use finite population corrections in its estimation procedures for cluster sampling. The STATA output generated from these commands is shown below:

Survey total estimation

pweight:	w		Number of obs	=	708
Strata:	< one >		Number of strata	=	1
PSU:	hospno		Number of PSUs	=	3
			Population size	=	23600

Total	Estimate	Std. Err.	[95% Conf. Inteval]		Deff
dxdead	499.3792	114.6776	5.961245	992.7971	.8059769

. svyratio dxdead lifethrt

Survey ratio estimation

pweight:	w		Number of obs	=	708
Strata:	< one >		Number of strata	=	1
PSU:	hospno		Population PSUs	=	3
			Population size	=	23600

Ratio	Estimate	Std Err.	[95% Conf. Interval]		Deff
dxdead/lifethrt	.1703017	.072273	−.140664	.4812674	3.247372

The following commands are used in SUDAAN to estimate the total and proportion discharged dead among persons having life-threatening conditions:

```
1 PROC DESCRIPT DATA=IL10PT2 FILETYPE=SAS DESIGN=WOR MEANS
   TOTALS;
2 NEST _ONE_ HOSPNO;
```

```
 3 WEIGHT W;
 4 TOTCNT M NI;
 5 VAR DXDEAD LIFETHRT;
 6 SETENV COLWIDTH = 13;
 7 SETENV DECWIDTH = 3;
 8 PROC RATIO DATA = IL10PT2 FILETYPE = SAS DESIGN = WOR;
 9 NEST _ONE_ HOSPNO;
10 WEIGHT W;
11 TOTCNT M NI;
12 NUMER DXDEAD;
13 DENOM LIFETHRT;
14 SETENV COLWIDTH = 13;
15 SETENV DECWIDTH = 3;
```

The output generated by SUDAAN is shown overleaf.

The estimated standard errors generated by three different methods of estimation (Text, STATA, and SUDAAN) are shown below. All three methods generate the same point estimates. It should be remembered that STATA does not make use of finite population corrections in its estimation procedure for cluster sampling.

Estimated Standard Errors of Estimates

Estimate	Point Estimate	Standard Error of Estimate from Formulas in Text Box 10.5	Standard Error of Estimate from STATA	Standard Error of Estimate from SUDAAN Assuming WOR Design	Standard Error of Estimate from SUDAAN Assuming WR Design
Total number of persons discharged dead	499.38	114.65	114.68	116.07	114.68
Proportion of patients discharged dead among those diagnosed with life-threatening condition	0.1703	0.072	0.072	0.064	0.072

As shown above, the estimated standard errors produced by the three methods are very close to each other.

Number of observations read: 708   Weighted count: 23600
Number of observations skipped: 0
Denominator degrees of feedom: 2

Variable		One 1
DXDEAD	Sample Size Weighted Size Total SE Total Mean SE Mean	708.000 23599.988 499.379 116.072 0.021 0.011
LIFETHRT	Sample Size Weighted Size Total SE Total Mean SE Mean	708.000 23599.988 2932.319 773.082 0.124 0.018

by: Variable, One.
Number of observations read: 708   Weighted count: 23600
Number of observations skipped: 0
Denominator degrees of freedom: 2

by: Variable, One.

Variable		One 1
DXDEAD/LIFETHRT	Sample Size Weighted Size Weighted X-Sum Weighted Y-Sum Ratio Est SE Ratio	708.000 23599.988 2932.319 499.379 0.170 0.064

10.2.4 Sampling Distribution of Estimates

To illustrate the sampling distributions of estimates in simple two-stage cluster sampling from clusters having unequal numbers of listing units, let us look at an example.

Illustrative Example. Suppose that we wish to estimate the total number X of patients discharged dead and the proportion R of all admissions discharged dead among the ten hospitals shown in Table 10.9 (it will be assumed for this example that the only deaths are among those individuals having life-threatening conditions). Suppose (for simplicity) that we will do this by a simple one-stage cluster sample of two hospitals. The sampling distributions of the estimated total discharged dead, x'_{clu} the estimated total admissions, y'_{clu}, and the estimated proportion, r_{clu}, of all patients discharged dead are shown in Table 10.11.

The mean, standard error, and coefficient of variation of the distribution of x'_{clu} and r_{clu}, obtained by enumeration over the 45 possible samples using the techniques of Chapter 2, are as follows:

$$E(x'_{clu}) = 651 \qquad E(r_{clu}) = .0134$$
$$X = 651 \qquad R = .0130$$
$$SE(x'_{clu}) = 623.313 \qquad SE(r_{clu}) = .0017$$
$$V(x'_{clu}) = .9575 \qquad V(r_{clu}) = .1308$$

Note that the estimated total discharged dead, x'_{clu}, has a very large standard error and a coefficient of variation of over 95%, whereas the estimated proportion of patients discharged dead, r_{clu}, has both a low standard error and a low coefficient of variation. This high variability among estimated totals x'_{clu} is seen clearly in its frequency distribution over the 45 samples (Table 10.12). Note that only two of the 45 samples yield values of x'_{clu} that fall into the interval 600–799 which contains the true total ($X = 651$). Note also that 9 of the 45 samples yield values of x'_{clu} that grossly overestimate the true total. ☐

The pattern shown in the distributions of x'_{clu} and r_{clu} in the example above is typical of what often happens when clusters having a great variability with respect to the number of listing units are sampled by simple random sampling. Those clusters containing large numbers of listing units have no greater chance of being selected than those having small numbers of listing units. The sampling procedure does not take into consideration the number of listing units. In our example, hospitals are the clusters and hospital medical records are the listing units. There is considerable variation among the ten hospitals with respect to numbers of admissions, with one hospital (hospital 5) admitting more patients than the combined total of the other nine hospitals. The number of patients discharged dead is highly correlated with the number of admissions, and so it too varies tremendously from hospital to hospital, with hospital 5 accounting for more than 50% of the total fatalities in the ten hospitals. Since the number of admissions in a given hospital is not taken into consideration either in the sampling plan or in the estimation procedure, the distribution of estimated hospital deaths shows very high variability.

Table 10.11   Sampling Distribution of x'_{clu}, y'_{clu}, and r_{clu}

Hospitals in Sample	y'_{clu}	x'_{clu}	r_{clu}
1,2	46,620	600	.0129
1,3	27,330	295	.0108
1,4	24,630	255	.0104
1,5	156,490	1900	.0121
1,6	27,050	295	.0109
1,7	32,110	395	.0123
1,8	30,560	300	.0098
1,9	44,800	550	.0123
1,10	32,210	345	.0107
2,3	31,070	475	.0153
2,4	28,370	435	.0153
2,5	160,230	2080	.0130
2,6	30,790	475	.0154
2,7	35,850	575	.0160
2,8	34,300	480	.0140
2,9	48,540	730	.0150
2,10	35,950	525	.0146
3,4	9,080	130	.0143
3,5	140,940	1775	.0126
3,6	11,500	170	.0148
3,7	16,560	270	.0163
3,8	15,010	175	.0117
3,9	29,250	425	.0145
3,10	16,660	220	.0132
4,5	138,240	1735	.0126
4,6	8,800	130	.0148
4,7	13,860	230	.0166
4,8	12,310	135	.0110
4,9	26,550	385	.0145
4,10	13,960	180	.0129
5,6	140,660	1775	.0126
5,7	145,720	1875	.0129
5,8	144,170	1780	.0123
5,9	158,410	2030	.0128
5,10	145,820	1825	.0125
6,7	16,280	270	.0166
6,8	14,730	175	.0119
6,9	28,970	425	.0147
6,10	16,380	220	.0134
7,8	19,790	275	.0139
7,9	34,030	525	.0154
7,10	21,440	320	.0149
8,9	32,480	430	.0132
8,10	19,890	225	.0113
9,10	34,130	475	.0139

Table 10.12 Frequency Distribution of Estimated Total x'_{clu} Over All Possible Samples of Two Hospitals

Estimated Total Number of Persons Discharged Dead, x'_{clu}	Frequency f_i
0–199	7
200–399	15
400–599	12
600–799	2
800–999	0
1000–1199	0
1200–1399	0
1400–1599	0
1600–1799	4
1800–1999	3
2000–2199	2
Total	45

On the other hand, the *proportion* of patients discharged dead is roughly the same among each of the ten hospitals and shows little correlation with number of admissions. Thus, in contrast to the estimated total x'_{clu}, the estimated proportion of patients discharged dead has a relatively small standard error.

In the next chapter we will discuss methods of modifying the estimation procedure and/or the sampling plan to yield estimated totals having lower standard errors when the number N_i of listing units varies greatly among the clusters and the level of the characteristic being estimated in the cluster is strongly related to the number of listing units in the cluster.

The theoretical standard errors of estimated totals, means, and ratios are given in Box 10.5 for cluster sampling in which clusters are chosen by simple random sampling and listing units are chosen within selected clusters also by simple random sampling.

These expressions reduce to those listed in Box 10.3 when all N_i are equal (i.e., $N_i = \bar{N}$).

Examining the formula for the standard error of an estimated total, we see that it has a term depending on σ^2_{1x}, the variance among clusters with respect to the total level in the cluster of the characteristics being measured, and a term depending on the variance among listing units within a given cluster with respect to the level of the characteristic. Again, when the cluster totals, X_i are strongly correlated with the number N_i of listing units in the cluster, and when there is a great diversity among clusters with respect to N_i, then σ^2_{1x} might be very large, and hence the standard error of the estimated total might be large (as we observed earlier).

BOX 10.5   THEORETICAL STANDARD ERRORS FOR POPULATION ESTIMATES FOR SIMPLE TWO-STAGE CLUSTER SAMPLING, UNEQUAL NUMBERS OF LISTING UNITS

Total, x'_{clu}

$$
SE(x'_{clu}) = \left\{ \left(\frac{M^2}{m} \right) \sigma_{1x}^2 \left(\frac{M-m}{M-1} \right) \right.
$$

$$
\left. + \left(\frac{M}{m} \right) \left[\sum_{i=1}^{M} \left(\frac{N_i}{n_i} \right) \left(\frac{N_i - n_i}{N_i - 1} \right) \sum_{j=1}^{N_i} (X_{ij} - \bar{\bar{X}}_i)^2 \right] \right\}^{1/2}
$$

Mean Per Cluster, $\bar{x}_{clu}$

$$
SE(\bar{x}_{clu}) = \left\{ \left(\frac{\sigma_{1x}^2}{m} \right) \left(\frac{M-m}{M-1} \right) \right.
$$

$$
\left. + \left(\frac{1}{Mm} \right) \left[\sum_{i=1}^{M} \left(\frac{N_i}{n_i} \right) \left(\frac{N_i - n_i}{N_i - 1} \right) \sum_{j=1}^{N_i} (X_{ij} - \bar{\bar{X}}_i)^2 \right] \right\}^{1/2}
$$

Mean Per Listing Unit, $\bar{\bar{x}}_{clu}$

$$
SE(\bar{\bar{x}}_{clu}) = \left(\frac{1}{N} \right) \left\{ \left(\frac{M^2}{m} \right) \sigma_{1x}^2 \left(\frac{M-m}{M-1} \right) \right.
$$

$$
\left. + \left(\frac{M}{m} \right) \left[\sum_{i=1}^{M} \left(\frac{N_i}{n_i} \right) \left(\frac{N_i - n_i}{N_i - 1} \right) \sum_{j=1}^{N_i} (X_{ij} - \bar{\bar{X}}_i)^2 \right] \right\}^{1/2}
$$

Ratio, r_{clu}

$$
SE(r_{clu}) = R \left\{ \left(\frac{\sigma_{1R}^2}{m\bar{X}^2} \right) \left(\frac{M-m}{M-1} \right) + \left(\frac{1}{m\bar{X}^2} \right) \sum_{i=1}^{M} \left(\frac{1}{N_i n_i} \right) \left(\frac{N_i - n_i}{N_i - 1} \right) \right.
$$

$$
\times \left[\sum_{j=1}^{N_i} (X_{ij} - \bar{\bar{X}}_i)^2 + R^2 \sum_{j=1}^{N_i} (Y_{ij} - \bar{\bar{Y}}_i)^2 \right.
$$

$$
\left. \left. - 2R \sum_{j=1}^{N_i} (X_{ij} - \bar{\bar{X}}_i)(Y_{ij} - \bar{\bar{Y}}_i) \right] \right\}^{1/2}
$$

The notation used here is defined in Boxes 10.1 and 10.3.

10.2.5 How Large a Sample Do We Need?

Suppose that we intend to take a two-stage cluster sample in which a simple random sample of clusters is taken at the first stage, followed by a simple random sample of n_i listing units from the N_i listing units within each sample cluster. In other words, we are assuming that the second-stage sampling fractions have already been decided upon. We then wish to know how many clusters m are needed in our sample for us to be virtually certain that the relative differences between our estimates and the true values are no more than ε. Formulas for the *number m of clusters* needed to meet the specifications stated above are given below.

For estimated *totals* (x'_{clu}) or *means* ($\bar{x}_{clu}$, $\bar{\bar{x}}_{clu}$):

$$m = \frac{\left(\dfrac{\sigma_{1x}^2}{\bar{X}^2}\right)\left(\dfrac{M}{M-1}\right) + \left(\dfrac{M}{N^2\bar{\bar{X}}^2}\right)\left[\Sigma_{i=1}^{M}\left(\dfrac{N_i}{n_i}\right)\left(\dfrac{N_i-n_i}{N_i-1}\right)\Sigma_{j=1}^{N_i}(X_{ij}-\bar{X}_i)^2\right]}{\dfrac{\varepsilon^2}{z_{1-(\alpha/2)}^2} + \dfrac{\sigma_{1x}^2}{\bar{X}^2(M-1)}}$$

$$(10.16)$$

and for estimated *ratios* ($r_{clu} = \bar{x}_{clu}/\bar{y}_{clu}$):

$$m = \frac{\left[\begin{array}{c}\left(\dfrac{\sigma_{1R}^2}{\bar{X}^2}\right)\left(\dfrac{M}{M-1}\right) + \left(\dfrac{M}{N^2\bar{X}^2}\right)\Sigma_{i=1}^{M}\left(\dfrac{1}{n_iN_i}\right)\left(\dfrac{N_i-n_i}{N_i-1}\right) \\ \times[\Sigma_{j=1}^{N_i}(X_{ij}-\bar{X}_i)^2 + R^2\Sigma_{j=1}^{N_i}(Y_{ij}-\bar{Y}_i)^2 - 2R\Sigma_{j=1}^{N_i}(X_{ij}-\bar{X}_i)(Y_{ij}-\bar{Y}_i)]\end{array}\right]}{\dfrac{\varepsilon^2}{z_{1-(\alpha/2)}^2} + \dfrac{\sigma_{1R}^2}{\bar{X}^2(M-1)}}$$

$$(10.17)$$

Illustrative Example. Let us suppose that we wish to be virtually certain of estimating the total number of persons discharged dead to within 30% of the true value and the proportion of deaths among persons admitted with life-threatening conditions to within 20% of the true value. Suppose that we take a second-stage sample of 20% (to the nearest integer) of all admissions from those hospitals selected at the first stage. Then from the population data in Table 10.9, we have

$$\sigma_{1x}^2 = 8741.69 \qquad \bar{X} = 65.1 \qquad \bar{\bar{X}} = .0130$$

$$\sum_{i=1}^{M}\left(\frac{N_i}{n_i}\right)\left(\frac{N_i-n_i}{N_i-1}\right)\sum_{j=1}^{N_i}(X_{ij}-\bar{X}_i)^2 = 5783.32$$

$$\sum_{i=1}^{M}\left(\frac{1}{n_i N_i}\right)\left(\frac{N_i - n_i}{N_i - 1}\right)\left[\sum_{j=1}^{N_i}(X_{ij} - \bar{X}_i)^2 + R^2 \sum_{j=1}^{N_i}(Y_{ij} - \bar{\bar{Y}}_i)^2\right.$$

$$\left. -2R\sum_{j=1}^{N_i}(X_{ij} - \bar{X}_i)(Y_{ij} - \bar{\bar{Y}}_i)\right] = .00064$$

$$\sigma_{1R}^2 = 81.39 \qquad N = 50{,}056 \qquad M = 10$$

Then from relation (10.16) with $\varepsilon = .30$, we have

$$m = \frac{\left(\frac{8741.69}{(65.1)^2}\right)\left(\frac{10}{10-1}\right) + \left(\frac{10}{(50{,}056)^2(.0130)^2}\right)(5783.32)}{\dfrac{(.30)^2}{9} + \dfrac{8741.69}{(65.1)^2(10-1)}} = 10.15 \approx 10$$

And from relation (10.17) with $\varepsilon = .3$, we have

$$m = \frac{\left(\frac{81.39}{(65.1)^2}\right)\left(\frac{10}{10-1}\right) + \left(\frac{10}{(50{,}056)^2(.0130)^2}\right)(.00064)}{\dfrac{(.30)^2}{9} + \dfrac{81.39}{(65.1)^2(10-1)}} = 1.76 \approx 2$$

Thus, we would need a sample of all ten hospitals to meet the specifications set for estimated total discharged dead (X_i), whereas we would need only two clusters to meet the specifications set for the ratio (R) of deaths to life-threatening illnesses. □

10.2.6 Choosing the Optimal Cluster Size $\bar{n}$ Considering Costs

Let us again assume that the clusters will be taken by simple random sampling and that within each cluster the second-stage sampling fraction n_i/N_i will be the same (within the limitations of the N_i discussed earlier) for each cluster selected. Suppose we define the average cluster size $\bar{n}$ as

$$\bar{n} = \frac{\sum_{i=1}^{m} n_i}{m}$$

and suppose that the *field costs* can be approximated by the function

$$C = C_1 m + C_2 m \bar{n} \tag{10.18}$$

Then the *optimal average cluster size* $\bar{n}$ that would yield estimated totals (x'_{clu}) or means ($\bar{x}_{\text{clu}}, \bar{\bar{x}}_{\text{clu}}$) having the lowest standard errors among all other estimates obtained at the same field costs from two-stage cluster sampling with a constant second-stage sampling fraction is given by

$$\bar{n} = \left[\left(\frac{C_1}{C_2} \right) \left(\frac{1 - \delta_x}{\delta_x} \right) \right]^{1/2} \tag{10.19}$$

where δ_x is a generalization of the intraclass correlation coefficient discussed earlier and is given by

$$\delta_x = \frac{[M/(M-1)]\sigma_{1x}^2 - \bar{N}\sigma_{2x}^2}{[M/(M-1)]\sigma_{1x}^2 + \bar{N}(\bar{N}-1)\sigma_{2x}^2} \tag{10.20}$$

and where

$$\bar{N} = \frac{\sum_{i=1}^{M} N_i}{M}$$

$$\sigma_{2x}^2 = \left(\frac{1}{N} \right) \sum_{i=1}^{M} \left(\frac{N_i}{N_i - 1} \right) \sum_{j=1}^{N_i} (X_{ij} - \bar{X}_i)^2 \tag{10.21}$$

For estimation of ratios, $r_{\text{clu}} = \bar{x}_{\text{clu}}/\bar{y}_{\text{clu}}$, the optimal cluster size $\bar{n}$ is given by

$$\bar{n} = \left[\left(\frac{C_1}{C_2} \right) \left(\frac{1 - \delta_R}{\delta_R} \right) \right]^{1/2} \tag{10.22}$$

where

$$\delta_R = \frac{[M/(M-1)]\sigma_{1R}^2 - \bar{N}\sigma_{2R}^2}{[M/(M-1)]\sigma_{1R}^2 + \bar{N}(\bar{N}-1)\sigma_{2R}^2} \tag{10.23}$$

$$\sigma_{1R}^2 = \sigma_{1x}^2 + R^2\sigma_{1y}^2 - 2R\sigma_{1xy}$$

and

$$\sigma_{2R}^2 = \frac{1}{N} \sum_{i=1}^{M} \left(\frac{N_i}{N_i - 1} \right) \left[\sum_{j=1}^{N_i} (X_{ij} - \bar{X}_i)^2 + R^2 \sum_{j=1}^{N_i} (Y_{ij} - \bar{Y})^2 \right.$$

$$\left. -2R \sum_{j=1}^{N_i} (X_{ij} - \bar{X}_i)(Y_{ij} - \bar{Y}_i) \right] \tag{10.24}$$

Illustrative Example.   To illustrate the use of these formulas, let us suppose that we wish to take a simple two-stage cluster sample from the population of ten hospitals shown in Table 10.9 for the purpose of estimating the total number of persons discharged dead (X) and the proportion discharged dead (R) among those admitted with life-threatening illnesses. Suppose that it would cost approximately \$500 in administrative and travel costs for every hospital sampled and approximately \$5.00 per admission record. In other words, $C_1 = 500$ and $C_2 = 5$. From Table 10.9 we calculate

$$\sigma_{1x}^2 = 8741.69 \qquad \sigma_{2x}^2 = \frac{642.37}{50,056} = .01283 \qquad \bar{N} = 5005.6$$

$$\delta_x = \frac{\frac{10}{9}(8741.69) - (5005.6)(.01283)}{\frac{10}{9}(8741.69) + (5005.6)(5004.6)(.01283)} = .02914$$

Therefore

$$\bar{n} = \left[\left(\frac{500}{5} \right) \left(\frac{1 - .02914}{.02914} \right) \right]^{1/2} = 57.75 \approx 58$$

Thus the optimal average cluster size for estimating the total number discharged dead is 58 admissions and the optimal second-stage sampling fraction would be $f_2 = 58/5005.6 = .011586$. Once the optimal second-stage sampling fraction has been determined, we would then use relation (10.16) to determine the number of clusters needed to meet the required specifications set on the estimate.

To illustrate the use of relation (10.22) for a ratio R, we have, from Table 10.9 and from formulas shown earlier

$$\sigma_{1R}^2 = 81.39$$
$$\sigma_{2R}^2 = \sigma_{2x}^2 + R^2 \sigma_{2y}^2 - 2R\sigma_{2xy}$$
$$\qquad = .01283 + (.09186)^2(.12081) - 2(.09186)(.01113) = .01180$$
$$\delta_R = \frac{\frac{10}{9}(81.39) - (5005.6)(.01180)}{\frac{10}{9}(81.39) + (5005.6)(5004.6)(.01180)} = .000106$$

Therefore,

$$\bar{n} = \left[\left(\frac{500}{5} \right) \left(\frac{1 - .000106}{.000106} \right) \right]^{1/2} = 971.234$$

Thus, the optimal second-stage sampling fraction for estimating the ratio of persons discharged dead to persons admitted with life-threatening conditions is

$$f_2 = \frac{971.234}{5005.6} = .194$$

We could then use relation (10.17) (with n_i set equal to $f_2 N_i$) to determine the number of clusters that should be sampled in order for the specifications set on the estimate to be met. $\quad\square$

It often happens (as it did in this example) that the optimal cluster sizes are not the same for each estimate needed. In practice, a compromise on the cluster size $\bar{n}$ is often made by some method such as computation of the mean of the optimal $\bar{n}$ over the most important estimates that are needed from the survey.

10.3 SYSTEMATIC SAMPLING AS CLUSTER SAMPLING

A systematic sample of 1 in M listing units beginning with a random start, as described in Chapter 4, is in reality a single-stage cluster sample in which only one PSU is sampled. This is evident if we consider the listing units (numbered as they appear on the list) as being grouped into the following M clusters:

Cluster	Listing Units
1	$1, 1+M, 1+2M, 1+3M, \ldots$
2	$2, 2+M, 2+2M, 2+3M, \ldots$
3	$3, 3+M, 3+2M, 3+3M, \ldots$
$\vdots$	$\vdots$
$M-1$	$M-1, 2M-1, 3M-1, 4M-1, \ldots$
M	$M, 2M, 3M, 4M, \ldots$

For simplicity, let us assume that the number N of listing units is exactly divisible by M so that each of the clusters above contains $\bar{N} = N/M$ listing units. Then if the number chosen to start the systematic sample is 1, the sample will consist of every listing unit in cluster 1; that is, listing units $1, 1+M, 1+2M, \ldots, 1+(\bar{N}-1)M$. Likewise, if the random number is 2, the sample will consist of all units in cluster 2, and so on. Thus the theory of systematic sampling with a random start is a special case of single-stage cluster sampling with $m = 1$ and $\bar{n} = \bar{N}$.

10.4 SUMMARY

In this chapter we developed methods for two-stage cluster sampling in which clusters are selected with equal probability at the first stage and, within each sample cluster, the second-stage sampling fractions are the same (or nearly the same). When the sampling at each stage is by simple random sampling, the sampling plan is known as *simple two-stage cluster sampling*, and we focused in this chapter on that sampling plan. The section was divided into two major subsections: one treating the scenario in which all clusters in the population have the same number of enumeration units; the other considering the more complex scenario in which there are differences among clusters with respect to the number of enumeration units. We discussed, for each of these two scenarios, methods of estimating population characteristics and of estimating standard errors of these estimates. In this chapter, we introduced the intraclass correlation coefficient as an index of the homogeneity among enumeration units within sample clusters with respect to characteristic $\mathscr{X}$ being measured. This index is an important determinant of the optimum number of enumeration units to be selected at the second stage within each cluster as well as a determinant of the sampling errors of estimates obtained from two-stage cluster sampling.

For specified second-stage sampling fractions, we discussed procedures for determining how many clusters should be sampled at the first stage in order to ensure that the standard errors of resulting estimates be below tolerances set for them. We also discussed determination of the optimal second-stage sampling fraction on the basis of cost and the intraclass correlation coefficient. Finally, we showed that systematic sampling is, in reality, simple one-stage cluster sampling with one cluster selected from the population.

EXERCISES

10.1 Suppose that Chicago is divided into 75 community areas and that each community area contains 20 retail pharmacies. Suppose that you wish to estimate the average prices charged for some standard prescription drugs by taking a simple random sample of eight community areas followed by a simple random sample of four pharmacies within each of the eight community areas selected.

   a. Prepare a simple cost function for estimating the overall survey cost including the field costs. Specify each of the cost components.

   b. How would the total cost indicated above be affected if 16 community areas and two pharmacies per community area were selected?

   c. Suppose it is guessed that the standard deviation σ among all stores in Chicago with respect to the price of a certain drug is $1.50 and that the average cost of this drug is $10.00. Using the cost function you specified in part (a), determine the optimum value of $\bar{n}$ if the intraclass correlation coefficient is equal to .35. What then would be the coefficient of variation of the estimate if six PSUs were used?

10.2 **a.** Suppose that the elementary schools in a city were grouped into 30 school districts, with each school district containing ten schools. Suppose that a simple random sample of three school districts

Sample School District	Sample School	Number of Children	Number of Color-Blind Children
1	1	130	2
	2	150	3
	3	160	3
	4	120	5
2	1	110	2
	2	120	4
	3	100	0
	4	120	1
3	1	89	4
	2	130	2
	3	100	0
	4	150	2

was taken and that within each sample school district a simple random sample of four schools was taken for purposes of estimating the number of school children in the city that are color-blind (as measured by a standard test). The data shown in the accompanying table were obtained from this sample. Estimate, and obtain a 95% confidence interval for, the total number of color-blind school children in the city.

b. Estimate, and obtain a 95% confidence interval for, the proportion of school children in the city who are color-blind.

10.3 A simple random sample requires 400 listing units in order for estimated means and totals to meet specifications of precision. If all PSUs have the same number $\bar{N}$ of listing units, how large a simple cluster sample with cluster size $\bar{n}$ equal to 4 would be needed to achieve the same precision when the intraclass correlation coefficient is equal to .6?

10.4 Suppose that during the peak season the number of visitors to a state park and the number of injuries occurring among these visitors are as given in the accompanying table by week and day (the park is closed on Fridays).

Suppose that a simple two-stage cluster sample was taken with weeks as clusters, days as listing units, $m = 4$, and $\bar{n} = 3$. Suppose further that at the first stage of sampling, clusters 2, 6, 8, and 10 are selected. At the second stage of sampling, let us suppose that listing units 2, 3, and 5 are selected within cluster 2; listing units 1, 3, and 6 are selected within cluster 6; listing units 3, 4, and 6 are selected within cluster 8; and

	Number of Visitors						Number of Injuries					
Week	Su	M	Tu	W	Th	Sa	Su	M	Tu	W	Th	Sa
1	200	150	130	140	150	190	2	3	1	4	3	8
2	120	105	111	103	111	130	1	0	0	1	0	3
3	310	200	180	130	125	208	4	0	1	0	1	3
4	200	107	101	98	103	137	3	0	2	0	1	8
5	170	160	130	121	107	114	3	0	0	1	0	5
6	250	237	209	212	231	180	2	0	0	0	0	1
7	380	378	325	330	306	331	4	3	0	8	0	2
8	495	400	315	302	350	395	4	0	3	2	2	4
9	206	200	108	95	107	190	1	2	3	0	1	4
10	308	300	293	206	200	300	0	0	1	2	0	3

listing units 2, 4, and 5 are selected within cluster 10. From this sample, estimate and give 95% confidence intervals for the following:

a. The total number of visitors during the peak season

b. The total number of injuries during the peak season

c. The total number of injuries and visitors per week

d. The total number of injuries and visitors per day

e. The number of injuries per visitor

10.5 Suppose that a simple one-stage cluster sample was selected from the population shown in Exercise 10.4 and that clusters two and eight were selected. From this sample compute the 95% confidence intervals for the characteristics given in parts (a)–(e) of Exercise 10.4.

10.6 From the population shown in Exercise 10.4, compute the intraclass correlation coefficient for the number of visitors to the park.

10.7 Using the intraclass correlation coefficient calculated in Exercise 10.6, and assuming $C_1^* = 2C_2^*$, what would be the optimal number of days to sample in a two-stage simple cluster sample with weeks as clusters?

10.8 A manufacturer of an orthopedic device would like to initiate a quality control program in which a sample of these devices would be sampled and tested for defects. After the units exit the assembly, they are grouped in batches of 20 boxes, with each box containing 10 units. It is desired to sample each batch and to reject the batch if the estimated proportion of defective units within the batch is above 5%. A pilot study was conducted in which all units within a batch were tested, and the results of this pilot are shown opposite:

Box	Proportion of Defective Units
1	.50
2	.00
3	.00
4	.40
5	.00
6	.00
7	.00
8	.00
9	.00
10	.00
11	.00
12	.10
13	.10
14	.00
15	.00
16	.00
17	.00
18	.10
19	.00
20	.00

Suppose that a two-stage cluster sampling plan were to be used with boxes serving as clusters, and that five units would be selected within each box. Based on the data shown above, how many boxes should be sampled in order that the specifications stated above be met with 95% confidence?

10.9 If in Exercise 10.8, the cost associated with testing the units were 15 times that associated with listing and sampling the boxes, how many units should be sampled within each selected box?

10.10 Would the data shown in Exercise 10.8 indicate a high or low intraclass correlation coefficient? State the reason for your answer and verify it by computing the intraclass correlation coefficient.

10.11 A study was initiated having as a major objective estimation of the number of patients with severe trauma seen during the calendar year 1974 in hospitals not designated as *trauma centers* in urban counties in Illinois outside of the Chicago area which have both Trauma Centers (T) and hospitals not designated as Trauma Centers (NT). The following data were available to the investigators:

County	Hospital	No. of Beds	Type
1	1	310	NT
	2	229	T
	3	367	NT
2	1	134	T
	2	198	NT
3	1	242	T
	2	300	NT
4	1	358	T
	2	410	NT
5	1	32	NT
	2	156	T
6	1	231	NT
	2	209	T
	3	44	NT
7	1	227	NT
	2	178	T
	3	61	NT
	4	59	NT
	5	223	NT
8	1	16	NT
	2	263	T
	3	295	NT
9	1	180	T
	2	152	NT
	3	256	NT
10	1	100	T
	2	65	NT
11	1	595	NT
	2	648	T
12	1	76	NT
	2	133	T
	3	117	NT
	4	117	NT
	5	254	NT
13	1	574	NT
	2	824	T
	3	304	NT
14	1	350	NT
	2	256	T
	3	275	NT
	4	150	NT
15	1	133	NT
	2	314	T

County	Hospital	No. of Beds	Type
	3	124	T
	4	188	NT
	5	212	NT
	6	143	NT
16	1	60	NT
	2	55	T
17	1	150	T
	2	50	NT
18	1	72	NT
	2	80	T
	3	38	NT
19	1	64	NT
	2	125	T
20	1	367	NT
	2	329	T
	3	312	T
	4	178	NT
	5	281	NT

A two-stage cluster sampling design with counties as primary sampling units and non-trauma center hospitals as listing units was chosen. Six counties were selected at the first stage and one non-trauma center hospital within each sample county was sampled at the second stage. The following data were obtained from this sample survey.

County	Hospital	Cases of Severe Trauma
1	1	14
7	5	10
14	1	6
15	6	0
19	1	1
20	1	24

Use a ratio estimate based on number of beds to estimate from the above sample the total number of cases of severe trauma among hospitals in these 20 counties not designated as trauma centers.

10.12 A sample survey of patient records is being planned in a city that has 25 local mental health centers. The objective of the survey is to estimate the total number of patients who were given diazepam (Valium) as part of their therapeutic regimen. The number of patients treated in each of the mental health centers is listed in the accompanying table. A sample of patients is to be selected by choosing a simple random sample of mental health centers and, within each sample mental health center, choosing a subsample of patients.

Health Center	No. of Patients	Health Center	No. of Patients
1	491	14	672
2	866	15	475
3	188	16	439
4	994	17	392
5	209	18	584
6	961	19	882
7	834	20	424
8	9,820	21	775
9	348	22	262
10	246	23	968
11	399	24	586
12	175	25	809
13	166		

A survey of 10% of all patients conducted the previous year in health centers 1, 3, 8, 12, and 15 yielded the following data:

Health Center	No. of Patients	No. Given Diazepam
1	46	14
3	13	5
8	942	340
12	15	1
15	42	20

a. Based on the data for these five health centers, calculate the intraclass correlation coefficient with respect to the number of patients given diazepam.

b. Based on the above calculated intraclass correlation coefficient, what would be the optimal average cluster size $\bar{n}$ for the proposed survey of the 25 health centers listed above if the cost component associated with clusters is one thousand times that associated with listing units?

10.13 Based on the average cluster size calculated above, how many health centers should be sampled if one wishes to be 95% certain of estimating the number of patients given diazepam to within 10% of the true value?

10.14 What would be the standard error of the estimated total number of patients given diazepam based on the cluster size $\bar{n}$ and number m of sample clusters determined in Exercises 10.12 and 10.13?

10.15 A household survey is to be conducted for purposes of estimating certain health status and health utilization variables. The survey research laboratory contracted to perform the study has access to U.S. Census Bureau lists of households and can define clusters of 18 households from which a sample of households can be taken. From a study conducted on similar lists the intraclass correlation coefficients were estimated (see the accompanying table). It estimated that the cost component associated with clusters is about one-fourth of that associated with listing units. On the basis of this information, choose between the three different types of clusters and determine the appropriate sample cluster size.

Variable	Intraclass Correlation (δ_x) for Various Cluster Sizes		
	$N_i = 6$	$N_i = 9$	$N_i = 18$
Number of bed-days in last 2 weeks	.022	.038	.011
Number of hospital discharges in past 12 months	.057	.069	.077

10.16 A list of hospitals in a rural geographic area is shown in the accompanying table, by county. A sample survey is planned using a sample design in which counties are clusters, hospitals are listing units, and one hospital is to be selected from each county. If it is assumed that the total expenses for a hospital are proportional to the number of admissions, how many counties should be selected in order to be 95% confident of estimating the total expenses per day among hospitals in that region to within 20% of the true value?

10.17 Suppose that a simple random sample of five clusters is selected from the population shown in Exercise 10.16 and that the clusters selected are 5, 8, 23, 30, and 36. Take a second-stage sample of 1 listing unit from each sample cluster and estimate from this sample the mean

County	Hospital	No. of Beds	Average No. of Admissions per Day in 1989
1	1	72	4.8
2	1	87	8.4
	2	104	9.4
	3	34	2.0
3	1	99	5.1
4	1	48	4.4
5	1	99	6.2
6	1	131	9.1
	2	182	15.9
7	1	42	2.4
8	1	38	2.8
9	1	34	2.3
10	1	42	4.9
11	1	39	4.0
	2	59	4.1
12	1	76	5.2
13	1	25	3.1
	2	80	5.3
14	1	50	4.9
15	1	88	7.1
16	1	50	4.4
17	1	63	5.1
18	1	45	3.9
19	1	75	8.5
20	1	17	3.8
	2	140	11.9
21	1	44	4.9
22	1	171	12.0
	2	85	4.6
23	1	48	3.8
	2	18	2.9
24	1	54	4.9
25	1	68	3.8
	2	68	5.5
26	1	44	3.5
27	1	32	1.0

County	Hospital	No. of Beds	Average No. of Admissions per Day in 1989
	2	90	6.1
28	1	35	2.9
29	1	72	5.2
30	1	104	6.6
31	1	86	6.4
	2	91	6.4
	3	53	4.5
32	1	108	6.4
33	1	50	4.9
34	1	45	3.8
35	1	65	4.3
36	1	48	4.9
37	1	61	5.7

number of admissions per hospital bed. (Use statistical software if available.)

10.18 From the sample taken in Exercise 10.17 estimate the total number of admissions for 1989 among the 37 counties in this region. What is the estimated standard error of this estimate? (Use appropriate statistical software if available.)

10.19 A simple random sample of five gasoline stations was taken in a medium-size city containing 30 such stations. Within each of these five sample stations, a mobile unit with equipment to collect urine and saliva specimens was set up, and a sample of 1 in 10 automobiles entering the station was taken. The driver of each sampled automobile was requested to participate in the survey which consisted of a short interview and submission of a urine and saliva specimen. Each participant was given a free tank of gasoline as an incentive and assured that the information obtained was strictly confidential. The major objective of the survey was to obtain estimates of the number of drivers who show evidence of substance abuse while driving. The following data were obtained.

Station	Number of Persons Tested	Number of Persons Showing Evidence of Substance Abuse
1	15	3
2	6	1
3	11	1
4	6	3
5	8	1

a. Based on these data, estimate the number of drivers in the city who show evidence of substance abuse.

b. Is the estimate used above unbiased? Show that it is/is not.

c. If it is not unbiased, what further information would be needed to construct an unbiased estimate?

BIBLIOGRAPHY

Virtually every textbook on sampling theory or sample survey methodology contains considerable material on two-stage cluster sampling. Recent review or expository articles relevant to this topic appearing in the Encyclopedia of Biostatistics *are listed below:*

1. Shimizu, I. M. Multistage sampling. In *Encyclopedia of Biostatistics*, Armitage, P. A., and Colton, T. D., Eds., Wiley, Chichester, U.K., 1998.

2. Brock, D. B., Beckett, L. A., and Bienias, A. L., Sample surveys. In *Encyclopedia of Biostatistics*, Armitage, P. A., and Colton, T. D., Eds., Wiley, Chichester, U.K, 1998.

3. Freeman, D. H., Optimum allocation in cluster sampling. In *Encyclopedia of Biostatistics*, Armitage, P. A., and Colton, T. D., Eds., Wiley, Chichester, U.K, 1998.

Since two-stage cluster sampling is one of the most common designs used in sample surveys, there is an immense number of published studies presenting substantive findings obtained from such studies. A few of these are mentioned below:

4. Goldberg, J., Levy, P. S., Gelfand, H. M., Mullner, R., Iverson, N., Lemeshow, S., and Rothrock, J., Factors affecting trauma center utilization in Illinois. *Medical Care*, **19**: 547, 1981.

5. Brenniman, G. R., Kojola, W. H, Levy, P. S., Carnow, B. W., and Namekata, T., High barium levels in public drinking water and its association with elevated blood pressure. *Archives of Environmental Health*, **36**: 28–32, 1981.

6. Barr, D., Hershow, R., Levy, P. S., Furner, F, and Handler, A., Assessing prenatal hepatitis B screening in Illinois using an inexpensive study design adaptable to other jurisdictions. *American Journal of Public Health*, January 1999.

The text by Hansen, Hurwitz, and Madow develops the use of ultimate cluster variance estimates.

7. Hansen, M., Hurwitz, W. and Madow W., *Sample Survey Methods and Theory*, Vol. 1, Wiley, New York, 1953.

CHAPTER 11

Cluster Sampling in Which Clusters are Sampled with Unequal Probabilities: Probability Proportional to Size Sampling

The cluster sampling methodology developed in both Chapters 9 and 10 has been confined exclusively to sampling designs in which the clusters are sampled with equal probability. In other words, in our discussion of cluster sampling so far, every cluster in the population has had the same probability of being chosen in the sample independent of its number of enumeration units or, for that matter, any other characteristic that it may possess. In this chapter, we demonstrate that such designs, in certain instances, can result in sample selections that are not feasible to implement, and to linear estimates (e.g., means, totals, proportions) that have very high standard errors. The particular scenarios that are most vulnerable to such problems are those in which there is considerable variability among the primary sampling units with respect to number of enumeration units. Such scenarios, unfortunately, are among those encountered most often in practice.

To avoid such problems, in this chapter we develop a methodology for cluster sampling in which all clusters in the population do not have the same probability of being selected in the sample. We focus particularly on a class of cluster sampling designs known as *probability proportional to size sampling* (generally abbreviated to *PPS sampling*). In this class of designs, the probability of a cluster being selected in the sample is proportional to some measure of its size—generally the number of enumeration units which it contains. Alternatively, some other variable related to the level of the variable being estimated could be used.

In developing the concepts involved in sampling clusters with unequal probability, we will use, in some instances for purposes of clarity, illustrative examples from single-stage cluster sampling, even though we recognize that it is much less widely used than two- and (and even higher) stage cluster sampling.

11.1   MOTIVATION FOR *NOT* SAMPLING CLUSTERS WITH EQUAL PROBABILITY

Let us consider the population of three hospitals shown in Table 11.1. Suppose that we were to take a simple one-stage cluster sample of two of these hospitals for purposes of estimating the total number of unnecessary outpatient surgical procedures among all three hospitals. The survey would entail abstracting information from each sample record, and the sample sizes are shown below for each of the three possible samples.

Hospitals in Sample	Number of Outpatient Records Sampled			
	Hospital 1	Hospital 2	Hospital 3	Total Sample Size
1 and 2	3000	4000	—	7,000
1 and 3	3000	—	10,000	13,000
2 and 3	—	4000	10,000	14,000

The table shown above clearly indicates that this one-stage simple cluster sampling design results in a very unpredictable total sample size (it can be as low as 7000 and as high as 14,000), and a very unequal abstracting burden among hospitals sampled (only 3000 records would have to be selected from hospital 1 if sampled, as opposed to 10,000 records from hospital 3). The inequality with respect to sample size among hospitals and lack of predictability with respect to the total sample size could seriously compromise the feasibility of conducting this survey.

In addition to the feasibility problems stated above, we see below (from use of the standard error formulas in Chapter 9) that a linear estimate such as an estimated population total would have considerable variability. The distri-

Table 11.1   Number of Outpatient Surgical Procedures Performed in 1997 in Three Community Hospitals

Hospital	Outpatient Surgical Procedures	Number of Unnecessary Outpatient Surgical Procedures
1	3,000	35
2	4,000	38
3	10,000	100
Total	17,000	173

bution over the three possible samples of the estimated total, y'_{clu}, of unnecessary outpatient surgical procedures is shown below:

Hospitals in Sample	Sample Total, y	Estimated Population Total, y'_{clu}
1,2	73	109.5
1,3	135	202.5
2,3	138	207

The expected value and standard error of the estimated total, y'_{clu}, along with its coefficient of variation, are given below:

$$E(y'_{clu}) = 173$$
$$SE(y'_{clu}) = 55.04$$
$$V(y'_{clu}) = 0.32$$

Note that this estimate has a large coefficient of variation when one considers that the sample included two-thirds of the clusters in the population. The reason for this is that the variable of interest, number of unnecessary outpatient surgical procedures, is mainly related to the number of outpatient surgical procedures, and there is considerable variability among hospitals with respect to total number of outpatient surgical procedures. In fact, hospital 3 has more outpatient surgical procedures, and hence more unnecessary outpatient surgical procedures, than hospitals 1 and 2 combined. Thus, the sample not including hospital 3 yields a gross underestimate of the number of unnecessary surgical procedures, whereas the two samples that do include hospital 3 yield overestimates of this total. In simple cluster sampling, as described in Chapters 9 and 10, each hospital has the same chance of getting into the survey regardless of any information known about the cluster. Also, the estimation procedures used in simple cluster sampling make no use of information about the characteristics of the cluster.

We shall show that it is possible to reduce the sampling error of an estimated total from a cluster sample by making use of known information about the cluster that may be correlated with the response variable. This information can be used both in the sampling procedure and in the estimation process.

Let us suppose that, instead of sampling clusters with equal probability, we take a sample in such a way that the probability of a hospital appearing in the sample is proportional to its number of outpatient surgical procedures. More specifically, let us describe a sampling procedure in which the sampling is without replacement, and the hospitals are drawn one at a time from a hypothetical "urn." Suppose that the probability of a hospital being selected at any drawing is proportional to its number of outpatient surgical procedures, and that once it is drawn, it is removed from the urn. Letting X_i equal the number of outpatient surgical procedures in the ith hospital, we see that the probability, P_i, of hospital i being selected at the first drawing is given by

$$P_i = \frac{X_i}{X}$$

where

$X_i =$ The number of outpatient surgical procedures in hospital i
$X =$ The total number of outpatient surgical procedures among the 3 hospitals

From the above, it follows from combinatorial theory that if two hospitals are sampled without replacement, then the probability, π_{ij}, that hospitals i and j are chosen in the sample is given by

$$\pi_{ij} = \frac{X_1 X_2}{X} \left(\frac{1}{X - X_1} + \frac{1}{X - X_2} \right) \tag{11.1}$$

For the data in Table 11.1, we then have the following selection probabilities:

Hospitals in Sample (i, j)	Probability of Hospitals i and j Appearing Together in Sample [from Relation (11.1)] π_{ij}
(1,2)	0.10472
(1,3)	0.37815
(2,3)	0.51713

For example, from relation (11.1)

$$\pi_{12} = \frac{3000 \times 4000}{17,000} \times \left[\frac{1}{17,000 - 3000} + \frac{1}{17,000 - 4000} \right] = .1047$$

Once the π_{ij} are obtained, we can then obtain the probability, π_i that hospital i appears in the sample:

$$\pi_i = \sum_j \pi_{ij}$$

For each of the three hospitals in the population, the probability, π_i, that it appears in the sample is shown below:

Hospital	Probability, π_i, of Being in Sample
1	.48287
2	.62185
3	.89528

Now, based on the sampling plan shown above, we construct the estimator, y'_{hte}, given by

$$y'_{hte} = \sum_{i=1}^{n} \frac{y_i}{\pi_i}$$

The initials "hte" stand for *Horvitz–Thompson estimator*, which is a class of estimators that we discuss in more general terms in a later section.

In contrast to the estimator, x'_{clu}, this estimator makes use of information about the cluster both in the sampling and the construction of the estimator. The chance of any hospital appearing in the sample is greater for those hospitals that have a greater number of outpatient surgical procedures, which is assumed to be related to the variable of interest—that is, the number of unnecessary outpatient surgical procedures. In the estimation procedure, each hospital is weighted by the inverse of its probability of being in the sample in order for the resulting estimator to be unbiased.

The distribution of y'_{hte} over all possible samples is shown below:

Hospitals in Sample	y'_{hte}	Probability of Sample Being Selected, π_{ij}
(1,2)	133.59	.10472
(1,3)	184.18	.37815
(2,3)	172.80	.51713

The expected value of y'_{hte} is shown below along with its standard error and coefficient of variation:

$$E(y'_{hte}) = \sum_{\substack{\text{all samples}}} y'_{hte}\pi_{ij} = 133.59 \times .10472 + 184.18 \times .37815$$

$$+ \, 172.80 \times .5171 = 173 = Y$$

$$SE(y'_{hte}) = \left(\sum_{\text{all samples}} (y'_{hte} - 173)^2 \pi_{ij} \right)^{1/2} = 14.49$$

$$V(y'_{hte}) = \frac{14.49}{173} = .084$$

It should be noted that the sampling procedure of taking clusters with unequal probability in combination with the use of the estimator y'_{hte} yields, in this example, a coefficient of variation of 8.4% which is much smaller than the coefficient of variation of 32% obtained from sampling the clusters with equal probability. Both procedures produce unbiased estimators of the population total.

We have demonstrated in the above example that by sampling clusters with unequal probability, it is possible to obtain an estimator having a standard error that is considerably lower than that obtained by sampling the clusters with equal probability. In later sections of this chapter, we show how such methods can be used in two-stage cluster sampling to obtain estimates that are valid and reliable, and are based on samples of approximately the same number of enumeration units within clusters. As stated earlier, it is often extremely important, for budgetary and feasibility reasons, for the total sample size to be predictable and for the sample to be evenly distributed among the clusters. In the next section, we develop some estimation methods used in sampling clusters with unequal probability.

11.2 TWO GENERAL CLASSES OF ESTIMATORS VALID FOR SAMPLE DESIGNS IN WHICH UNITS ARE SELECTED WITH UNEQUAL PROBABILITY

The literature on unequal probability sampling has evolved primarily around two general classes of estimators; namely, the *Horvitz–Thompson estimator*, which was illustrated in the previous section, and an earlier estimator, known as the *Hansen–Hurwitz estimator*. These are discussed in more detail in this section.

11.2.1 The Horvitz–Thompson Estimator

The Horvitz–Thompson estimator was originally proposed in 1952 as an estimator of a total that can be constructed for any sampling design, with or without replacement [8]. For a single-stage cluster sampling design, its form is given by

$$y'_{hte} = \sum_{i=1}^{v} \frac{Y_i}{\pi_i} \tag{11.2}$$

where

Y_i = the total for the ith sample cluster
π_i = the probability of the ith cluster being selected in the sample
v = the number of distinct clusters sampled

Clearly, when the sampling is without replacement, $v = m$, where m is the total number of clusters sampled. It can be shown that for any single-stage cluster sampling design, y'_{hte} is an unbiased estimator of Y with standard error given by:

$$SE(y'_{hte}) = \sqrt{\sum_{i=1}^{M} \frac{1 - \pi_i}{\pi_i} Y_i^2 + \sum_{i=1}^{M}\sum_{j \neq i} \left(\frac{\pi_{ij} - \pi_i\pi_j}{\pi_i\pi_j}\right) Y_i Y_j} \qquad (11.3)$$

where M is the number of clusters in the population, and π_{ij} is the probability that clusters i and j are both included in the sample.

For the illustrative example shown in the previous section, we have

$$\sum_{i=1}^{M} \frac{1 - \pi_i}{\pi_i} Y_i^2 = 3359.71$$

$$\sum_{i=1}^{M}\sum_{j \neq i} \left(\frac{\pi_{ij} - \pi_i\pi_j}{\pi_i\pi_j}\right) Y_i Y_j = -3149.79$$

and

$$SE(y'_{hte}) = \sqrt{3359.71 + (-3149.79)} = 14.49$$

Note that this agrees with the results obtained earlier by use of the definitional formula.

The following estimator, $\widehat{Var}(y'_{hte})$, is an unbiased estimator of the variance $Var(y'_{hte})$ for a single-stage cluster sampling design:

$$\widehat{Var}(y'_{hte}) = \sum_{i=1}^{v} \frac{1 - \pi_i}{\pi_i} Y_i^2 + \sum_{i=1}^{v}\sum_{j \neq i} \left(\frac{\pi_{ij} - \pi_i\pi_j}{\pi_i\pi_j}\right) \frac{Y_i Y_j}{\pi_{ij}} \qquad (11.4)$$

This estimator has some difficulties in that it is often unstable and can be negative. Other estimators that are less problematic have been developed and are discussed elsewhere [2]–[4].

The importance of the Horvitz–Thompson estimator is that it is an unbiased estimator that can be computed for any sampling design so long as one can assess the probability, π_i, of any unit being included in the sample. This is often feasible even for very complex sampling schemes. Its generalization to any sampling design has made it extremely important in the development and unification of sampling theory. Its disadvantage in many practical situations is that its variance depends not only on the inclusion probabilities, π_i, but on the joint probability, π_{ij}, of any two units being included together in the sample. In practice, especially when sampling is without replacement, it is often difficult and inconvenient to assess the values of these π_{ij}, which makes estimation of sampling errors problematic. In the next section, we discuss an alternative estimator that is often easier to use in practice.

11.2.2 The Hansen–Hurwitz Estimator

This estimator, shown below for single-stage cluster sampling, was proposed in 1943 by Hansen and Hurwitz [7] as an estimator of a total, Y, that is unbiased when sampling is *with replacement*:

$$y'_{hh} = \frac{1}{m} \sum_{i=1}^{m} \frac{Y_i}{\pi'_i} \tag{11.5}$$

where π'_i is the probability of selecting the ith unit at any drawing of the sample. The standard error of this estimate is given by

$$SE(y'_{hh}) = \sqrt{\frac{1}{m} \sum_{i=1}^{M} \left(\frac{Y_i}{\pi'_i} - Y\right)^2 \pi'_i} \tag{11.6}$$

and an estimator of the standard error is given by

$$\widehat{SE}(y'_{hh}) = \sqrt{\frac{\sum_{i=1}^{m} \left(\frac{Y_i}{\pi'_i} - y'_{hh}\right)^2}{m(m-1)}} \tag{11.7}$$

It should be noted that the expression under the square root sign in Equation (11.7) is an unbiased estimator of the variance of the estimator for any single-stage cluster sampling design.

Illustrative Example. Let us illustrate the use of this estimator with the following example, shown in Table 11.2. A community contains four nursing homes, and a sample of two of them is to be taken with replacement for purposes of estimating the total number, Y, of women over 90 years of age admitted to nursing homes in 1997. For purposes of illustrating the Hansen–Hurwitz estimator, let us assume that the sampling is with replacement and that at each drawing of a nursing home, the probability of a particular nursing home being selected is equal to its number of beds, X_i, divided by the total

Table 11.2 Number of Women Over 90 Years of Age Admitted to Nursing Homes in a Community During 1997

Nursing Home	Number of Beds (X_i)	Number, Y_i, of Women over 90 yr Admitted in 1997	Probability, π_i' of Selecting Nursing Home in Sample at any Drawing
1	35	3	.12727
2	75	7	.27273
3	140	24	.50909
4	25	1	.09091
Total	275	35	1.00000

number of beds, X, over all four nursing homes in the community. For each nursing home selected, the number of persons over 90 years of age admitted during 1997 is determined from admission records.

In this scenario, the number, M, of nursing homes in the community is equal to 4; the number, m, of units sampled is equal to 2; and the number of possible samples with replacement is equal to $4^2 = 16$. The distribution of values of the Hansen–Hurwitz estimated total, y_{hh}', is shown in Table 11.3.

From the definitional formulas, we see that the Hansen–Hurwitz estimator is an unbiased estimator of Y:

Table 11.3 Distribution of the Hansen–Hurwitz Estimator, y_{hh}', Over All Possible Samples of Two Nursing Homes Drawn with Replacement

Sample r	Nursing Homes in Sample (i, j)	Probability, $P(r)$, of Sample r Being Selected $(\pi_i' \times \pi_j')$	$y_{hh}'(r)$
1	(1,1)	.01620	23.57143
2	(1,2)	.03471	24.61905
3	(1,3)	.06479	35.35714
4	(1,4)	.01157	17.28571
5	(2,1)	.03471	24.61905
6	(2,2)	.07438	25.66667
7	(2,3)	.13884	36.40476
8	(2,4)	.02479	18.33333
9	(3,1)	.06479	35.35714
10	(3,2)	.13884	36.40476
11	(3,3)	.25917	47.14286
12	(3,4)	.04628	29.07143
13	(4,1)	.01157	17.28571
14	(4,2)	.02479	18.33333
15	(4,3)	.04628	29.07143
16	(4,4)	.00826	11.00000

$$E[y'_{hh}] = \sum_r y'_{hh}(r)P(r) = 23.57143 \times .016198 + \cdots + 29.07143 \times .008264$$
$$= 35 = Y$$

and it can also be seen from the data in Table 11.3 that its standard error (as obtained from the definitional formula) is numerically equal to what would be calculated from expression (11.6). Specifically, we have:

$$SE(y'_{hh}) = 9.16$$

The Horvitz–Thompson estimator, y'_{hte}, can also be used in this example, since it is an unbiased estimator of the population total in sampling with replacement as well as in sampling without replacement. The construction of this estimator and its sampling distribution is shown in Tables 11.4 and 11.5.

Again, one can see from applying the definitional formula to the data in Table 11.5 that $E(y'_{hte}) = 35 = X$, and that $SE(y'_{hte}) = 10.82$, slightly higher in this particular instance than the standard error of the Hansen–Hurwitz estimator. The standard errors of both of these estimators, however, are considerably smaller than the standard error of the ordinary inflation estimator $(x'_{clu} = (M/m)x)$. The standard error of that estimator is 25.6418. □

11.3 PROBABILITY PROPORTIONAL TO SIZE SAMPLING

In the previous sections, we observed that in two examples use of unequal probability sampling resulted in estimated totals that had standard errors that were considerably lower than what would have been obtained by estimation based on equal probability sampling of the clusters. In both of these examples, the sampling of clusters was based on a known characteristic of the clusters that was assumed to be related to the variable of interest (e.g., number of beds in a nursing home was assumed to be associated with the

Table 11.4 Number of Women over 90 Years of Age Admitted to Nursing Homes in a Community During 1997

Nursing Home	Number of Beds (X_i)	Number, Y_i, of Women over 90 yr Admitted in 1997	Probability, π_i, of Selecting Nursing Home in Sample
1	35	3	.238347
2	75	7	.471074
3	140	24	.759008
4	25	1	.173554
Total	275	35	

Table 11.5 Distribution of the Horvitz–Thompson Estimator, y'_{hte}, Over All Possible Samples of Two Nursing Homes Drawn with Replacement

Sample r	Nursing Homes in Sample (i, j)	Probability, $P(r)$, of Sample r Being Selected $(\pi'_i \times \pi'_j)$	$y'_{hte}(r)$
1	(1,1)	.01620	12.58669
2	(1,2)	.03471	27.44633
3	(1,3)	.06479	44.20689
4	(1,4)	.01157	18.34859
5	(2,1)	.03471	27.44633
6	(2,2)	.07438	14.85965
7	(2,3)	.13884	46.47986
8	(2,4)	.02479	20.62155
9	(3,1)	.06479	44.20689
10	(3,2)	.13884	46.47986
11	(3,3)	.25917	31.62021
12	(3,4)	.04628	37.38211
13	(4,1)	.01157	18.34859
14	(4,2)	.02479	20.62155
15	(4,3)	.04628	37.38211
16	(4,4)	.00826	5.76190

number of women over 90 years of age admitted during a given time period). In general, this is a strategy that is widely used in the design of sample surveys, and we will discuss it in more detail in this section.

We define *probability proportional to size sampling* (abbreviated *PPS sampling*) as a class of unequal probability sampling in which the probability of a unit being sampled is proportional to the level in that unit of some known variable. Some examples of PPS sampling are given below:

- A city contains 35 grocery stores, and a sample survey is to be conducted for purposes of estimating the total amount of cat food sold in the past week. The design calls for a sample of 10 stores to be selected with the probability of a store's being selected proportional to its total gross revenue the previous year.
- A large health maintenance organization (HMO) has filed claims in the last two years for 329 Medicare beneficiaries. The purpose of the survey is to estimate the total amount of money overpaid by Medicare to the HMO. The claims are organized on computer by beneficiary. A sample of 25 beneficiaries is to be taken, with the probability of a beneficiary being sampled proportional to the total number of claims filed on behalf of the beneficiary.

- A two-stage cluster sample is to be taken in which city blocks are selected at the first stage with the probability of any block being sampled proportional to the known number of households in the block. At the second stage a sample of 10 households is to be taken within each city block selected at the first stage.

In the ensuing discussion of PPS sampling, we focus primarily on its use in two-stage cluster sampling. As indicated above, when clusters differ widely with respect to the number of enumeration units contained in them, unequal probability sampling of clusters will often result in estimates of population characteristics, especially population totals, that have lower standard errors than those obtained from sampling clusters with equal probability.

Among various ways of sampling clusters with unequal probability, it makes sense to sample with probability proportional to the level of some known characteristic of a cluster that is associated with the variable of interest in the sample survey. A heuristic and idealized demonstration of this is seen by the following scenario. Suppose we are trying to estimate the total, Y, of some variable in a population, and that we know that it is proportional to the known population total, X, of another variable. In other words, $Y = cX$, where c is unknown. Suppose that this relationship also holds within each cluster i, that is, $Y_i = cX_i$. If we take a sample of one cluster with probability proportional to the known total, X_i, in that cluster, then the Hansen–Hurwitz estimate of Y is given by

$$y'_{hh} = \frac{Y_i}{\left(\frac{X_i}{X}\right)} = Y_i\left(\frac{X}{X_i}\right) = \left(\frac{Y_i}{X_i}\right)X$$

But

$$\frac{Y_i}{X_i} = \frac{Y}{X} = c$$

and therefore,

$$y'_{hh} = \left(\frac{Y}{X}\right)X = Y$$

Therefore, no matter what cluster is sampled, one obtains an estimator of Y that is without error.

Clearly, the demonstration shown above assumes a perfect deterministic relationship between Y and X that is rarely, if ever, seen in practice. However, if there is a strong correlation between Y and X within each cluster, then an estimator based on PPS sampling will be relatively unaffected by the particular clusters sampled, and hence will have low sampling error compared to an estimation procedure which does not use PPS sampling. It should be noted that the reasons why PPS sampling produces estimates having relatively low sampling errors are very similar to those that make ratio estimators very reliable.

11.3.1 Probability Proportional to Size Sampling with Replacement: Use of the Hansen–Hurwitz Estimator

As noted above, PPS sampling is a general class of sample designs based on unequal probability sampling in which the probability of a unit being sampled is proportional to some known variable, X. The sampling plan itself can be with or without replacement and can be any form of probability sampling (e.g., simple random sampling, systematic sampling, etc.). In this subsection, we develop for two-stage cluster sampling a particular form of PPS sampling having the following properties:

1. At the first stage, a sample of m clusters is taken with replacement and with probability proportional to the level in the cluster of some known variable $\mathcal{X}$ that is assumed to be related to the variable of interest, $\mathcal{Y}$.
2. From each of the m clusters selected at the first stage, a simple random sample of $\bar{n}$ enumeration units is taken from the N_i enumeration units in the cluster.
3. The estimated population total, y'_{ppswr}, is given by

$$y'_{\text{ppswr}} = \frac{1}{m} \sum_{i=1}^{m} \frac{N_i}{\bar{n}\pi'_i} y_i \tag{11.8}$$

where

$$\pi'_i = \frac{X_i}{X}$$

$$y_i = \sum_{j=1}^{\bar{n}} y_{ij} = \text{the sample total of the } i\text{th sample cluster}$$

$\bar{n} = $ the number of enumeration units sampled per cluster

The estimator shown in Equation (11.8) is the generalization of the Hansen–Hurwitz estimator appropriate for two-stage cluster sampling. If the measure of size variable, X_i, is the number, N_i, of enumeration units in the cluster, then the estimator is equal to

$$y'_{ppswr} = \frac{N}{n} \sum_{i=1}^{m} y_i \qquad (11.9)$$

Analogous to the expression given in Equation (11.7) for the standard error of the Hansen–Hurwitz estimator for single-stage cluster sampling, the following can be used in two-stage PPS sampling as an estimator of the standard error of y'_{ppswr}:

$$\widehat{SE}(y'_{ppswr}) = \sqrt{\frac{\sum_{i=1}^{m}\left(\dfrac{N_i X y_i}{\bar{n} X_i} - y'_{ppswr}\right)^2}{m(m-1)}} \qquad (11.10)$$

Illustrative Example. Let us consider the population of ten hospitals shown in Table 10.9 (data repeated below).

Suppose that we wish to estimate the total number of patients discharged dead from a two-stage cluster sample in which, at the first stage, a random sample of two hospitals is selected with replacement and with probability proportional to the number, N_i, of admissions (known from administrative data), and at the second stage, a simple random sample of 50 patient admissions is taken from each sample hospital.

Suppose that the two hospitals chosen are hospitals 6 and 9; that the 50 admission records sampled from hospital 6 yield 10 individuals with life-

Table 10.9   Total Admissions with Life-Threatening Conditions, and Total Admissions Discharged Dead from Ten Hospitals, 1987

Hospital	Total Admissions, N_i	Probability of Hospital Being Selected at any Drawing, $\pi'_i = N_i/N$	Total with Life-Threatening Conditions	Total Discharged Dead Among Those with Life-Threatening Conditions
1	4,288	.085664	501	42
2	5,036	.100607	785	78
3	1,178	.023534	213	17
4	638	.012746	173	9
5	27,010	.539596	3404	338
6	1,122	.022415	217	17
7	2,134	.042632	424	37
8	1,824	.036439	246	18
9	4,672	.093335	778	68
10	2,154	.043032	346	27

threatening conditions of whom 0 was discharged dead; and that the 50 sampled from hospital 9 yield 10 admitted with life-threatening conditions and 2 were discharged dead.

From Equations (11.9) and (11.10) we have the following:

$$m = 2 \qquad N = 50,056 \qquad \bar{n} = 50$$
$$y_1 = 0 \qquad N_1 = 1122$$
$$y_2 = 2 \qquad N_2 = 4672$$
$$y'_{ppswr} = \frac{50,056}{2 \times 50} \times (0 + 2) = 1001.12$$
$$\widehat{SE}(y'_{ppswr}) = \sqrt{\frac{(0 - 1001.12)^2 + (2002.24 - 1001.12)^2}{2(2 - 1)}} = 1001.12$$

$\square$

Illustrative Example. Let us now consider a second example based on the data from Table 10.9. Suppose that we take a PPS sample in which five hospitals are drawn with replacement and with probability proportional to the number, N_i, of admissions. From each drawing of hospitals we then take a simple random sample of 10 admissions. From this sample, we wish to estimate the total number of persons admitted with life-threatening diseases, and the proportion of persons discharged dead among these persons admitted with life-threatening conditions. As in the previous example, we will use the generalization of the Hansen–Hurwitz estimator.

The five drawings resulted in selection of hospitals, 2, 5, 5, 5, and 9, and the findings are shown below in Table 11.6.

We see that $m = 5, \bar{n} = 10$, and from Equation (11.9):

$$x'_{ppswr} = \frac{50,056}{50} \times 6 = 6006.72$$

Table 11.6 Results of the PPS Sample

Hospital	Probability of Selection at any Drawing (π'_i)	Number of Admissions Sampled ($\bar{n}$)	Number of Patients with Life-Threatening Conditions (x_i)	Number of Patients Discharged Dead (y_i)
2	5,036/50,056	10	1	1
5	27,010/50,056	10	1	0
5	27,010/50,056	10	2	0
5	27,010/50,056	10	1	0
9	4,672/50,056	10	1	1

and

$$y'_{ppswr} = \frac{50,056}{50} \times 2 = 2002.24$$

To estimate the standard errors of these estimated totals, we note that when the measure of size variable is the number, N_i, of enumeration units, the formula for the estimated standard error shown in Equation (11.10) reduces to the following:

$$\widehat{SE}(y'_{ppswr}) = \sqrt{\frac{\sum_{i=1}^{m}\left(\frac{Ny_i}{\bar{n}} - y'_{ppswr}\right)^2}{m(m-1)}} \qquad (11.11)$$

From Equation (11.11), we compute the following standard errors:

$$\widehat{SE}(x'_{ppswr}) = 1001.12$$

and

$$\widehat{SE}(y'_{ppswr}) = 1226.17$$

Finally, the proportion discharged dead among those admitted with life-threatening diseases is estimated by the ratio estimate given by

$$r_{ppswr} = \frac{y'_{ppswr}}{x'_{ppswr}} = \frac{2002.24}{6006.72} = .33$$

An estimate of the standard error of this ratio estimator can be obtained by linearization methods, and will be shown below in our discussion of software analysis for this design.

We will now demonstrate the use of SUDAAN and STATA in obtaining estimates for this particular PPS design.

The data file used for SUDAAN consists of 50 records, with each record containing information from an admission record sampled at the second stage following selection of a hospital at the first stage. Thus, the data file consists of 50 admission records—10 for each of the 5 drawings of hospitals. For SUDAAN, the data file is a SAS PC file, *hospslct.ssd*. The data in the file are shown in Table 11.7 and the variables in the file are described below:

drawing is the variable that denotes the particular drawing of a hospital at the first stage. Since there were 5 separate and independent drawings, the value of that variable ranges from 1 to 5.

Table 11.7   Data File for Use in Illustrative Example

drawing	hospno	admiss	lifethrt	dxdead	wstar
1	2	5036	1	1	1001.12
1	2	5036	0	0	1001.12
1	2	5036	0	0	1001.12
1	2	5036	0	0	1001.12
1	2	5036	0	0	1001.12
1	2	5036	0	0	1001.12
1	2	5036	0	0	1001.12
1	2	5036	0	0	1001.12
1	2	5036	0	0	1001.12
1	2	5036	0	0	1001.12
2	5	27010	1	0	1001.12
2	5	27010	0	0	1001.12
2	5	27010	0	0	1001.12
2	5	27010	0	0	1001.12
2	5	27010	0	0	1001.12
2	5	27010	0	0	1001.12
2	5	27010	0	0	1001.12
2	5	27010	0	0	1001.12
2	5	27010	0	0	1001.12
2	5	27010	0	0	1001.12
3	5	27010	1	0	1001.12
3	5	27010	1	0	1001.12
3	5	27010	0	0	1001.12
3	5	27010	0	0	1001.12
3	5	27010	0	0	1001.12
3	5	27010	0	0	1001.12
3	5	27010	0	0	1001.12
3	5	27010	0	0	1001.12
3	5	27010	0	0	1001.12
3	5	27010	0	0	1001.12
4	5	27010	1	0	1001.12
4	5	27010	0	0	1001.12
4	5	27010	0	0	1001.12
4	5	27010	0	0	1001.12
4	5	27010	0	0	1001.12
4	5	27010	0	0	1001.12
4	5	27010	0	0	1001.12
4	5	27010	0	0	1001.12
4	5	27010	0	0	1001.12
5	9	4672	1	1	1001.12
5	9	4672	0	0	1001.12
5	9	4672	0	0	1001.12
5	9	4672	0	0	1001.12

Table 11.7   Data File for Use in Illustrative Example (continued)

drawing	hospno	admiss	lifethrt	dxdead	wstar
5	9	4672	0	0	1001.12
5	9	4672	0	0	1001.12
5	9	4672	0	0	1001.12
5	9	4672	0	0	1001.12
5	9	4672	0	0	1001.12
5	9	4672	0	0	1001.12

hospno denotes the particular hospital from which the admission record was sampled (can have values from 1 to 10, since there are 10 hospitals in the population).

admiss denotes the number of admissions that occurred during that year in the hospitals from which the admission records was drawn.

lifethrt indicates whether the particular record represents an admission of a patient with a life-threatening condition—takes on the value 1 if "yes"— 0 if "no."

dxdead indicates whether the patient admitted was discharged dead—1 if "yes"; 0 if "no."

wstar is the sampling weight—in this instance, it is equal to N/n, or $50,056/50 = 1,001.12$.

The SUDAAN commands used for this estimation are shown below:

```
proc descript data = hospslct filetype = SAS design = wr means totals;
nest drawing/psulev = 1;
weight wstar;
var lifethrt dxdead;
proc ratio data = hospslct filetype = SAS design = wr;
nest drawing /psulev = 1;
weight wstar;
numer dxdead;
denom lifethrt;
```

The first command indicates the particular SUDAAN module to be used; the data file and file type; the particular SUDAAN design (WR or with replacement sampling in this instance); and the computation of both means and totals. The second command describes the clustering, indicating that the primary sampling unit identification is in the variable *drawing*. It should be noted carefully that the variable, *hospno*, which indicates the hospital identification, is *not* the primary sampling unit. In PPS sampling with replacement, a given cluster (i.e., hospital, in this instance) can be sampled more than once, and each drawing of a cluster is considered a primary sampling unit. The third command indicates the sampling weight, and the fourth command indicates the variable for which totals and means are to be estimated. The remaining commands are those used for the ratio estimation. They are self-explanatory.

The corresponding SUDAAN output for this estimation is shown below:

by: Variable, One.		
Variable		One 1
LIFETHRT	Sample Size Weighted Size Total SE Total Mean SE Mean	50 50056.00 6006.72 1001.12 0.12 0.02
DXDEAD	Sample Size Weighted Size Total SE Total Mean SE Mean	50 50056.00 2002.24 1226.12 0.04 0.02
by: Variable, One.		
Variable		One 1
DXDEAD/LIFETHRT	Sample Size Weighted Size Weighted X-sum Weighted Y-sum Ratio Est SE Ratio	50.0000 50056.0000 6006.7200 2002.2400 0.3333 0.2324

The equivalent analysis can be performed using STATA by means of the following commands:

```
use "a:\hospslct.dta", clear
. svyset pweight wstar
. svyset psu drawing
. svytotal lifethrt dxdead
. svyratio dxdead lifethrt
```

which yield the following output:

Survey total estimation					
pweight: wstar			Number of obs	=	50
Strata: <one>			Number of strata	=	1
PSU: drawing			Number of PSUs	=	5
			Population size	=	50056

total	Estimate	Std. Err.	[95% Conf. Interval]		Deff
lifethrt	6006.72	1001.12	3227.165	8786.275	.1856061
dxdead	2002.24	1226.117	−1402.005	5406.485	.765625

.svyratio dxdead lifethrt

Survey ratio estimation					
pweight: wstar			Number of obs	=	50
Strata: <one>			Number of strata	=	1
PSU: drawing			Number of PSUs	=	5
			Population size	=	50056

Ratio	Estimate	Std. Err.	[95% Conf. Interval]		Deff
dxdead/lifethrt	.3333333	.2324056	−.3119279	.9785946	1.429167

□

11.3.2 PPS Sampling When the Measure of Size Variable is not the Number of Enumeration Units

We are sometimes in a situation in which it is neither possible nor desirable to use the number, N_i, of enumeration units within a cluster as the measure of size variable in PPS sampling. Often, the number of enumeration units is not known in advance of the sampling. Sometimes, however, the number of enumeration units within a cluster may not be particularly related to the response variable, and there would thus be little to be gained by using it as the measure of size variable. For example, if hospitals are clusters, and it is desired to estimate some characteristic of melanoma patients, the number of melanoma patients admitted to a particular hospital is likely to be more closely related to the size and quality of the hospital's oncology and dermatology sections than it is to the overall size of the hospital as characterized by the overall number of admissions to that hospital.

In situations where the measure of size variable used in generating the PPS sample is not the number of enumeration units, the appropriate formulas for estimation of the population total and estimation of the standard error of this estimated total are, respectively, Equations (11.8) and (11.10). In both situations, the estimated total is a weighted sum of the individual sample observations having the form $y'_{\text{ppswr}} = \sum_{i=1}^{m} \sum_{j=1}^{\bar{n}} w_i y_{ij}$. In the situation discussed earlier where the measure of size variable is proportional to the number, N_i, of enumeration units in the cluster, the weight, w_i, is equal to N/n, and is therefore the same for each sample observation independent of the cluster from which it was sampled. In the situation in which the measure of size variable is not the number of enumeration units in the cluster, the weight, w_i, is equal to $(N_i X)/(n X_i)$, and is therefore not the same for each cluster.

In the illustrative example discussed above, if the measure of size variable used in the PPS sampling of clusters were the number, X_i, of admissions to a hospital with life-threatening conditions, then the same sample data shown in Table 11.7 would yield the following estimates (SUDAAN commands and output are shown below):

```
proc descript data = hspslct2 filetype = sas means totals;
nest drawing/psulev = 1;
weight w2star;
var lifethrt dxdead;
proc ratio data = hspslct2 filetype = sas;
nest drawing/psulev = 1;
weight w2star;
numer dxdead;
denom lifethrt;
```

where the variable, *w2star*, is equal to $(N_i X)/(n X_i)$.

The output for estimation of totals follows:

LIFETHRT	Sample Size	50
	Weighted Size	51344.99
	Total	6259.18
	SE Total	1277.32
	Mean	0.12
	SE Mean	0.02
DXDEAD	Sample Size	50
	Weighted Size	51344.99
	Total	1760.47
	SE Total	1079.04
	Mean	0.03
	SE Mean	0.02

Output for the Estimated Ratio

Variable		One
		1
DXDEAD/LIFETHRT	Sample Size	50
	Weighted Size	51344.99
	Weighted X-Sum	6259.18
	Weighted Y-Sum	1760.47
	Ratio Est.	0.28
	SE Ratio	0.21

11.3.3 How to Take a PPS Sample with Replacement

Operationally, it is very easy to take a two-stage PPS sample with replacement. We illustrate this method again using the population of hospitals shown in Table 10.9. Again we assume that the number, N_i, is the measure of size variable to be used in taking the sample. We first cumulate the measure of size variable (in this instance, the N_i) and associate random numbers with each cluster, as shown in Table 11.8. The number of random numbers associated with each cluster is equal to N_i, as shown in the table.

If m clusters are to be sampled and $\bar{n}$ enumeration units sampled at each drawing of a cluster, the procedure involves (1) taking a random number between 1 and N; (2) identifying the cluster corresponding to the random number; (3) taking a simple random sample without replacement of $\bar{n}$ enumeration units within that cluster; and (4) repeating this procedure until m clusters and $n = m\bar{n}$ enumeration units have been chosen.

To illustrate this, suppose $m = 5$, and $\bar{n} = 6$. We first take a random number between 00001 and 50056 and suppose this is 36207. This corresponds to hospital 5. We then take 6 random numbers between 0001 and 27010 without replacement, and the admissions corresponding to these numbers are sampled for that particular drawing of a cluster. We then take a second random number between 00001 and 50056 for purposes of drawing our second hospital. Suppose this random number is 42751. This corresponds to Hospital 8, which has 1824 admissions; we then take 6 random numbers without replacement between 0001 and 1824 for purposes of sampling 6 admissions from this hospital. We continue this process until samples of six admissions have been selected from five hospitals. From Table 11.8, we see that for this illustration, hospital 5 was drawn three times and hospitals 2 and 8 were each drawn once. The particular admissions sampled at the second stage are shown in the sixth column of Table 11.8.

11.3.4 How Large a Sample is Needed for a Two-Stage Sample in Which Clusters are Selected PPS with Replacement

In two-stage cluster sampling, the standard error of an estimated parameter is determined not only by the total number, n, of enumeration units sampled but

Table 11.8 Procedure for PPS Sampling with Replacement

Hospital	Total Admissions, N_i	Cumulative Admissions	Random Numbers	Random Numbers Chosen for First Stage	Random Numbers Chosen for Second Stage
1	4,288	4,288	00001–04288		
2	5,036	9,324	04289–09324	08589	0480, 2368, 4130, 2167, 3475, 3553
3	1,178	10,502	09325–10502		
4	638	11,140	10503–11140		
5	27,010	38,150	11141–38150	36207	09429, 10365, 07119, 02368, 01011, 07056
				18602	16631, 16815, 20206, 05300, 22164, 24369
				18738	19687, 11052, 19746, 14349, 00697, 19124
6	1,122	39,272	38151–39272		
7	2,134	41,406	39273–41406		
8	1,824	43,230	41407–43230	42751	1624, 1601, 1284, 0119, 1805, 0903
9	4,672	47,902	43231–47902		
10	2,154	50,056	47903–50056		

also by the two factors composing n, namely the number, m, of clusters sampled and the average number, $\bar{n}$, of enumeration units sampled per cluster. Thus, for example, an estimated population total obtained from a two-stage sample of 80 enumeration units consisting of 10 sample clusters, each having 8 sample enumeration units, is likely to have a standard error that is different from an estimate obtained from a sample of 20 clusters, each having 4 sample enumeration units. More often than not, however, the number, $\bar{n}$, of enumeration units to be sampled is determined in advance on the basis of cost and intraclass correlation considerations (such as those discussed in Chapter 10), so that the issue of sample-size determination reduces to that of determining the number, m, of clusters to be sampled, given that $\bar{n}$ enumeration units will be sampled per sample cluster. In our formulation of the issue of how large a sample is needed in PPS sampling with replacement, we then make the following assumptions:

1. The number, $\bar{n}$, of enumeration units to be sampled within each cluster will be the same for each sample cluster and has already been determined.
2. A "preliminary" estimate is available from a PPS cluster sample of the level of the variable of interest (in our discussion, this is a population total for that variable) as well its standard error. (Hence, we know the coefficient of variation of the estimate.)
3. We wish to determine with $100 \times (1 - \alpha)\%$ confidence, the number of sample clusters needed in order to estimate the total level of a particular variable in the population to within $100 \times \varepsilon\%$ of its true value.

Let us assume that the measure of size variable for the PPS sampling is the number of enumeration units within each cluster, which implies that the preliminary estimate of the standard error is given by the formula in Equation (11.11). Note that this estimate is of the form:

$$\widehat{SE}(y'_{\text{ppswr}}) = \sqrt{\frac{G(y_1, y_2, \ldots, y_m)}{m}}$$

where

$$G(y_1, y_2, \ldots, y_m) = \frac{\sum_{i=1}^{m} \left(\frac{N y_i}{\bar{n}} - y'_{\text{ppswr}} \right)^2}{m - 1}$$

From this, we have

$$m = \frac{z^2_{1-\alpha/2} G(y_1, y_2, \ldots, y_m)}{(y'_{\text{ppswr}})^2 \varepsilon^2} \tag{11.12}$$

and the estimated number, m, of clusters required to meet the specifications stated above is approximately equal to that shown in Equation (11.12).

Illustrative Example. Again, let us consider the population of 10 hospitals shown in Table 10.9. Suppose that we wish to take a PPSWR sample in which the first stage will consist of m independent drawings of a hospital in which, at each drawing, a simple random sample without replacement is taken of 10 enumeration units. Suppose further that we have taken a pilot survey of 5 hospitals (using the same PPSWR design that will be used in the main survey). Finally, let us suppose that the data obtained in that pilot study are the data described in our earlier discussion of that survey. We now wish to use these data to compute the number, m, of clusters that we will have to sample in order to be 95% confident that the resulting estimate, y'_{ppswr}, of the total number, Y, admitted with life-threatening conditions is within 30% of the true value.

The data obtained in that preliminary survey needed for estimating the required number, m, of sample clusters are shown below:

$$y'_{\text{ppswr}} = 6,006.72$$
$$\widehat{\text{SE}}(y'_{\text{ppswr}}) = 1,001.12$$
$$m^* = 5 \text{ (the number of clusters sampled in the preliminary survey)}$$
$$G(y_1, \ldots, y_m) = (1001.12 \times \sqrt{5})^2 = (2238.572)^2 = 5,011,206.272$$
$$\bar{n} = 10$$
$$\varepsilon = .3$$
$$z_{1-(\alpha/2)} = 1.96$$

Entering the above values into Equation (11.12), we have

$$m = 5.9 \approx 6$$

Thus, we would require six drawings of hospitals (60 total sample admissions) to meet the specifications set for the estimated total number admitted with life-threatening conditions.   □

11.3.5 Telephone PPS Sampling: The Mitofsky–Waksberg Method of Random Digit Dialing

Telephone sampling has become so important in survey methodology that we devote an entire chapter (Chapter 15) to cover this topic in detail. It appears in the present chapter as an example of PPS sampling, and we show that a widely used technique known as the *Mitofsky–Waksberg Method of Random Digit Dialing* is, in fact, a form of PPS sampling.

The use of telephone interviewing in sample surveys has increased greatly in recent years, primarily because field costs involved in personal visits to households are often prohibitive. If it is recognized that not all households have telephones, and if the totality of households having telephones is acceptable as a target population, then telephone interviewing very often is used as an alternative to personal household visits.

In telephone surveys, households can be chosen in several ways for inclusion in the sample. For instance, the telephone directory of the target area can be used as the sampling frame. However, telephone directories contain neither unlisted numbers nor numbers assigned to households since the publication of the latest directory. Exclusion of these households may be a source of serious bias since households having unlisted numbers or new numbers might form a substantial percentage of households with telephones.

An alternative sampling frame for telephone surveys is a list of all possible four-digit numbers within existing telephone exchanges. A telephone number consists of ten digits. The first three digits designate the *area code*, the next three designate the *telephone exchange*, and the last four digits identify the particular *phone listing*. For example, to dial the Dean of the School of Public Health at the University of Illinois at Chicago, you would first dial area code 312 (the area code for Chicago), followed by the number 996 (the particular exchange for all University of Illinois at Chicago numbers), followed by 6623 (the Dean's private line). Verify this by dialing the ten digits: 3129966623. The present Dean is an especially gregarious individual and welcomes such calls. The use of these digits as the sampling frame is known as *random digit dialing* and avoids many of the biases often associated with telephone directories. Our ensuing discussion of random digit dialing is based primarily on methods originally developed by Mitofsky [9] and later refined and expanded by Waksberg [10].

A list of area codes and exchanges for the target area of a survey can be obtained from the local telephone company office. Thus, within a given area code (e.g., 312) and exchange (e.g., 996), only the last four digits of a telephone number need to be chosen randomly. However, it turns out that a relatively large proportion (approximately 80%) of all telephone numbers within designated area codes and exchanges either are not used at all or else are assigned to businesses, institutions, or other nonhouseholds. In other words, the process of taking random, four-digit numbers within given area codes and exchanges would be wasteful since we would expect to dial approximately five telephone numbers for every household obtained. Mitofsky and Waksberg suggest an alternative procedure that increases the yield of numbers corresponding to households. In this procedure the telephone numbers are grouped into clusters defined by the first 8 (rather than the first 6) digits. For example, if the target population includes those households in area code 312, exchanges 996 and 835, the numbers are grouped into 200 clusters as follows based on the first 8 digits:

312-835-00 to 312-835-99 (100 clusters)
312-996-00 to 312-996-99 (100 clusters)

The clusters are identified (e.g., 1 to 200, as above) and sampled as follows. A random cluster is taken (e.g., 312-996-47) and a random number between 00 and 99 is taken (e.g., 60). The telephone number (e.g., 312-996-4760) is then dialed. If the number is a household, the cluster is retained and additional two-digit numbers are taken until a total of $\bar{n}$ residences (including the first one dialed) are reached. If the original number is not a residence, the cluster is rejected. This procedure is continued until a total of m clusters are sampled, which would result in a total of $m\bar{n}$ interviews.

The Mitofsky–Waksberg procedure yields a great improvement in the proportion of households dialed because of a tendency for residential numbers to be clustered within "banks" of sequential numbers. The sample design described above is that of PPS sampling since the initial phone call made in the cluster determines whether the cluster is or is not included in the sample, and the probability of this initial phone call yielding a household depends on the proportion of the 100 numbers in the cluster that are associated with households.

11.4 FURTHER COMMENT ON PPS SAMPLING

In discussing PPS sampling, we focused on a particular sampling plan and estimation procedure. The sampling plan involved drawing clusters by simple random sampling with replacement and then taking a simple random sample (without replacement) of enumeration units in each sample cluster each time that cluster was drawn. The estimation procedure involved use of the Hansen–Hurwitz estimator. This type of PPS sampling is used quite often in surveys, perhaps because estimates of standard errors can be obtained relatively easily since the clusters are drawn independently of each other. The Hansen–Hurwitz estimator is used in combination with this type of sampling, because it is much easier to compute than the Horvitz–Thompson estimator.

There are, however, other types of PPS sampling that are also sometimes used in practice. For example, clusters can be selected by simple random sampling without replacement or by some other form of sampling without replacement. Since the Hansen–Hurwitz estimator can only be used if the sampling is done with replacement, PPS sampling in which the clusters are selected without replacement often use some form of the Horvitz–Thompson estimator. Standard errors of the resulting estimates are not easily obtainable from such designs, although various methods have been proposed [1].

In PPS sampling designs, if the same number of enumeration units is selected within each first-stage sample cluster, then the probability of any enumeration unit being sampled is the same, no matter which cluster the enumeration unit belongs to. In other words, the sample is *self-weighting* in the sense that every enumeration unit in the sample represents the same number of enumeration units in the population. This is not generally true in simple two-stage cluster sampling unless all clusters have the same number, N_i, of enumeration units.

11.5   SUMMARY

In this chapter, we showed by way of examples that simple two-stage cluster sampling can yield estimates that have excessively high sampling errors, especially if there is considerable diversity among the clusters with respect to the number, N_i, of enumeration units within clusters. This is especially true in the estimation of population totals. We also demonstrated that use of a sample design in which clusters are sampled with probability proportional to some characteristic of the cluster (e.g., number of enumeration units in the cluster) can lead to estimates having sampling errors that are much lower than those obtained from sampling clusters with equal probability. Two general classes of estimators, the Horvitz–Thompson estimator, and the Hansen–Hurwitz estimator are discussed and can be used in combination with unequal probability sampling. We focused our discussion of PPS sampling on the scenario in which clusters are selected by simple random sampling with replacement and with selection probabilities proportional to some measure of the size of the cluster. At each drawing of a cluster, a simple random sample of enumeration units is selected without replacement, and estimation is done by use of the Hansen–Hurwitz estimator. Using illustrative examples, we showed how samples are taken by this procedure; how parameters are estimated, and how standard errors are obtained. Formulas for determination of sample size for this design were also developed. Finally, we also discussed the use of PPS sampling in random digit dialing telephone surveys.

EXERCISES

Let us consider again the population of 25 local mental health centers of Exercises 10.12–10.15 (table reproduced opposite):

Health Center	No. of Patients	Health Center	No. of Patients
1	491	14	672
2	866	15	475
3	188	16	439
4	994	17	392
5	209	18	584
6	961	19	882
7	834	20	424
8	9820	21	775
9	348	22	262
10	246	23	968
11	399	24	586
12	175	25	809
13	166		

11.1 Suppose that you wish to take a two-stage PPS sample with replacement of health centers for purposes of estimating the total number of patients currently taking Prozac. Suppose further that the measure of size variable for the PPS sampling is the number of patients, and that the random numbers chosen are 11,052 and 12,614.

  a. Which two health centers are sampled?

  b. Suppose that a simple random sample of 20 patients is taken at each drawing from the health center selected at that drawing. Suppose further that the sample corresponding to the random number, 11,052, contains 12 patients on Prozac, and that the sample corresponding to the random number, 12,614, contains 6 persons on Prozac. Use the Hansen–Hurwitz estimator to estimate the total number of persons on Prozac. What is the estimated standard error of that estimate?

11.2 It is desired to estimate the number of Koreans living in a particular city. The city encompasses six telephone exchanges, and examination of the latest telephone directory showed the following frequencies of the two most common Korean surnames—Kim and Park.

Exchange	Population of Geographic Area Corresponding to Exchange	No. of Kims and Parks in Directory
832	5231	21
856	3012	8
935	2123	7
936	1256	35
937	2569	17
983	8321	10

It is thought that approximately 60% of all Koreans in that area have either "Kim" or "Park" as surnames, and that the average Korean household comprises four persons.

a. If you were to use exchanges as clusters, what method of sampling the clusters should be used?

b. Use this method to take a sample of three exchanges. Show in detail how the sample was selected.

11.3 From the population of counties shown in Exercise 10.16, a PPS sample with replacement of 5 counties is taken, and for every selection of a county at the first stage, a sample of 1 hospital is taken at the second stage. The sampling is performed as follows:

a. The procedure for taking a PPS sample of counties is that described in Section 11.3.3.

b. The measure of size variable for sampling a county is the total number of hospitals within the county.

c. The random numbers chosen for selection of the sample are as follows:

Selection Sequence	Random Number for Selection of Counties at First Stage	Random Number for Selection of Hospital at Second Stage
1	38	1
2	24	1
3	24	1
4	42	3
5	08	1

From the above information, determine the sample counties and hospitals.

11.4 From the sample selected in the previous exercise, determine the total number of hospital admissions during 1989 in the 37 county region. Also, determine the standard error of this estimated total.

11.5 (For those having access to software such as STATA or SUDAAN.) Estimate the total number of admissions per bed from the sample selected in Exercise 11.3. Also, determine the standard error of this estimate.

BIBLIOGRAPHY

The text by Brewer referenced below gives a very comprehensive treatment of sampling designs and estimators based on unequal probability sampling.

1. Brewer, K. R. W., and Hanif, M., *Sampling with Unequal Probabilities*, Springer-Verlag, New York, 1983.

The following recent texts give excellent discussions of the Horvitz–Thompson and Hansen–Hurwitz estimators and of the various types of PPS Sampling.

2. Hedayat, A. S., and Sinha, B. K., *Design and Inference in Finite Population Sampling*, Wiley, New York, 1991.

3. Lehtonen, R., and Pahkinen, E. J., *Practical Methods for Design and Analysis of Complex Surveys*, Rev. Ed., Wiley, Chichester, U.K., 1997.

4. Thompson, S. K., *Sampling*, Wiley, New York, 1992.

The following expository review in the Enclyclopedia of Statistical Sciences *gives an excellent overview of PPS sampling and contains a long list of useful references on the topic.*

5. Skinner, C. J., Probability proportional to size (PPS) sampling. In *The Encyclopedia of Statistical Sciences*, Johnson, N., and Kotz, S., Eds., Wiley, New York, 1983.

The following entry in the Encyclopedia of Biostatistics *provides a very detailed discussion of practical aspects of PPS sampling including its strengths and weaknesses.*

6. Czaja, R., Sampling with probability proportionate to size. In *Encyclopedia of Biostatistics*, Armitage, P. A., and Colton, T. D., Eds., Wiley, Chichester, U.K., 1998.

The two original papers on the Hansen–Hurwitz and Horvitz–Thompson estimators are referenced below.

7. Hansen, M. H., and Hurwitz, W. N., On the theory of sampling from finite population. *Annals of Mathematical Statistics*, **14**: 333–362, 1943.

8. Horvitz, D. G., and Thompson, D. J., A generalization of sampling without replacement from a finite universe. *Journal of the American Statistical Association*, **47**: 663–685, 1952.

The following two articles are the seminal papers on the Mitofsky–Waksberg method of telephone sampling.

9. Mitofsky, W., *Sampling of Telephone Households* (Unpublished CBS Memorandum), 1970.

10. Waksberg, J., Sampling methods for random digit dialing. *Journal of the American Statistical Association*, **73**: 40–46, 1978.

CHAPTER 12

Variance Estimation in Complex Sample Surveys

In previous chapters, we have presented methods for estimating the variances of estimated characteristics for most of the various sample designs that have been discussed. In many of these designs, the theoretical variance of the particular estimator is a linear function of population parameters. For example, in simple random sampling, the variance of an estimated total, x', is given by

$$\text{Var}(x') = \frac{N^2}{n} \, \sigma_x^2 \left(\frac{N-n}{N-1} \right)$$

Clearly, because the above expression is a linear function of the population variance σ_x^2, an unbiased estimate can be obtained by substituting into the expression for $\text{Var}(x')$ given in Chapter 2, the unbiased estimate, $\hat{\sigma}_x^2$ of σ_x^2.

For many sample designs that are used in practice, however, the estimation process may involve stratification, several stages of cluster sampling, ratio or regression estimation, poststratification to known totals, and other procedures, with the result that the variance of the resulting estimate may not be a linear or even a known function of the population parameters. This is true in many of the sample surveys conducted by the U.S. Bureau of the Census, the National Center for Health Statistics, the Bureau of Labor Statistics, and other agencies.

In order to estimate the variances of estimates obtained from sample surveys involving complex sampling and estimation procedures, it is necessary to use one of two general classes of methods that have been developed expressly for this purpose: *linearization* and *replication* methods.

The technique of *linearization* was developed for sample surveys by Keyfitz [1], Woodruff [2], and others, and is based on a Taylor series approximation. In the late 1970s, investigators at the Research Triangle Institute began development of what eventually became user-friendly software based on linearization [3]. This software was the precursor of SUDAAN and went through considerable evolution to the now widely used package discussed and demonstrated throughout this book. The availability and appeal of this and other software has made linearization perhaps now the most widely used method of variance estimation for complex surveys.

Replication is a general class of methods in which an estimate of the variance of an estimated population parameter is obtained by expressing the estimated population parameter as a sum or mean of several statistics, each of which is based on a subset of the sample observations. The variance of the estimated population parameter can then be estimated by obtaining an estimate of the variance of these "part sample" statistics. A simple example of this technique was demonstrated in Chapter 4 with respect to the estimated variance of an estimated population characteristic under repeated systematic sampling. Variants of this class of techniques have been used for many years. In their textbook written in the early 1950s, Hansen et al. [5] referred to these techniques as *random group methods*. These methods were refined by McCarthy [6], [7] in the 1960s and became widely used at the National Center for Health Statistics and at other federal agencies. There have been studies by Frankel [8], Bean [9], and several publications by Lemeshow and collaborators [10]–[16] attempting to evaluate these methods.

The purpose of this chapter is to present the rationale behind the algorithms used in the various software packages now available for estimating variances of estimates obtained from sample surveys having complex designs. In the ensuing discussion, we focus on linearization and replication methods, which are currently the two most widely used methods of variance estimation.

12.1 LINEARIZATION

In complex sample surveys, estimation of the variances of estimated population characteristics can be difficult either because of the way the sample was taken or because of the way the estimates of population characteristics were constructed. For example, an estimated total based on several stages of cluster sampling, ratio adjustment, and poststratification often may not readily yield an appropriate variance estimator. In such situations, the technique of linearization can be used to construct an approximation to the functional form of the estimated population characteristic that is a linear function of the original observations and hence is amenable to construction of a variance estimator.

The discussion of linearization methodology that follows is essentially a selection and condensation of material presented in the technical appendix of the SUDAAN manual that accompanies the personal computer version of that software product [3].

For simplicity, let us suppose that we have a population that consists of observations, x_i and y_i, on the ith enumeration unit. Suppose further that it is desired to estimate some population characteristic, θ, and that there exists an estimator, $\hat{\theta}$, which is a function, $f(x, y)$ of variables x and y which are both linear functions of sample observations. The function, $f(x, y)$, however, is not a linear function of sample observations.

To illustrate, $\hat{\theta}$ might be the ratio, $\bar{x}/\bar{y}$, of the sample means, $\bar{x}$ and $\bar{y}$. Clearly, $\bar{x}$ and $\bar{y}$ are linear functions of the sample observations, whereas $f(\bar{x}, \bar{y})$ is a nonlinear function of the two sample means, and hence is nonlinear in the sample observations.

The computation of the variance of $\hat{\theta}$ by the linearization method is a two-step procedure. The first step or linearization step involves approximating $f(x, y)$ by a first order Taylor series. This would result in an approximation that is linear in the sample statistics, $\bar{x}$ and $\bar{y}$, and hence linear in the sample observations. Once this first-order Taylor series approximation to $\hat{\theta}$ is obtained, the second step involves use of design-based methods such as those described in Chapters 3–11 to estimate its variance. We describe below how this is done mechanically.

We define the entity, z_i, called the *linearized value* of $f(\bar{x}, \bar{y})$ for observation i as follows:

$$z_i = (\partial f_{\bar{X}})x_i + (\partial f_{\bar{Y}})y_i$$

where

$$\partial f_{\bar{X}} = \frac{\partial f(\bar{x}, \bar{y})}{\partial \bar{x}} \text{ evaluated at the point } (\bar{X}, \bar{Y})$$

and

$$\partial f_{\bar{Y}} = \frac{\partial f(\bar{x}, \bar{y})}{\partial \bar{y}} \text{ evaluated at the point } (\bar{X}, \bar{Y})$$

(where $\bar{X}$ and $\bar{Y}$ are the unknown population parameters, of which $\bar{x}$ and $\bar{y}$ are unbiased estimators).

For example, if $\hat{\theta} = \bar{x}/\bar{y}$, then

$$\partial f_{\bar{X}} = \frac{1}{\bar{Y}}, \qquad \partial f_{\bar{Y}} = -\frac{\bar{X}}{\bar{Y}^2} \quad \text{and} \quad z_i = \frac{1}{\bar{Y}}x_i - \frac{\bar{X}}{\bar{Y}^2}y_i$$

The first-term Taylor series expansion of $\hat{\theta}$ is given by

$$\hat{\theta} = f(\bar{x}, \bar{y}) \approx (\partial f_{\bar{X}})(\bar{x} - \bar{X}) + (\partial f_{\bar{Y}})(\bar{y} - \bar{Y})$$
$$= (\partial f_{\bar{X}})\bar{x} + (\partial f_{\bar{Y}})\bar{y} - ((\partial f_{\bar{X}})\bar{X} + (\partial f_{\bar{Y}})\bar{Y})$$

and

$$\text{Var}(\hat{\theta}) \cong \text{Var}((\partial f_{\bar{X}})\bar{x} + (\partial f_{\bar{Y}})\bar{y})$$

since the term $((\partial f_{\bar{X}})\bar{X} + (\partial f_{\bar{Y}})\bar{Y})$ is a constant. But

$$(\partial f_{\bar{x}})\bar{x} + (\partial f_{\bar{y}})\bar{y} = (\partial f_{\bar{x}})\sum_{i=1}^{n}\frac{x_i}{n} + (\partial f_{\bar{y}})\sum_{i=1}^{n}\frac{y_i}{n} = \sum_{i=1}^{n}\frac{z_i}{n} = \bar{z}.$$

Thus, the problem of finding the approximate variance of $\hat{\theta}$ reduces to that of determining the variance of a linear combination of the sample observations, and can be obtained by identifying the sample design and using the appropriate formula. For example, if the design is simple random sampling, then the variance of $\hat{\theta}$ is estimated by

$$\widehat{\text{Var}}(\hat{\theta}) = \frac{\sum_{i=1}^{n}(\tilde{z}_i - \bar{\tilde{z}})^2}{n(n-1)}\left(\frac{N-n}{N}\right) \tag{12.1}$$

where

$$\tilde{z}_i = (\partial f_{\bar{x}})x_i + (\partial f_{\bar{y}})y_i$$

$$\partial f_{\bar{x}} = \frac{\partial f(\bar{x}, \bar{y})}{\partial \bar{x}} \text{ evaluated at } (\bar{x}, \bar{y})$$

and

$$\partial f_{\bar{y}} = \frac{\partial f(\bar{x}, \bar{y})}{\partial \bar{y}} \text{ evaluated at } (\bar{x}, \bar{y})$$

(since $\bar{X}$ and $\bar{Y}$ are unknown parameters).

Illustrative Example. We take a very small simple example to illustrate exactly how linearization works. Suppose we are doing an audit of Medicaid costs for a patient and take a simple random sample of 10 claims from a total of 65 claims made on behalf of the patient. The data from this audit are shown in Table 12.1. We wish to estimate the proportion of total dollars paid on behalf of this patient that are overpayments.

From the data, we have $\bar{x} = 106.5$ and $\bar{y} = 275.6$. Since we are using a ratio estimate, the linearized variable

$$\tilde{z}_i = \frac{1}{275.6}x_i - \frac{106.5}{(275.6)^2}y_i$$

would be obtained as described above. For example, $\tilde{z}_1 = (1/275.6) \times 210 - (106.5/275.6^2) \times 210 = .4675$, and the $\tilde{z}_i$ are shown in the fourth column of Table 12.1. With $N = 65$ and $n = 10$, we calculate from

Table 12.1 Medicaid Payments and Overpayments for 10 Sample Claims Submitted on Patient

Claim	Payment (y) $	Overpayment (x) $	Linearized Observation $\tilde{z}_i$
1	210	210	.4675
2	78	0	−.1094
3	343	123	−.0346
4	298	157	.1518
5	349	0	−.4894
6	210	210	.4675
7	536	0	−.7516
8	289	135	.0846
9	98	0	−.1374
10	345	230	.3508

Equation (12.1) the standard error of the ratio estimate, r, which is equal to .1158. $\square$

Both SUDAAN and STATA use linearization to estimate variances of estimated statistics. To use either of these, we would need to add to each record in the data set shown in Table 12.1 the variables $N (= 65)$ and $w (= 65/10 = 6.5)$. We would not need the variable, $\tilde{z}_i$, since that would be computed by the program. The resulting data set for use by either SUDAAN or STATA is shown below:

claim	payment	ovpaymnt	N	w
1	210	210	65	6.5
2	78	0	65	6.5
3	343	123	65	6.5
4	298	157	65	6.5
5	349	0	65	6.5
6	210	210	65	6.5
7	536	0	65	6.5
8	289	135	65	6.5
9	98	0	65	6.5
10	345	230	65	6.5

The following STATA commands are used to estimate the ratio, x/y, and its standard error:

```
use "a: \exmp12_2.dta", clear
. svyset fpc N
. svyset pweight w
. svyratio ovpaymnt/payment
```

These commands generate the following output:

Survey ratio estimation			
pweight: W		Number of obs	= 10
Strata: <one>		Number of strata	= 1
PSU: <observations>		Number of PSUs	= 10
FPC: N		Population size	= 65

Ratio	Estimate	Std. Err.	[95% Conf. Interval]	Deff
ovpaymnt/payment	.3864296	.1158187	.1244294 .6484298	1

Finite population correction (FPC) assumes simple random sampling without replacement of PSUs within each stratum with no subsampling within PSUs.

The following commands are used for estimation with SUDAAN:

```
1   PROC RATIO DATA = EXMP12_2 FILETYPE = SAS DESIGN = WOR;
2   NEST _ONE_;
3   WEIGHT W;
4   TOTCNT N;
5   NUMER OVPAYMNT;
6   DENOM PAYMENT;
7   SETENV COLWIDTH = 15;
8   SETENV DECWIDTH = 3;
```

These commands yield the following output:

Number of observations read :	10	Weighted count : 65
Number of observations skipped :	0	
(WEIGHT variable nonpositive)		
Denominator degrees of freedom :	9	

by: Variable, One.

Variable		One 1
OVPAYMNT/PAYME- NT	Sample Size	10.000
	Weighted Size	65.000
	Weighted X-Sum	17914.000
	Weighted Y-Sum	6922.500
	Ratio Est.	0.386
	SE Ratio	0.116

12.2 REPLICATION METHODS

Replication methods (sometimes called *resampling methods*) estimate the sampling variance of a statistic by computing the statistic for subsets of the sample and examining its variability over the subsets. The two general approaches to replication that have been developed over the past three decades are the *jackknifing* approach, and the *balanced repeated replication* approach (also known as the *balanced half-sample approach*). In this discussion of replication techniques, we will focus primarily on balanced repeated replication (BRR) methods, since historically they have been more widely used in sample survey work than jackknifing.

12.2.1 The Balanced Repeated Replication Method

The BRR method is most applicable to the widely used class of sample designs in which primary sampling units (PSUs) are grouped into L strata, random samples of two PSUs are selected from each stratum, and independent estimates of stratum characteristics are obtained from each PSU.

More specifically, let us illustrate the BRR method by showing how the variance of a ratio estimate would be estimated by this procedure. Suppose that $x'_{h1}, x'_{h2}, y'_{h1}$, and y'_{h2} are estimates from each of the two PSUs of the stratum parameters X_h and Y_h in each of the L strata. (For this discussion, let us assume that each stratum has equal weight in determining population estimates.) It follows that the ratio estimate r of the population ratio R based on all $2L$ estimates would be given by

$$r = \frac{x'}{y'}$$

where

$$x' = \sum_{h=1}^{L} \sum_{i=1}^{2} (x'_{hi}/2)$$

and

$$y' = \sum_{h=1}^{L} \sum_{i=1}^{2} (y'_{hi}/2)$$

We define a *half sample estimate* of the ratio R as follows:

$$r_{(k)} = \frac{\sum_{h=1}^{L} [\delta_{kh} x'_{h1} + (1 - \delta_{kh}) x'_{h2}]}{\sum_{h=1}^{L} [\delta_{kh} y'_{h1} + (1 - \delta_{kh}) y'_{h2}]}$$

where $(\delta_{k1}, \ldots, \delta_{kL})$ is an L-dimensional vector whose elements are equal to unity or zero. In other words, each $r_{(k)}$ is an estimate of R formed by taking one of the two estimates from each stratum. Clearly, there are 2^L possible vectors (δ_k) having the form shown above, and hence a total of 2^L possible half sample estimates $r_{(k)}$. An appropriate estimate of the variance of r computed from the 2^L possible half samples would be

$$\widehat{\text{Var}}(r) = \left(\frac{1}{2^L}\right) \sum_{k=1}^{2^L} (r_{(k)} - \bar{r})^2.$$

Usually 2^L is so large that it is impractical to compute all of the possible $r_{(k)}$. A subset of K half sample estimates (where $K \leq 2^L$) can be constructed by obtaining the δ_{ij} from an orthogonal matrix of the type described by Plackett and Burman [17]. The details of this procedure are discussed by McCarthy [6], who showed that it is possible to select, in a rigidly prescribed manner, a small subset of the half samples and still obtain satisfactory variance estimates. In fact, he showed for linear estimates such as means and totals that the use of the small subset gives precisely the same variance estimate as would be obtained from all 2^L half samples. The resulting set of half sample estimates is referred to as being *balanced* since between-strata contributions to the variance are shown to cancel out. Suppose that we take a balanced set consisting of K such half sample estimates, and define our final estimate $\bar{r}$ as follows:

$$\bar{r} = \frac{1}{K} \sum_{k=1}^{K} r_{(k)}. \tag{12.2}$$

An estimator of the variance of this ratio estimate $\bar{r}$ is given by

$$\widehat{\text{Var}}(\bar{r}) = \left(\frac{1}{K}\right) \sum_{k=1}^{K} (r_{(k)} - \bar{r})^2. \tag{12.3}$$

The rationale for and statistical properties of this balanced half sample variance estimator are detailed by McCarthy [6] and by Bean [9] and Lemeshow and Levy [10]. We give a heuristic rationale for this variance estimator in the Technical Appendix to this chapter. We now illustrate the use of this method with a simple example.

Illustrative Example. A city is divided into three emergency service areas, with each emergency service area containing five ambulance stations. It is desired to estimate, for the city as a whole, the proportion arriving alive at a hospital among all persons who had suffered a cardiac arrest and were seen by paramedics from one of the 15 ambulance stations described above. A sample survey was conducted in which two random ambulance stations from each of the three emergency service areas were sampled. In each of the six ambulance stations sampled, records were reviewed and estimates were made for the service area of the number of cardiac arrests and the number and proportion of these arrests that reached the hospital alive. The results of this sample survey are shown below:

Emergency Service Area (ESA)	Ambulance Station	Estimate for ESA of Number of Cardiac Arrests y'_{hi}	Estimate for ESA of Number Reaching Hospital Alive x'_{hi}
1	1	120	25
	2	78	24
2	1	185	30
	2	228	49
3	1	670	80
	2	530	70

It should be emphasized that the x'_{hi} and y'_{hi} shown above are estimates based on data from the particular ambulance station of the number of cardiac arrests and number successfully reaching the hospital alive.

Clearly, the design of this sample survey features stratification by emergency service area and estimation for each emergency service area from two randomly sampled ambulance stations.

The following $2^3 = 8$ half sample replications can be constructed from three strata:

Replication (k)	δ_{k1}	$1 - \delta_{k1}$	δ_{k2}	$1 - \delta_{k2}$	δ_{k3}	$1 - \delta_{k3}$
1	1	0	1	0	1	0
2	1	0	1	0	0	1
3	1	0	0	1	1	0
4	1	0	0	1	0	1
5	0	1	1	0	1	0
6	0	1	1	0	0	1
7	0	1	0	1	1	0
8	0	1	0	1	0	1

For example, replication 1 would yield the following value of $r_{(k)}$:

$$r_{(1)} = \frac{\sum_{h=1}^{3}(\delta_{ih}x'_{h1} + (1 - \delta_{ih})x'_{h2})}{\sum_{h=1}^{3}(\delta_{ih}y'_{h1} + (1 - \delta_{ih})y'_{h2})} = \frac{135}{975} = .1385$$

The eight replications yield the following values of $r_{(k)}$:

k	$x'_{(k)}$	$y'_{(k)}$	$r_{(k)}$
1	135	975	.1385
2	125	835	.1497
3	154	1018	.1513
4	144	878	.1640
5	134	933	.1436
6	124	793	.1564
7	153	976	.1568
8	143	836	.1711

From the data shown above, we see that the estimated ratio $\bar{r}$ and its estimated variance, $\widehat{\text{Var}}(\bar{r})$, based on the eight replications are given by

$$\bar{r} = \frac{1}{8}\sum_{k=1}^{8} r_{(k)} = .1539$$

and

$$\widehat{\text{Var}}(\bar{r}) = .000098$$

Plackett and Burman [17] presented $m \times m$ matrices of dimension $m = \{4, 8, 12, \ldots, 100\}$ excluding $m = 92$. The dimension of the matrix to be used in a given problem would depend on the number of strata. McCarthy [6] used matrices in which m is a multiple of 4 and $L \leq m \leq L + 3$, where, in all cases with $L > 2$, $m \ll 2^L$. Once the $m \times m$ matrix is selected, all rows but only the first L columns are used.

A *balanced* set of four replications can be obtained from the set of eight possible replications by taking replications 1, 4, 6, and 7 as shown below:

Replication k	δ_{k1}	$1 - \delta_{k1}$	δ_{k2}	$1 - \delta_{k2}$	δ_{k3}	$1 - \delta_{k3}$
1	1	0	1	0	1	0
4	1	0	0	1	0	1
6	0	1	1	0	0	1
7	0	1	0	1	1	0

Note that in this set, each stratum estimate x'_{hk} or y'_{hk} appears the same number of times (twice in this small example), and appears with every other estimate the same number of times (once in this example). Let us examine the estimate $\bar{r}$ and its variance $\widehat{\text{Var}}(\bar{r})$ for this set of four replications:

$$\bar{r} = (r_{(1)} + r_{(4)} + r_{(6)} + r_{(7)})/4 = .1539$$

and

$$\widehat{\mathrm{Var}}(\bar{r}) = .000088$$ □

Since each half sample stratum estimate appears the same number of times in the set of K balanced half samples, the estimate $\bar{r}$ will be equal to that obtained from a complete set of 2^L half samples. Also, McCarthy [6] has shown that the stability of the variance estimator from a set of balanced half sample replications is approximately that of the variance estimator constructed from the full set of 2^L half sample replications.

It should be noted that often surveys are designed in which there are $2L$ strata and one PSU is selected from each. In order to apply the BRR technique, the PSUs are paired to form L "pseudostrata" and the estimation process goes on as previously described. Care is generally exercised in this pairing to keep the PSUs as similar as possible with respect to known demographic information.

USE OF SUDAAN TO OBTAIN BRR ESTIMATES. The most recent release of SUDAAN at the time of this writing (Release 7.5) can obtain BRR estimates of standard errors as well as estimates from linearization. In the example shown above in which a balanced set of four of the eight possible replications is used to estimate the proportion of cardiac arrests arriving at the hospital alive, the data set required for analysis by SUDAAN is shown below:

ESA	AMBSTAT	CARDARRS	ALIVE	WT	REPWT1	REPWT4	REPWT6	REPWT7
1	1	120	25	2.5	5	5	0	0
1	2	78	24	2.5	0	0	5	5
2	1	185	30	2.5	5	0	5	0
2	2	228	49	2.5	0	5	0	5
3	1	670	80	2.5	5	0	0	5
3	2	530	70	2.5	0	5	5	0

Note that there are six records in the file, one for each sample point, and nine variables. The first two variables, *ESA* and *AMBSTAT*, identify the emergency service area and ambulance station. The next two variables, *CARDARRS* and *ALIVE* represent, respectively, the number of cardiac arrests serviced at each sample ambulance station and the number of these reaching the hospital alive. The variable, *WT*, is the sample weight, N/n, given to each ambulance station. In this example, $N = 15$, $n = 6$, and $WT = 2.5$ for each sample record. The variable, *REPWT1*, specifies the weight given in balanced half sample 1 to each sample observation used in the half sample. Since balanced half sample 1 includes only three sample points, $REPWT1 = 15/3 = 5$ for the 3 sample points used to obtain that half sample estimate and would equal 0 for the 3 sample points not included in that half sample. The other three variables *REPTW4*, *REPWT6*, and *REPWT7* are defined analogously.

The following SUDAAN commands are used to obtain the BRR estimates:

```
PROC RATIO DATA = AMBLNCE2 FILETYPE = SAS DESIGN = BRR;
WEIGHT WT;
REPWGT REPWT1 REPWT4 REPWT6 REPWT7;
NUMER ALIVE;
DENOM CARDARRS;
SETENV COLWIDTH = 14;
SETENV DECWIDTH = 5;
```

The first command indicates the name and type of the data file and that ratio estimation is to be performed by BRR. The second command indicates the variable containing the sampling weights, and the third command indicates, for each balanced half sample, the variables containing the sampling weights for that half sample. The remaining commands state the variables containing the numerator and denominator of the ratio and the format of the output. The resulting output is shown below:

Variance Estimation Method: BRR
by: Variable, One.

Variable		One - -
ALIVE/CARDARRS	Sample Size	6.00000
	Weighted Size	15.00000
	Weighted X-Sum	4527.50000
	Weighted Y-Sum	695.00000
	Ratio Est.	0.15351
	SE Ratio	0.00943

The SUDAAN estimate of the ratio and its standard error agrees with that shown earlier (except for differences in the third decimal place due to rounding error).

We now compare the estimates obtained above using SUDAAN with estimates obtained from the same data by use of linearization. The design is a stratified random sample with Emergency Service Areas as strata and a sample of 2 ambulance stations taken from the population of 5 ambulance stations in each emergency service area. The data file for obtaining linearization estimates is shown opposite:

ESA	AMBSTAT	CARDARRS	ALIVE	WT	NAMBSTAT
1	1	120	25	2.5	5
1	2	78	24	2.5	5
2	1	185	30	2.5	5
2	2	228	49	2.5	5
3	1	670	80	2.5	5
3	2	530	70	2.5	5

Note that the variable, *NAMBSTAT* is added to each record. This is needed since the sampling is without replacement within Emergency Service Areas and indicates that the population size is equal to five for each stratum. The commands used to generate the estimates are shown below:

```
PROC RATIO DATA = AMBLNCE2 FILETYPE = SAS DESIGN = STRWOR;
NEST ESA;
TOTCNT NAMBSTAT;
WEIGHT WT;
NUMER ALIVE;
DENOM CARDARRS;
SETENV COLWIDTH = 14;
SETENV DECWIDTH = 5;
```

The design statement *design = strwor*, indicates that the design is a single-stage stratified random sample with enumeration units selected without replacement.

The output resulting from this set of commands is shown below:

Variance Estimation Method: Taylor Series (STRWOR) by: Variable, One.		
Variable		One - -
ALIVE/CARDARRS	Sample Size	6.00000
	Weighted Size	15.00000
	Weighted X-Sum	4527.50000
	Weighted Y-Sum	695.00000
	Ratio Est.	0.15351
	SE Ratio	0.00760

Note that the standard error of the estimated ratio obtained by linearization is smaller than that obtained by the BRR method. This is not unexpected, since the linearization method takes into consideration that the sampling is without replacement (and therefore uses a finite population correction), whereas the BRR method does not. If we had used the linearization method, but indicated a stratified sampling with replacement design (design statement would be *design = strwr*) we would have obtained an estimated standard error of the estimated ratio equal to .00981, which is very close to the standard error of .00943 obtained by the BRR method.

12.2.2 Jackknife Estimation

Jackknifing is another method used for estimating the standard errors of estimates obtained from complex sample surveys. Like the BRR method, it involves computation of the estimate of interest (e.g., a total, mean, ratio) for several part-samples, and then computation of the variance of these estimates over the set of part-samples. Jackknife estimation has had a long history going back to a paper by Quenouille in the 1950s [20], and there are a great many variations of this estimate. We will describe for a ratio estimate the particular jackknife methodology currently used in SUDAAN and then demonstrate the SUDAAN estimation methodology, again using the sample of ambulance stations.

Let us suppose that we have L strata and n_h sample PSUs within stratum h $(h = 1, \ldots, L)$. We wish to estimate the standard error of a ratio estimate r, where

$$r = \frac{\displaystyle\sum_{h=1}^{L}\sum_{i=1}^{n_h} x_{hi}'}{\displaystyle\sum_{h=1}^{L}\sum_{i=1}^{n_h} y_{hi}'}$$

and x_{hi}' and y_{hi}' are estimates based on data from the particular PSU.

For each PSU in the data set, we obtain an estimate $r_{(hi)}$ of the population ratio based on all observations *except* those in PSU, *hi*. For a ratio estimate, $r_{(hi)}$ is given by

$$r_{(hi)} = \frac{\displaystyle\sum_{h'\neq h}\sum_{i=1}^{n_h} x_{h'i}' + \sum_{i'\neq i}\frac{n_h}{n_h - 1} x_{hi'}'}{\displaystyle\sum_{h'\neq h}\sum_{i=1}^{n_h} y_{h'i}' + \sum_{i'\neq i}\frac{n_h}{n_h - 1} y_{hi'}'}$$

Note that the estimate, $r_{(hi)}$, consists of stratum estimates from all PSUs except PSU *hi*, and that the stratum estimate from that PSU is based on the estimates from the other PSUs within that stratum appropriately adjusted by the factor $(n_h/(n_h - 1))$ to reflect the absence of the data from that PSU.

Once the $r_{(hi)}$ are computed, the estimated standard error of r is given by

$$\widehat{SE}(r) = \sqrt{\sum_{h=1}^{L} \sum_{i=1}^{n_h} \frac{n_h - 1}{n_h} (r_{(hi)} - r)^2} \tag{12.4}$$

Illustrative Example. Considering again the previous illustrative example, we have the following data.

ESA (h)	AMBSTAT (i)	x'_{hi}	y'_{hi}	$r_{(hi)}$	r	$(r_{(hi)} - r)^2/2$
1	1	692.5	4422.5	.156586	.153506	4.74×10^{-6}
1	2	697.5	4632.5	.150567	.153506	4.32×10^{-6}
2	1	742.5	4635.0	.160194	.153506	2.24×10^{-5}
2	2	647.5	4420.0	.146493	.153506	2.46×10^{-5}
3	1	670.0	4177.5	.160383	.153506	2.36×10^{-5}
3	2	720.0	4877.5	.147617	.153506	1.73×10^{-5}
Total						9.7×10^{-5}

The x'_{hi}, y'_{hi}, and $r_{(hi)}$ are obtained as illustrated for x'_{11}, y'_{11}, and $r_{(11)}$:

$$x'_{11} = 2.5 \times (2 \times 24 + 30 + 49 + 80 + 70) = 692.5$$
$$y'_{11} = 2.5 \times (2 \times 78 + 185 + 228 + 670 + 530) = 4422.5$$
$$r_{(11)} = \frac{692.5}{4422.5} = .156586$$

As shown before, $r = .153506$, and from Equation (12.4), we have

$$\widehat{SE}(r) = \sqrt{9.7 \times 10^{-5}} = .009849 \qquad \square$$

This estimation can be performed using SUDAAN with the following commands:

```
PROC RATIO DATA = AMBLNCE2 FILETYPE = SAS DESIGN = JACKKNIFE;
NEST ESA;
WEIGHT WT;
NUMER ALIVE;
DENOM CARDARRS;
SETENV COLWIDTH = 14;
SETENV DECWIDTH = 7;
```

which yields the following output:

Variance Estimation Method: Jackknife
by: Variable, One.

Variable		One
		- -
ALIVE/CARDARRS	Sample Size	6.0000000
	Weighted Size	15.0000000
	Weighted X-Sum	4527.5000000
	Weighted Y-Sum	695.0000000
	Ratio Est.	0.1535064
	SE Ratio	0.0098492

Note that the estimated standard error of the ratio agrees with that obtained by direct use of Equation (12.4). Its value of .009842 is very similar to that obtained earlier for the BRR method (estimated standard error of r is equal to .00943). Both are similar to the estimated value of .00943 obtained by linearization under assumptions of a with replacement sampling design, but larger than that obtained by linearization under assumptions of without replacement sampling (estimated standard error of r is equal to .00760).

The basic assumption for use of either the BRR or jackknife variance estimation procedures for single-stage sampling is that the sampling is either with replacement or that the sampling fraction is small (i.e., below 10%). For multistage sampling, the sampling at the first stage should also be with replacement (or sampling fraction small). Sampling without replacement is permitted at subsequent stages.

12.2.3 Estimation of Interviewer Variability by Use of Replicated Sampling Designs (Interpenetrating Samples)

Replication methods can also be used to estimate that portion of the variability that is attributable to differences in the measurement process among individuals responsible for collecting the data. A method known as *interpenetrating samples* is sometimes used to measure this "interviewer" variability. This method can perhaps be best explained for the relatively simple situation in which a simple random sample of n elements is selected from a population of N elements. If the data are to be collected by M interviewers, then instead of taking a simple random sample of n elements, we select M independent simple random samples, each containing $\bar{n} = n/M$ elements, and each set of $\bar{n}$ elements is allocated to a particular interviewer by some random process which gives an interviewer an equal probability of being assigned any of the M samples.

Under this design, each interviewer would provide a separate estimate, $\bar{x}_i$, of the mean level $\bar{X}$ of characteristic $\mathscr{X}$ in the population, and the variance, σ_x^2, of the distribution of $\mathscr{X}$ could be estimated by s_{bx}^2 under the assumption that there were no differences among interviewers in the measurement process:

$$s_{bx}^2 = \frac{\bar{n}\Sigma_{i=1}^M (\bar{x}_i - \bar{x})^2}{M - 1}$$

where $\bar{x}$ is the mean of the $\bar{x}_i$.

Another estimate of σ_x^2, valid whether or not there are interviewer effects, is given by

$$s_{wx}^2 = \frac{\Sigma_{i=1}^M s_{ix}^2}{M}$$

where

$$s_{ix}^2 = \frac{\Sigma_{j=1}^{\bar{n}} (x_{ij} - \bar{x}_i)^2}{\bar{n} - 1}$$

for $i = 1, \ldots, M$. Under the null hypothesis that there are no interviewer effects the ratio s_{bx}^2/s_{wx}^2 would follow the F distribution with $(M - 1)$ and $(n - M)$ degrees of freedom, and this test statistic could be used to test that hypothesis.

Under this replicated sample design, each interviewer can also be considered as a cluster of $\bar{n}$ observations. With this interpretation, the intraclass correlation can be used as an indicator of the proportion of the total variance that is attributable to variability among interviewers with respect to the measurement process. An estimator δ_x of the intraclass correlation coefficient suggested by Kalton [19] and others is as follows:

$$\delta_x = \frac{\left(\dfrac{s_{bx}^2}{s_{wx}^2} - 1\right)}{\left(\dfrac{s_{bx}^2}{s_{wx}^2} - 1 + \bar{n}\right)} \tag{12.5}$$

Illustrative Example. Suppose that a sample of 20 users of an accounting software package was taken from a list of persons registered with the company that manufactures the package. The 20 users were allocated randomly, 5 each to 4 interviewers who conducted telephone interviews with each user in his/her assigned list. The main variable of interest was satisfaction with the package rate on a five-point scale, with "1" indicating unsatisfied and "5" indicating very satisfied. Data for each of these 4 interviews are shown overleaf:

	Interviewer			
	1	2	3	4
	1	2	3	4
	1	2	3	3
	2	2	4	5
	3	3	4	5
	2	4	5	5
$\bar{x}_i$	1.80	2.60	3.80	4.40
s_{ix}^2	.70	.80	.70	.80

With $M = 4$ and $\bar{n} = 5$, we have

$$\bar{x} = 3.15 \qquad s_{bx}^2 = 6.85 \qquad s_{wx}^2 = 0.75.$$

The F ratio is given by

$$\frac{s_{bx}^2}{s_{wx}^2} = \frac{6.85}{0.75} = 9.133$$

which with 3 and 16 degrees of freedom is highly significant. The intraclass correlation coefficient, δ_x, is given by

$$\delta_x = \frac{9.133 - 1}{9.133 - 1 + 5} = .6192.$$

Thus, one would estimate that more than 61% of the total variance is explained by interviewer effects. □

12.3 SUMMARY

In this chapter we discussed issues pertaining to estimation of the variances or standard errors of statistics obtained from complex sample surveys. Specifically, we discussed in some detail and provided examples of variance estimates derived from three widely used methods, *linearization*, *balanced repeated replication*, and *jackknifing*. Empirical studies have found that no method has performed consistently better than the others and that each method can provide reasonably reliable variance estimates, provided that the sample sizes involved are sufficiently large.

EXERCISES

12.1 Let $\bar{x}$ be an estimate of the mean level of a variable $\mathscr{X}$, and $\bar{y}$ be an estimate of the mean level of a variable $\mathscr{Y}$, where both are obtained from simple random sampling. Let $\bar{z} = \bar{x}\bar{y}$. Use linearization to find an expression for the estimated variance of the distribution of $\bar{z}$.

12.2 In a large state there are 34 counties that are not in metropolian areas. For purposes of estimating the total number of admissions during the calendar year 1990 to hospitals in this 34-county area with acquired immune deficiency syndrome (AIDS), these counties are grouped into six strata, and a simple random sample of two counties is selected within each stratum. Within each of the sample counties, a simple random sample of one hospital is taken, and within each sample hospital, all hospital medical records of patients having a discharge diagnosis of AIDS are reviewed, abstracted, and enumerated. The following table lists the hospitals by stratum, county, and number of beds.

Stratification for AIDS Admission Survey

Stratum	County	Hospital	Beds
1	1	1	72
1	2	1	87
1	2	2	104
1	2	3	34
1	3	1	17
1	3	2	140
1	4	1	104
2	1	1	44
2	2	1	99
2	3	1	86
2	3	2	91
2	3	3	53
2	4	1	48
3	1	1	171
3	1	2	85
3	2	1	108
3	3	1	99
3	4	1	131
3	4	2	182
4	1	1	48
4	1	2	18
4	2	1	50

Stratification for AIDS Admission Survey (*continued*)

Stratum	County	Hospital	Beds
4	3	1	42
4	4	1	38
5	1	1	42
5	2	1	54
5	3	1	45
5	4	1	34
6	1	1	39
6	1	2	59
6	2	1	76
6	3	1	68
6	3	2	68
6	4	1	65

a. Show how you would estimate the number of AIDS admissions for the 34-county area, taking into consideration number of beds.

b. The hospitals actually sampled are shown in the accompanying table along with the number of AIDS admissions enumerated at each sample hospital. From these data, estimate the total number of AIDS admissions for the 34-county area.

Hospitals in Sample

Stratum	County	Hospital	Beds	Total AIDS
1	1	1	72	20
1	2	1	87	49
2	2	1	99	38
2	4	1	48	23
3	3	1	99	38
3	4	1	131	78
4	3	1	42	7
4	4	1	38	28
5	1	1	42	26
5	4	1	34	9
6	1	1	39	18
6	2	1	76	20

c. Use a set of balanced half samples to estimate the standard error of the estimated total number of AIDS admissions for the 34-county area. The following Plackett–Burman matrix can be used to construct the half sample estimates (McCarthy [6, p. 17]):

Stratum

Rep.	1	2	3	4	5	6
1	+	−	−	+	−	+
2	+	+	−	−	+	−
3	+	+	+	−	−	+
4	−	+	+	+	−	−
5	+	−	+	+	+	−
6	−	+	−	+	+	+
7	−	−	+	−	+	+
8	−	−	−	−	−	−

    d. Use the jackknife method to obtain the standard error of the estimated total number of AIDS admissions for the 34-county area. Compare this to the BRR estimate obtained in part (c).

12.3 A sample survey of video stores was taken for purposes of estimating the proportion of these stores that offer incentives to customers based on prepaid membership plans. A simple random sample of 48 such establishments was taken and each of 6 interviewers was randomly allocated 8 such stores for a telephone interview. The following data were obtained:

Interviewer	Number Having Prepaid Membership Plans
1	7
2	1
3	0
4	8
5	7
6	0

Is there evidence of an interviewer effect? If "yes," how great is this effect?

12.4 Use the jackknife method to estimate the standard error of the overpayment proportion for the data in Table 12.1. How does this compare with that obtained by the linearization method?

TECHNICAL APPENDIX

Let X'_{h1} and X'_{h2} be independent unbiased estimates from two PSUs of a para-meter X_h (e.g., mean, total) for stratum $h(h = 1, \ldots, L)$ and let $X'_{(1)}, \ldots, X'_{(K)}$ be a balanced set of half sample estimates. Let us assume that L is divisible by K, and let us define the estimate $\hat{X}$ as follows:

$$\hat{X} = \frac{\Sigma_{k=1}^{K} X'_{(k)}}{K}$$

$$= \left(\frac{1}{K}\right) \sum_{h=1}^{L} \frac{K}{2}(X'_{h1} + X'_{h2})$$

$$= \sum_{h=1}^{L} \frac{(X'_{h1} + X'_{h2})}{2}$$

Let us define $\widehat{\text{Var}}(\hat{X})$ as follows:

$$\widehat{\text{Var}}(\hat{X}) = \frac{\Sigma_{k=1}^{K}(X_{(k)} - \hat{X})^2}{K}$$

We will show that $\widehat{\text{Var}}(\hat{X})$ is an unbiased estimate of $\text{Var}(\hat{X})$.
   Note the following five results:

1.
$$E(X'_{h1} - X'_{h2})^2 = \text{Var}(X'_{h1} - X'_{h2}) + E^2(X'_{h1} - X'_{h2})$$
$$= \text{Var}(X'_{h1} - X'_{h2})$$
$$= \text{Var}(X'_{h1}) + \text{Var}(X'_{h2})$$

2.
$$E\left[\sum_{h=1}^{L}(X'_{h1} - X'_{h2})^2\right] = \sum_{h=1}^{L}[\text{Var}(X'_{h1}) + \text{Var}(X'_{h2})]$$

(This follows from Result 1.)

3.
$$E(\hat{X}) = \left(\frac{1}{K}\right) \sum_{k=1}^{K} \sum_{h=1}^{L} E[\delta_{kh}X'_{h1} + (1 - \delta_{kh})X'_{h2}]$$

$$= \left(\frac{1}{K}\right) \sum_{k=1}^{K} \sum_{h=1}^{L} X_h$$

$$= \left(\frac{1}{K}\right) K \times X$$

$$= X$$

4. $$\mathrm{Var}(\hat{X}) = \left(\frac{1}{K^2}\right)\mathrm{Var}\left(\sum_{k=1}^{K}\sum_{h=1}^{L}[\delta_{kh}X'_{h1} + (1 - \delta_{kh})X'_{h2}]\right)$$

$$= \left(\frac{1}{K^2}\right)\sum_{k=1}^{K}\sum_{h=1}^{L}\mathrm{Var}[\delta_{kh}X'_{h1} + (1 - \delta_{kh})X'_{h2}]$$

(This last expression is true because in a balanced set of half samples, the cross product terms sum to zero)

$$= \left(\frac{1}{K^2}\right)\sum_{h=1}^{L}\mathrm{Var}\left[\left(\frac{K}{2}\right)X'_{h1} + \left(\frac{K}{2}\right)X'_{h2}\right]$$

(since in a set of balanced half samples, each of the two stratum estimates would appear an equal number of times $[= K/2]$)

$$= \left(\frac{1}{4}\right)\sum_{h=1}^{L}(\mathrm{Var}(X'_{h1}) + \mathrm{Var}(X'_{h2}))$$

5. $$E\left[\sum_{k=1}^{K}(X'_{(k)} - \hat{X})^2\right] = \sum_{k=1}^{K}E(X'_{(k)} - \hat{X})]^2]$$

$$= \sum_{k=1}^{K}[\mathrm{Var}(X'_{(k)} - \hat{X}) + [E(X'_{(k)} - \hat{X})]^2]$$

$$= \sum_{k=1}^{K}[\mathrm{Var}(X'_{(k)} - \hat{X}) + 0]$$

(from Result 3 and from the fact that $E(X'_{(k)}) = X$)

$$= \sum_{k=1}^{K}\mathrm{Var}\left[\sum_{h=1}^{L}\left(\delta_{kh}X'_{h1} + (1 - \delta_{kh})X'_{h2} - \frac{X'_{h1} + X'_{h2}}{2}\right)\right]$$

$$= \sum_{k=1}^{K}\mathrm{Var}\left[\sum_{h=1}^{L}\left(\left(\delta_{kh} - \frac{1}{2}\right)X'_{h1} + \left(\delta_{kh} - \frac{1}{2}\right)X'_{h2}\right)\right]$$

$$= \sum_{k=1}^{K}\sum_{h=1}^{L}\left(\delta_{kh} - \frac{1}{2}\right)^2\mathrm{Var}(X'_{h1} - X'_{h2})$$

$$= \sum_{k=1}^{K} \frac{1}{4} \sum_{h=1}^{L} \text{Var}(X'_{h1} - X'_{h2})$$

$$= \frac{K}{4} \sum_{h=1}^{L} [\text{Var}(X'_{h1}) + \text{Var}(X'_{h2})]$$

$$= K \times \text{Var}(\hat{X})$$

Therefore,

$$E[\text{Var}(\hat{X})] = E\left[\left(\frac{1}{K}\right) \sum_{k=1}^{K} (X'_{(k)} - \hat{X})^2 \right]$$

$$= \left(\frac{1}{K}\right) \times K \times \text{Var}(\hat{X})$$

$$= \text{Var}(\hat{X})$$

We have shown for this particular case that $\widehat{\text{Var}}(\hat{X})$ is an unbiased estimator of $\text{Var}(\hat{X})$. Although nonlinear estimates such as ratio and product estimators are not unbiased, their bias is often small and the argument demonstrated above would often hold approximately for these nonlinear estimates, which motivates the use of the balanced half sample variance estimator for these nonlinear estimators.

BIBLIOGRAPHY

The following publications develop linearization methodology.
1. Keyfitz, N., Estimates of sampling variance where two units are selected from each stratum. *Journal of the American Statistical Association*, **52**: 503, 1957.
2. Woodruff, R. S., A simple method for approximating the variance of a complicated estimate. *Journal of the American Statistical Association*, **66**: 411, 1971.

The following publications are relevant to software for implementation of the linearization method.
3. Research Triangle Institute, *SUDAAN: Professional Software for SUrvey DAta ANalysis*, Research Triangle Institute, Research Triangle Park, N.C., 1989.
4. SAS Institute, Inc., *SAS Users Guide: Statistics*, SAS Institute Inc., Cary, N.C., 1982.

The following publications are relevant to the discussion of replication methods in this chapter.
5. Hansen, M. H., Hurwitz, W. N., and Madow, W. G., *Sample Survey Methods and Theory*, Vol. 1, Wiley, New York, 1953.
6. McCarthy, P. J., *Replication: An Approach to the Analysis of Data from Complex Surveys*, Vital and Health Statistics Series 2, No. 14, DHEW PUb No. (HSM) 73-

1260, Health Services and Mental Health Administration, U.S. Government Printing Office, Washington, D.C., 1966.

7. McCarthy, P. J., Pseudo-replication: Half samples. *Review of the International Statistical Institute*, **37**: 239, 1969.

8. Frankel, M. R., *Inference from Sample Surveys: An Empirical Investigation*, Institute for Social Research, Ann Arbor, MI., 1971.

9. Bean, J. A., *Distribution and Properties of Variance Estimators for Complex Multistage Probability Samples: An Empirical Distribution*, Vital and Health Statistics Series 2, No. 65, DHEW Pub. No. (HRA) 75-1339, Health Resources Administration, U.S. Government Printing Office, Washington, D.C., 1975.

10. Lemeshow, S., and Levy, P. S., Estimating the variances of ratio estimates in complex sample surveys with two primary sampling units per stratum—A comparison of balanced replication and jackknife techniques. *Journal of Statistical Computation and Simulation*, **8**: 191, 1979.

11. Lemeshow, S., Half-sample techniques. In *Encyclopedia of Statistical Sciences*, Vol. 3, Wiley, New York, 1983.

12. Lemeshow, S., and Stoddard, A. M., A comparison of alternative estimation strategies for estimating the slope of a linear regression in sample surveys. *Communications in Statistics B: Simulation and Computation*, **13**: 153, 1984.

13. Lemeshow, S., and Epp, R., Properties of the balanced half-sample and jackknife variance estimtion techniques in the linear case. *Communications in Statistics: Theory and Methods*, **A6**(13): 1259, 1977.

14. Stanek, E., and Lemeshow, S., The behavior of balanced half-sample variance estimates for linear and combined ratio estimates when strata are paired to form pseudo-strata. *Estadistica*, **32**: 71, 1978.

15. Lemeshow, S., The use of unique statistical weights for estimating variances with the balanced half-sample technique. *Journal of Statistical Planning and Inference*, **3**: 315, 1979.

16. Lemeshow, S., Hosmer, D. W., and Hislop, D., The effect of non-normality on estimating the variance of the combined ratio estimate. *Communications in Statistics: Simulation and Computation*, **B9**(4): 371, 1980.

17. Plackett, R. L., and Burman, J. P., The design of optimal multifactorial experiments. *Biometrika*, **33**: 305, 1946.

The following references contain discussions of the replicated sample designs or interpenetrating samples.

18. Deming, W. E., *Sample Design in Business Research*, Wiley, New York, 1960.

19. Kalton, G., *Introduction to Survey Sampling*, Sage Publications, Newbury Park, New York, 1983.

The following is considered the original article on jackknife estimation.

20. Quenouille, M. H., Note on bias in estimation. *Biometrika*, **43**, 353–360, 1956.

The following recent review articles are relevant to topics covered in this chapter.

21. Frankel, M. R., Resampling procedures in estimation of sampling error. In *Encyclopedia of Biostatistics*, Armitage, P. A., and Colton, T. D., Eds., Wiley, Chichester, U.K., 1998.

22. Carlson, B. L., Software for statistical analysis of sample survey data. In *Encyclopedia of Biostatistics*, Armitage, P. A., and Colton, T. D., Eds., Wiley, Chichester, U.K., 1998.

23. Shah, B. V., Linearization methods of variance estimation. In *Encyclopedia of Biostatistics*, Armitage, P. A., and Colton, T. D., Eds., Wiley, Chichester, U.K., 1998.

24. Ghosh, S., Interpenetrating samples. In *Encyclopedia of Biostatistics*, Armitage, P. A., and Colton, T. D., Eds., Wiley, Chichester, U.K., 1998.

The following articles show consequences of not using appropriate methods of analysis when analyzing sample survey data.

25. Brogan, D., Pitfalls of using standard statistical software packages for sample survey data. In *Encyclopedia of Biostatistics*, Armitage, P. A., and Colton, T. D., Eds., Wiley, Chichester, U.K., 1998.

26. Lemeshow, S., Letenneur, L., Lafont, S., Orgogozo, J. M., and Commenges, D., An Illustration of Analysis Taking into Account Complex Survey Considerations: The Association Between Wine Consumption and Dementia in the PAQUID study. *The American Journal of Epidemiology*, 148 No 3., 298–306, 1998.

In addition to the above literature, Dr Alan Zaslafsky of Harvard University maintains a home page on the Worldwide Web which features information on software for analysis of data from complex sample surveys. The address of this site is:

http://www/fas.harvard.edu/~stats/survey-soft/survey-soft.html/

PART 3

Selected Topics in Sample Survey Methodology

CHAPTER 13

Nonresponse and Missing Data in Sample Surveys

Once the sample is selected, the field work then begins and an attempt is made to collect the desired data from all the enumeration units selected in the sample. Unfortunately, it is rarely possible to achieve total success in obtaining complete data from all of the units sampled. For some units, the sample survey may have obtained no information at all, and for other units, the survey may have obtained information on some, but not all of the items ascertained. The former type of nonresponse is called *unit nonresponse*, while the latter is called *item nonresponse*.

Both unit nonresponse and item nonresponse pose major threats to the accuracy of estimates obtained from sample surveys, and both types of non-response are very difficult to avoid in the sampling of populations. In many surveys it may take a considerable amount of effort and resources to achieve a response rate even as high as 50% of all units originally selected in the sample. This could be true even when the survey protocol calls for the revisiting of households in which respondents were not at home at the time of the initial visit; for telephone callbacks in telephone surveys; or for second or third mailings in the case of mail surveys.

The increase over the years in the use of sample surveys to provide information for purposes of decision making, and the increasing difficulty of obtaining high response rates in sample surveys, has resulted in considerable attention paid to this problem and has led to the development of a wide variety of techniques for dealing with nonresponse and missing values in sample surveys. In this chapter, we will discuss the impact of nonresponse on the accuracy of estimates obtained from sample surveys and will then discuss some of the methods that have been used to reduce unit nonresponse and some of the methods that have been used to handle missing data in situations of item nonresponse.

13.1 EFFECT OF NONRESPONSE ON ACCURACY OF ESTIMATES

The purpose of most surveys is to estimate, with the greatest possible accuracy and reliability, such population parameters as means, totals, and proportions. Each of the sampling procedures described in this book can provide unbiased (or at least consistent) estimates of such parameters, provided that a response rate of 100% is obtained for each particular item. Clearly, this will rarely be the case, and therefore resulting estimates will no longer be unbiased. In fact, as the nonresponse rate increases, the amount of bias will increase as well.

To examine this idea more formally, let us define the following entities:

N = the total number of enumeration units in the population

N_1 = the total number of potential responding units in the population

N_2 = the total number of potential nonresponding units in the population (i.e., $N_2 = N - N_1$)

$\bar{X}_1$ = the mean level of a characteristic $\mathscr{X}$ among the N_1 potential responding enumeration units

$\bar{X}_2$ = the mean level of a characteristic $\mathscr{X}$ among the N_2 potential nonresponding enumeration units.

$\bar{X} = \dfrac{N_1\bar{X}_1 + N_2\bar{X}_2}{N}$ = the mean level of $\mathscr{X}$ among the total population of

N enumeration units

If we take a simple random sample of n enumeration units, and if no attempt is made to obtain data from the potential nonresponders, we are effectively estimating the mean level of characteristic $\mathscr{X}$ for the subgroup of N_1 responding enumeration units rather than from the totality of N enumeration units in the population. From our discussion of estimates for subgroups from simple random sampling (Chapter 3), we know that if our sample of n enumeration units (EU) yields n_1 responding EUs, and if $\bar{x}$ denotes the mean level of $\mathscr{X}$ among these n_1 responding EUs, then the mean value of $\mathscr{X}$ is given by

$$E(\bar{x}) = \bar{X}_1$$

and the bias of $\bar{x}$ is given by

$$B(\bar{x}) = \bar{X}_1 - \bar{X} = \left(\frac{N_2}{N}\right)(\bar{X}_1 - \bar{X}_2) \tag{13.1}$$

Upon examination of relation (13.1), we see that the bias due to nonresponse is independent of the number n_1 of units successfully sampled. Clearly it cannot be reduced by an increase in sample size, and other measures must be used to reduce the bias. One of these measures is to reduce the proportion N_2/N of potential nonrespondents, and this will be discussed in a later section. Thus, the effect of nonresponse depends on the proportion of nonrespondents and the difference between the means of the potential nonrespondents and respondents. Unfortunately, the parameters N_2, $\bar{X}_1$, and $\bar{X}_2$ are rarely known. Let us illustrate these ideas in an example.

Illustrative Example. Suppose that a sample survey of 100 households obtained from simple random sampling is to be conducted in a rural area containing 2000 households for purposes of estimating the proportion of all households that do not have flush toilets. Suppose further that 20% (400) of the 2000 households would refuse to cooperate in the survey or else would not be reachable if selected in the sample (this, of course, would not be known in advance of the survey). Thus the 2000 households in the population consist of 400 potential nonresponding households and 1600 potential responding households. Suppose, finally, that 100 (or 25%) of the 400 potential nonresponding households do not have flush toilets, whereas 160 (or 10%) of the 1600 potential responding households do not have flush toilets. Thus, in the entire population of 2000 households, 260 (or 13%) of all households do not have flush toilets.

If, in the survey procedure, no attempt is made to obtain data from the potential nonresponding households, the distribution of estimated proportions not having flush toilets that could be obtained from the sample survey would center around .10 (the proportion not having flush toilets among the 1600 potential responding households), whereas the target value is .13. In other words, the exclusion of potential nonresponders would result in biased estimation. In this example, we have

$$N_1 = 1600 \qquad \bar{X}_1 = 0.10 \qquad N_2 = 400 \qquad \bar{X}_2 = 0.25 \qquad N = 2000$$

From relation (13.1), we have

$$B(\bar{x}) = \left(\frac{400}{2000}\right)(.10 - .25) = -.03 \qquad \square$$

13.2 METHODS OF INCREASING THE RESPONSE RATE IN SAMPLE SURVEYS

We can see from relation (13.1) that one of the ways in which the bias due to nonresponse can be decreased is by use of methodology that would result in reduction in the number of potential nonresponding enumeration units. In this section we list, for household surveys, some methods of decreasing the potential number of nonresponding households.

13.2.1   Increasing the Number of Households Contacted Successfully

In household surveys using direct interviews, lack of contact will occur when nobody is at home. Since in many households, both parents work during the day and the children are at school, it is not likely that attempts to make contact with individuals in the household during the day will be successful. In the survey design, provision should be made to revisit these households during the evening or, if the information can be obtained in a reasonably short time, to telephone the household during the evening.

In mail surveys of households, lack of contact may occur if the family no longer lives at the address at which the name was listed and the mail is not forwardable. If the listing unit is the address rather than the particular family living there, a visit to the address might be necessary in order to obtain the name of its current resident. Since nearly one in every five American families moves every year, this type of problem is potentially large in mail surveys when the frame from which the name obtained is not current. Another method of reducing this difficulty is to label the envelope "Mr. and Mrs. John Smith or current occupant."

13.2.2   Increasing the Completion Rate in Mail Questionnaires

In mail questionnaires, the response rate often can be increased by a good-looking packaging of the questionnaire. The material sent to the household should contain a carefully worded covering letter explaining the purpose of the survey, identifying the organization responsible for the conduct of the survey, and stating that the information elicited from the respondent will be held in strict confidentiality and used in aggregate form for statistical purposes only. The statement of confidentiality is especially important if the information given by the respondent is potentially embarrassing or damaging.

The survey materials sent to the respondent should be of high quality and should be sent by first class mail; the return envelope also should contain first class postage. Organizations that conduct surveys have found, almost universally, that persons are more likely to respond to a mail questionnaire that has an attractive, professional appearance rather than one that has an unprofessional appearance. In addition, inordinately long questionnaires requiring 30 minutes or more for completion run a higher risk of refusal than do shorter questionnaires. Mullner et al. [12] report the findings of a controlled experiment designed to show the effects of a covering letter and questionnaire format on the response rate to a survey mailed to hospital administrators.

Mail surveys that incorporate in their design provisions for personal interviews of a subsample of nonrespondents are considered in Section 13.3.

13.2.3 Decreasing the Number of Refusals in Face-to-Face or Telephone Interviews

It is very easy for a designated respondent to refuse to complete a questionnaire sent by mail, since the respondent has no direct contact with the organization conducting the survey. It is somewhat more difficult for the respondent to refuse a telephone interview, since there is voice contact, and it is most difficult for the respondent to refuse a face-to-face interview, since there is eye-to-eye contact between respondent and interviewer.

In either telephone or face-to-face surveys (as well as in mail surveys), the nonresponse rates can often be reduced if an effective publicity campaign is initiated in advance of the survey. This, however, is not easily accomplished, especially in large metropolitan areas. For instance, the local news and broadcast media would probably be reluctant to use prime time or space to announce a coming survey of the frequency of utilization of branch libraries when more exciting news (such as the daughter of the mayor being caught by the police selling crack cocaine) has taken place.

Nonresponse rates might also be reduced, particularly in personal interviews, if the interviewer is provided with the proper credentials. This is especially true in large metropolitan areas where a fear of crime exists.

13.2.4 Using Endorsements

The response rate in household surveys might be increased if the survey is endorsed by an official agency or organization whose sphere of interest includes the subject matter of the survey. For example, a household health survey might benefit from the endorsement of a local medical society. In mail surveys the endorsement could be in the form of a covering letter sent with the survey material to the respondent. The covering letter should bear the logo of the endorsing agency and should be signed by a high official of the agency in order to have maximum impact.

Endorsement by an appropriate agency is especially important in surveys of institutions. For example, in a survey of hospitals, the likelihood of success would increase if the project had a strong endorsement from the state hospital association. Sometimes an endorsement from the appropriate organization can be obtained more easily if the organization is included as a collaborator or as part of a steering committee for the study. One then gains the additional benefit of having the expertise and experience of the organization as part of the resources of the study.

The reward given to a respondent for participating in a survey is called an *incentive.* Cash incentives, which are widely used in mail surveys, but less widely used in personal interview or telephone surveys, have been found to be effective in increasing response rates. For example, response rates might be increased if the covering letter includes a shiny 25 cent piece or a brand new dollar bill. Incentives other than cash may also be used, but the problem of bias arises with nonmonetary incentives, because they may be more likely to attract special subgroups of the population than would money, which has a more universal appeal. In a controlled study, the National Center for Health Statistics has shown that a $10.00 honorarium (at the 1971 valuation of the dollar) promised to the designated sample persons if they would participate in a rather long physical examination and interview resulted in a high response rate [13]. An excellent discussion of the use of incentives is found in the book by Erdos on mail surveys [10].

13.3 MAIL SURVEYS COMBINED WITH INTERVIEWS OF NONRESPONDENTS

Mail surveys are generally less expensive than household surveys conducted by personal interview. However, it is often difficult to obtain a response rate from mail surveys that is high enough to meet specifications pertaining to the validity and reliability of the resulting estimates. If the initial response rate to the mailed questionnaire is low, the resulting estimates may be seriously biased. To overcome this problem, it is possible to use a two-stage sampling procedure in which the first stage is a mail survey and the second stage is a telephone and/or personal interview of a subsample of those who did not respond to the mail questionnaire. This procedure often can yield estimates having high reliability and can be done at a reasonable cost. This type of sample design is described in some detail in the next example.

Illustrative Example. Suppose that in a community containing 300 physicians a questionnaire is sent to a simple random sample of 100 physicians; the questionnaire asks whether the physician accepts patients who cannot pay for their services either directly or indirectly. Of the 100 questionnaires sent out, let us suppose that 30 are returned. Let us suppose further that, from the 70 physicians who did not respond to the mail questionnaire, a simple random sample of 20 is selected, that intensive efforts are made by telephone and personal visit to obtain responses from these 20 physicians, and that, as a result of these intensive efforts, 15 of the 20 are successfully interviewed. Finally, let us suppose that the data shown in Table 13.1 are obtained from the respondents.

To generalize, let us introduce the following notation as representing this situation:

N = the number of EUs in the population

n = the number of EUs initially sampled by mail

n_1 = the number of EUs responding to the initial mailing

$n_2 = n - n_1$ = the number of EUs not responding to the initial mailing

Table 13.1 Data for the Survey of Physicians

	Number	Number Responding "Yes"
Physicians returning mail questionnaire	30	20
Physicians responding to telephone or visit	15	3

$n_2^* = $ the number of the n_2 nonresponding EUs selected for intensive effort (e.g., telephone or personal interview)

$n_2' = $ the number of these n_2^* EUs for which responses are obtained successfully

$\bar{x}_1 = \dfrac{\sum_{i=1}^{n_1} x_i}{n_1} = $ the mean level of $\mathscr{X}$ among the n_1 EUs successfully contacted at the first mailing

$\bar{x}_2 = \dfrac{\sum_{i=1}^{n_2'} x_i}{n_2'} = $ the mean level of $\mathscr{X}$ among the n_2' EUs successfully contacted through intensive efforts

An estimator which we will denote by $\bar{x}_{\text{dub}}$ (since it is based on a double sample), can be used to estimate the unknown population mean $\bar{X}$. This estimator is given by

$$\bar{x}_{\text{dub}} = \frac{n_1 \bar{x}_1 + n_2 \bar{x}_2}{n} \tag{13.2}$$

For this example we have

$$N = 300 \qquad n = 100 \qquad n_1 = 30 \qquad n_2 = 70 \qquad n_2^* = 20 \qquad n_2' = 15$$

$$\bar{x}_1 = \tfrac{20}{30} = .67 \qquad \bar{x}_2 = \tfrac{3}{15} = .20$$

and thus

$$\bar{x}_{\text{dub}} = \frac{30(.67) + 70(.20)}{100} = .34$$

If the number n_2' of the initial nonresponding EUs successfully contacted through intensive effort is numerically close to n_2^*, the number chosen for intensive effort, then the estimator, $\bar{x}_{\text{dub}}$, is a nearly unbiased estimator of the unknown population mean $\bar{X}$. ☐

The results of this example can be generalized to any appropriate survey.

13.3.1 Determination of Optimal Fraction of Initial Nonrespondents to Subsample for Intensive Effort

Suppose that we have decided on the two-stage sampling procedure consisting of an initial mail questionnaire followed by an intensive effort to obtain responses from a subsample of those enumeration units that do not respond to the initial mail questionnaire. An important decision to make is how large a sample of n_2^* to take from the n_2 enumeration units not responding to the mail questionnaire. To make this decision, we propose a strategy which yields optimal allocation for subsampling, taking into consideration the field costs and expected nonresponse rate.

First, let us discuss the unit costs associated with this sample design. Suppose the following *cost components* are defined:

C_0 = cost per mailing of initial questionnaires

C_1 = cost per returned questionnaire of processing those questionnaires returned by mail

C_2 = cost per questionnaire of obtaining data from those initial non-responding enumeration units designated for intensive effort and of processing the data once they are obtained.

The cost component C_0 consists of the cost of materials used in the questionnaire (e.g., stamps, envelopes, etc.) plus labor required for preparation of these materials for mailing. The cost component C_1 consists of labor involved in editing and coding the data and other data preparation work plus data processing costs such as computer time and computer programming. The component C_2 is a combination of field costs and data-preparation and processing costs.

An estimate of the *total field and processing costs* of the survey is given by

$$C = C_0 n + C_1 n_1 + C_2 n_2' \tag{13.3}$$

Finally, if it is anticipated that a proportion P_1 of those initially sampled will respond to the initial mailing, then the *optimum number n_2^* that should be sampled* is given by

$$n_2^* = n_2 \times \left(\frac{C_0 + C_1 P_1}{C_2 P_1} \right)^{1/2} \tag{13.4}$$

Illustrative Example. For the previous example let us suppose that the cost components are given by

$C_0 = \$1.50$ per questionnaire (initial mailing costs)

$C_1 = \$15.00$ per questionnaire (unit preparation and processing costs)

$C_2 = \$45.00$ per enumeration unit (unit cost of obtaining interview and processing data for nonrespondent EUs)

Then P_1, the observed response rate, is

$$P_1 = \frac{30}{100} = .30$$

and the optimum number to subsample is

$$n_2^* = 70 \times \left[\frac{1.50 + (15)(.30)}{45(.30)}\right]^{1/2} = 70 \times \tfrac{2}{3} \approx 47$$

Thus we should take a subsample of two-thirds or 47 of the 70 initial nonrespondents. $\qquad\qquad\square$

13.3.2 Determination of Sample Size Needed for a Two-Stage Mail Survey

Suppose we were starting from scratch with the survey of physicians and wish to know how many questionnaires to send out initially. Assuming that 30% of the physicians would respond to the mailing and assuming the cost components used in the previous section, we already know that we should subsample two-thirds of the initial nonrespondents for intensive effort (i.e., $n_2^*/n_2 = 2/3$).

To determine the required number of physicians to sample for initial mailing, we first determine the number n' that would be needed if there were a 100% response to the mailing. Since we are using simple random sampling in this case, we use the expression in Box 3.5 (for proportion) to obtain n'. Suppose we guess that 80% of all physicians accept patients who cannot pay for their services, and that we wish to be virtually certain of estimating this percentage to within 30% of its true value. Then from Box 3.5 with $\varepsilon = .30, p = .80$, and $N = 300$, we have

$$n' = \frac{9 \times 300 \times .8 \times .2}{9 \times .8 \times .2 + 299 \times .3^2 \times .8^2} = 23 \text{ physicians}$$

Thus, if there were a 100% response rate, we would need a sample of only 23 physicians in order to be virtually certain that the estimated proportion is within 30% of the true proportion.

However, we anticipate only a 30% response to the mailed questionnaire, and because of this, the estimate is subject to more variability. Hence, we need a larger sample size. In fact, the required number, n, of questionnaires needed can be obtained by multiplying n' (from Box 3.4) by a factor that takes nonresponse into consideration. This factor is shown in the following formula for n:

$$n = n' \left\{ 1 + (1 - P_1) \left[\left(\frac{C_2 P_1}{C_0 + C_1 P_1} \right)^{1/2} - 1 \right] \right\} \qquad (13.5)$$

Thus, for our previous example, from results shown above and earlier, we have

$$\left(\frac{C_2 P_1}{C_0 + C_1 P_1} \right)^{1/2} = \frac{3}{2} \qquad P_1 = .30 \qquad n' = 23$$

and hence

$$n = 23 \times \left[1 + .7 \left(\frac{3}{2} - 1 \right) \right] = 31.05 \approx 31$$

Thus, we would take a simple random sample of 31 physicians for the initial mailing in order to be virtually certain of meeting the specifications set for the estimate.

13.4   OTHER USES OF DOUBLE SAMPLING METHODOLOGY

The two-stage sampling methodology proposed in the previous section as a device for lowering bias due to nonresponse is often referred to as *double sampling* and is generalizable to situations in which biases are due to mechanisms other than nonresponse. In essence, the double sampling methodology involves a preliminary data collection (e.g., a mail questionnaire), followed by a grouping of elements into two strata (e.g., respondents and nonrespondents to the mail questionnaire). A sample of individuals in one of the strata (e.g., nonrespondents to the mailed questionnaire) is then taken, and the final estimator is a weighted combination of the two individual stratum estimates [e.g., relation (13.2)]. We show below an application of this double sampling procedure in which nonresponse is not involved.

Illustrative Example.   This example comes from an analysis performed by Rich et al. [14] of chest radiograph data collected from the Second National Health and Nutrition Examination Survey (NHANES II), a cross-sectional survey conducted from 1976 to 1980 by the National Center for Health Statistics on a sample of approximately 28,000 persons aged 6 months to 74 years residing in the United States. The survey included a battery of interviews, medical examinations, and laboratory tests. Chest radiographs were performed on approximately 10,000 subjects aged 25 years and above. Each radiograph was screened by two radiologists for a large number of items indicating possible lung disease. One of the items on a checklist of abnormalities was "enlargement of the pulmonary arteries." Such enlargement could be indicative of pulmonary hypertension, a severe condition which is often the end stage of chronic obstructive lung disease and other pulmonary abnormalities.

Of the 10,153 chest radiographs of survey respondents 25–74 years of age screened by the two radiologists, 326 had pulmonary artery enlargement checked by one or both radiologists. However, in only 30 (9.2%) of these, did *both readers* agree that there was enlargement. Because agreement among the two radiologists was so low, it was decided to have a third reader do a more careful measurement not only on the 326 chest radiographs read as having pulmonary artery enlargement by one or both of the original readers but also on a sample of 288 chest radiographs selected from the 9827 (10,153 − 326) read as *not* having pulmonary artery enlargement by both of the original readers.

If one ignores the fact that NHANES II is a complex sample survey and assumes that both the original and second samples were obtained by simple random sampling, one would have the following estimate of the prevalence of persons having enlarged pulmonary arteries.

$$p_{dub} = \frac{N_1 p_1 + N_2 p_2}{N_1 + N_2}$$

where

$N_1 =$ number of chest radiographs screened as positive by one or both of original readers

$= 326$

$N_2 =$ number of chest radiographs screened as negative by both of the original readers

$= 9827$

$p_1 = \dfrac{x_1}{N_1}$

$p_2 = \dfrac{x_2}{n_2}$

$x_1 =$ number confirmed positive by third reader among N_1 originally screened as positive by one or both readers

$n_2 =$ number sampled among N_2 originally screened as negative by both readers

$= 288$

$x_2 =$ number determined to be positive by third reader among n_2 originally screened negative by both first and second readers and sampled for confirmation by third reader

Based on the third reader's result, we obtained

$$p_1 = .675 \qquad p_2 = .257$$

Thus, our estimate of the prevalence of pulmonary artery enlargement from this double sample would be

$$p_{\text{dub}} = \frac{326(.675) + 9827(.257)}{10,153} = .2704 \text{ or } 27.04\%$$

Note that if the discordance among the original readers was not taken into consideration, the estimated prevalence would have been $326/10,153 = 3.2\%$, which would in all likelihood be a gross underestimate of the prevalence. $\square$

13.5   ITEM NONRESPONSE: METHODS OF IMPUTATION

One of the most difficult problems confronting investigators who analyze data from sample surveys is that of dealing with item nonresponse. As defined above, item nonresponse refers to missing data elements and can also include values of data elements that are clearly erroneous and cannot be used in the analysis process. Item nonresponse presents many problems when the data collected in a survey are subject to statistical analysis. Many statistical procedures, such as multiple regression analysis and factor analysis, cannot be immediately used if there are any missing values, and methods that allow for missing values are often difficult to use and interpret without considerable expertise on the part of the analyst.

In this section, we first discuss mechanisms by which missing values arise, and then present some strategies that can be followed by dealing with such problems. Much of this discussion is based on the methodology developed since the beginning of the 1980s. For a more detailed discussion of issues relating to missing values, we refer the reader to the books by Rubin [1] and by Little and Rubin [2], and to the recent review articles by Little [6] and by Barnard, Rubin, and Schenker [7].

13.5.1   Mechanisms by Which Missing Values Arise

Understanding of the stochastic mechanisms by which missing values arise is important because it impacts both on the type of analytic strategy that would be employed and the validity of the inferences resulting from the analysis. The following notation is used by Little [6] to describe patterns of missing data and to classify the mechanisms underlying these patterns.

Let $Y = (y_{ij})$ be the hypothetical n by k matrix consisting of the values of the set of k variables for the n units sampled. The y_{ij} may be recorded or missing (in the latter situation, they would not be known). Let $\mathbf{M} = (m_{ij})$ be the corresponding n by k matrix of 1's and 0's where 1 denotes that the particular y_{ij} is missing. The mechanism for the occurrence of missing values is characterized by the distribution of the random matrix, **M**, of missing values given the matrix, Y, of true values. In particular, we define three of the most common mechanisms below.

Missing Completely at Random. If the distribution of **M** conditional on Y is independent of Y, then we say that the mechanism of item nonresponse is *missing completely at random (MCAR)*.

Missing at Random. If the distribution of **M** conditional on Y is dependent on the observed values of Y, but not on the missing values of Y, then we say that the mechanism of item nonresponse is *missing at random (MAR)*.

Nonignorable Missing Values. If the distribution of **M** conditional on Y is dependent on the missing values of Y, then we say that the mechanism of item nonresponse is *nonignorable*.

Illustrative Example. A simple random sample is taken of the files of 3000 members of a large HMO. The objective of the survey is to estimate, from data originally collected at the initial evaluation of each member, information characterizing the membership on the following variables:

1. ID (Member identification number)
2. AGE
3. SEX
4. NSEXPART (Number of sexual partners during past 12 months)
5. HBSAG (Presence or absence of Hepatitis B Surface Antigen (HBsAG))
6. PSA (Abnormally high level of Prostate-Specific Antigen. High levels of PSA possibly indicate presence of a malignancy on the prostate gland.)

To illustrate some of the issues that will be discussed in this section, we generated an artificial dataset, *mcardemo.dta* (formatted for STATA). Using random number generators, we constructed 3000 records with complete data on all of the 6 variables described above. For the variables *NSEXPART, HBSAG*, and *PSA*, we then generated missing values according to the scenario described below. (We assumed that there would be no missing values for the variables *AGE* and *SEX*.)

HBSAG. To create a scenario in which only a random sample of members was measured for HBsAG, we generated missing values for that variable for a simple random sample of approximately 50% of the sample members using random numbers having a uniform distribution between 0 and 1.

PSA. We initially generated values of PSA equal to 0 for all women (since they do not have prostate glands) and, using random numbers following a logistic distribution with AGE as the independent variable, values designed to be monotonically increasing with age for men (since prostate cancer incidence increases steeply with age). Assuming that neither women nor men under 50 would be measured for the variable, *PSA*, we then generated missing values for all women and for men under 50.

NSEXPART. The original values for this variable were constructed using random-number generators to be slightly higher in males than in females; to decrease slightly with age; and to be slightly higher in those who were positive for HBsAG. Although we assumed that the entire membership was queried on number of sexual partners during the past 12 months, we also assumed that many of the individuals having a large number of partners would choose not to answer that question. To simulate this, we generated missing values for this variable using random numbers having a logistic distribution with parameters that would render the probability of a member having a missing value on the variable, *NSEXPART*, to be greater if she/he had a relatively high number of sex partners.

From the above description, we see that the mechanism for "missingness" with respect to the variable, *HBSAG*, is MCAR because the conditional probability of a sample element having this variable missing depends neither on the true value of that variable nor the value of any other variable in the data set. In contrast, the conditional probability of a sample element having a missing value for the variable, *PSA*, does not depend on the true value of that variable, but does depend on the value of the variables *SEX* and *AGE*. The mechansim for missing values for the variable, *PSA*, is therefore MAR (but not MCAR). Finally, the mechanism of missing values for the variable, *NSEXPART*, is neither MCAR nor MAR because the conditional probability of a sample element having a missing value for that variable depends on the actual value of that variable (since number of sex partners is likely a very sensitive question). Thus, missingness for this variable would be *nonignorable*.

The mean values of these variables along with the mean values if there were no missing values is shown below:

Variable	Survey Observations on Variable	Prevalence or Mean from Survey Data	True Prevalence or Mean
Prevalence of HBsAG	1,489	4.8%	5.1%
Number of sex partners in past year	2,343	1.29	1.60
Prevalence of elevated PSA (males > 50)	580	38.3	38.3
Prevalence of elevated PSA (all males)	580	38.3	27.1

From the above, we see that the prevalence of HBsAG observed in the survey is close to the value that would have been obtained had all individuals been measured. This is as expected, since HBsAG is MCAR. The mean number of sex partners, on the other hand, underestimates the true mean by nearly 20%, which is also not unexpected since the mechanism for generating missing values renders the subjects having higher numbers of sex partners more likely to have missing values. Finally, the prevalence of elevated PSA is equal (by construction) to the true prevalence in males over 50, but overestimates the true prevalence if this age group were taken to represent *all* males. □

Many methods for handling data imply that the data are either MCAR or MAR and can lead to biased estimates for variables that are neither MAR nor MCAR. For example, if the analysis were confined only to those elements for which there were no missing values on *any* variables, estimation of the prevalence of HBsAG would be unbiased (since it is MCAR), but estimation of the prevalence of abnormal PSA would be biased, since the resulting data set would exclude all males under 50 years of age who are less likely to have abnormal values of PSA. Estimation of the mean number of sexual partners seen in the past year would also be subject to bias, since those with a high number would be the most likely not to respond to this item.

The reader is referred to Little and Rubin [2] and to Little [6] for a more complete discussion of the effect that the mechansim for missing values has on the validity of estimates.

13.5.2 Some Methods for Analyzing Data in the Presence of Missing Values

Little and Rubin [2] list the following four generic classes of procedures for performing statistical analysis in the presence of item nonresponse.

- *Complete Case Methods.* These methods discard all units which have missing values on any variables used in the particular analysis. This is perhaps the most popular method of dealing with incomplete data. It entails deletion of all analysis units that have any data items missing that are being used in the particular analysis. Although this practice is widely used and permits immediate use of statistical methods that require complete data, there are several reasons why it is not generally considered a good procedure. First of all, with the deletion of all units having any missing data, the available sample size could shrink considerably, resulting in a concomitant loss in precision. Second, if the individuals who were dropped from the analysis are very different from those who remain, the resulting estimates may be highly biased. Third, in some complex sampling schemes, individuals are assigned statistical weights, W, which may reflect, among other things, their probabilities of selection. Deletion of units on the basis of missing values would be very likely to negate the validity of this weighting scheme.

- *Imputation-Based Methods.* These methods "fill in" or *impute* all values that are missing on the basis of certain information, generally on variables thought to be related to the missing values. Once the missing values are imputed, methods of analysis that require complete data on all variables (e.g., multiple regression, correlation) are then used to analyze the data. Imputation-based methods have been well accepted and widely used over the years in major nationwide surveys as well as in smaller surveys and, in our subsequent discussion, we will focus on this class of methods.

- *Reweighting Methods.* These methods attempt to adjust for missing values by adjusting the sampling weights to compensate for nonresponse. While this is most often done for unit nonresponse, it can also be used for item nonresponse by modeling the probability of a sample unit responding to a particular item as a function of a set of variables. This is done generally using a probit or a logistic regression model with the dependent variable equal to "1" for units having recorded values on the variable and "0" for those units having missing values on that item. The independent variables used in this regression are those thought to be associated with missingness in the item of interest, and the result of this regression would be to produce, for each sample unit, the estimated probability of that unit responding to the item of interest. The resulting analysis would use only those units having recorded (nonmissing) values for the item of interest, and would weight each unit by the inverse of the estimated probability of that unit responding to the item (in addition to any other sampling weights that would normally be used). The rationale for this is that each unit that is sampled and has responded to the item represents W units in the population, where $W =$ the inverse of the probability of the unit being sampled and responding to the item.

- *Model-Based Methods.* These procedures were developed for the most part in the last 10–15 years and analyze data having missing values by modeling the likelihood function of the incomplete data and using maximum likelihood procedures. Methods have been developed for MAR missing values as well as for nonignorable missing values. Many of these methods are discussed in the book by Little and Rubin [2], and in the more recent review by Little [6]. Because of the relatively high statistical sophistication required to understand and use these methods intelligently, we will not cover them in this text.

13.5.3 Some Imputation Methods

We describe below a few of the most commonly used methods of imputation:

> *Substitution of the Mean.* One of the most commonly used methods of imputation involves the assignment of the mean value, $\bar{y}$, of all individuals whose values on a particular variable, $\mathscr{Y}$, is present to any individual who has a missing value for that data item. This method results in an estimate of the population mean for that variable that is the same as would be obtained if the mean were computed only for those individuals who have that data item present. The advantage of this method is that it replaces the missing value with an "expected" value that has a relatively high degree of stability. A disadvantage is that variances computed using data imputed by this method will be understated, and correlations among variables will also be misleading. A refinement of this method involves classification of individuals into subgroups and imputation of subgroup means rather than grand means. This modification allows use of information on differences among subdomains with respect to mean levels of the variables that are to be imputed.
>
> *The Hot Deck Method.* This method, widely used by the U.S. Bureau of the Census, avoids to a large degree the underestimation of variances inherent in imputation methods that fill in missing values with grand means of subdomain means. In the hot deck method, the original data file is sorted in such a way that the order of the individual records corresponds to the structure of the sample design (e.g., individuals from the same cluster might be together in the file). Cells are established based on the values of selected demographic or other variables. For each cell, a register is set up containing the record of an individual on whom all variables are recorded. In a single pass through the data file each individual's cell is identified, and, if the variable of interest for that individual is missing, the value for that cell's register is substituted for the missing value. On the other hand, if the individual's record is complete, the complete record for that individual is substituted for the one previously serving as the register. In some surveys having much missing data, there may be little change in the registers of certain cells; hence, the same values will be imputed repeatedly. To avoid this problem, it is possible to have multiple cases in the registers that are rotated. This method is illustrated in the following example.

Illustrative Example. The following are data collected on a sample of 20 women 75 years of age at last birthday selected from persons residing in three retirement communities for elderly persons. Variables for which missing values are to be imputed are *education* (1 = elementary school; 2 = high school; 3 = some college; 4 = college graduate) and *score on the Mini Mental State Examination (MMSE)*, which is a screening test for cognitive impairment.

Retirement Community	Building	Subject	Education	MMSE
1	1	1	2	17
1	1	2	–	18
1	1	3	2	20
1	2	1	4	–
1	2	2	3	27
1	3	1	3	20
1	3	2	2	18
2	1	1	1	11
2	1	2	1	–
2	1	3	2	13
2	1	4	2	15
2	2	1	–	–
2	2	2	2	16
3	1	1	3	24
3	1	2	3	26
3	2	1	–	15
3	2	2	2	17
3	3	1	4	26
3	3	2	3	–
3	3	3	3	21

□

Let us establish cells based on retirement community. Based on this categorization the initial registers are:

Retirement Community	Education	MMSE
1	2	17
2	1	11
3	3	24

The first missing value is education in the second subject in housing development 1. From the above register, the imputed value would be "2". The next record is complete, and so the value for that record on the variable education "2" and MMSE "20" would replace the initial value for that register. The next record is also in the first retirement community and has MMSE missing. From the register for that cell "20" would be imputed. The next record having a missing value is the second record from housing development number 2. At that point, the register for that cell contains the value "11" for MMSE, and that value would be imputed. The remaining missing values are imputed in a similar way, and the procedure yields the data set shown below (imputed values are in boldface):

Retirement Community	Building	Subject	Education	MMSE
1	1	1	2	17
1	1	2	**2**	18
1	1	3	2	20
1	2	1	4	**20**
1	2	2	3	27
1	3	1	3	20
1	3	2	2	18
2	1	1	1	11
2	1	2	1	**11**
2	1	3	2	13
2	1	4	2	15
2	2	1	**2**	**15**
2	2	2	2	16
3	1	1	3	24
3	1	2	3	26
3	2	1	**3**	15
3	2	2	2	17
3	3	1	4	26
3	3	2	3	**26**
3	3	3	3	21

□

There are many variations of the hot deck method. In one variation, the registers contain values from more than one complete record at any time, and these values are rotated in the imputation process. This variation is useful when there is much missing data since registers constructed in the unmodified hot deck method contain, at any one time, values from only one complete record, and when many of the records are not complete, the registers would have infrequent turnover, which would result in the same values being imputed repeatedly. Another variation, known as the *cold deck* method, identifies cells as in the hot deck procedure, but the cell's registers are composed of records generally compiled in a survey other than the current one. Often this other survey may be an earlier one of the same population. There must at be at least one case available from the former survey in each of the established cells. When there are multiple records available in a cell, the selection of one for imputation to the current survey is done at random. The cold deck method has the disadvantage that it does not use data from the current survey for imputation, and for this reason it appears to be less appealing than the hot deck method.

Imputation from Randomly Selected Individuals.   This method is similar to the hot deck method, except that values from a randomly selected individual are substituted for those missing from the incomplete record. Even if the random selection occurs within cells similar to those established in the hot deck method, the procedure lacks an attractive feature of the hot deck method, namely its taking advantage of the intrinsic ordering of the file in the imputation process. This enables the hot deck method to take advantage of important regional and geographic features that may not have been used in the construction of register cells. Also, with respect to computational ease, the hot deck method is more convenient.

Subjective Regression. As the name implies, this is an intuitively deductive process which relies solely on the analyst's judgment based on the available evidence. For example, if the sex of a sample respondent is the missing value, data recorded on the survey instrument concerning age at menarche would lead the analyst to impute "female". Similarly, an analyst familiar with physical anthropometry could assign a reasonable estimate of height given the presence of other data such as age and sex.

Objective Regression. Finally, we discuss a method that may be termed "objective regression." In this method regression equations are generated from a data set consisting of complete records with the variable to be imputed serving as the dependent variable. The resulting equation may be of the form

$$y = b_0 + b_1 x_1 + b_2 x_2 + \cdots + b_k x_k$$

where y is the variable to be imputed for a given individual and $x_1, \ldots, x_k$, are covariates known for the individual. The values to be imputed in this manner may be superior to those derived from the previously described methods, since relevant information thought to be related to the variable to be imputed is utilized. This method also allows the imputed value to be "harmonious" with the rest of the subject's record. It can also allow random error to be incorporated by using the regression equation to estimate the value, but then generating a normally distributed random variable having that mean and error variance present in the data. This preserves the inherent error structure in the data.

13.6 MULTIPLE IMPUTATION

The methods discussed above replace each missing value by a single imputed value, and the resulting analysis treats the imputed value in the same way as truly measured values. The analysis does not take into consideration uncertainty about this missing value. In part, because of this problem, a techique called *multiple imputation* has been developed over the past decade by Rubin [1] and by other investigators. This method fills in each missing value with two or more imputed values and analyzes each resulting data set by complete data methods. By combining the results of these analyses, the resulting inferences can take into consideration the uncertainty about the missing values. The method has the advantage of being thoroughly grounded in statistical theory and of having considerable practical use since it can take advantage of contemporary computing methods. Although it is a method of imputation, because it differs so greatly from the methods discussed earlier, we present it here as a "stand-alone" topic. Consider the following simple illustrative example.

Illustrative Example. Let us consider the same example shown in Section 13.5.3.

Retirement Community	Building	Subject	Education	MMSE
1	1	1	2	17
1	1	2	–	18
1	1	3	2	20
1	2	1	4	–
1	2	2	3	27
1	3	1	3	20
1	3	2	2	18
2	1	1	1	11
2	1	2	1	–
2	1	3	2	13
2	1	4	2	15
2	2	1	–	–
2	2	2	2	16
3	1	1	3	24
3	1	2	3	26
3	2	1	–	15
3	2	2	2	17
3	3	1	4	26
3	3	2	3	–
3	3	3	3	21

Suppose that we wish to impute the four missing values of MMSE, and that we can replace the missing value with the value of that variable for any subject in the same primary sampling unit (PSU) (building). The missing values for subject 1 in PSU 2 of stratum 1 (denoted subject A) can be replaced by the value from one other subject since there are only two sampled subjects in that PSU. The missing value for subject 2 in PSU 1 of stratum 2 (denoted subject B) can be replaced by values from the three other subjects in that PSU not having missing values on that variable. The missing value for subject 1 in PSU 2 of stratum 2 (denoted subject C) can be replaced by only one other value, and the missing value for subject 2 in PSU 3 of stratum 3 (denoted subject D) can be replaced by values from the two other subjects having complete data for that variable in that PSU. Thus, the number of combinations of different subjects whose values can be used in the imputation is given by $1 \times 3 \times 1 \times 2 = 6$. These 6 choices are shown below:

		Subjects		
Combination	A	B	C	D
1	27	11	16	26
2	27	11	16	21
3	27	13	16	26
4	27	13	16	21
5	27	15	16	26
6	27	15	16	21

Suppose that we take a simple random sample of three of these combinations (e.g., 2, 3, and 5). The complete data set for the MMSE variable for each of these combinations with the missing value imputed is given below:

		Combination	
Subject	1	2	3
1	17	17	17
2	18	18	18
3	20	20	20
4	27	27	27
5	27	27	27
6	20	20	20
7	18	18	18
8	11	11	11
9	11	13	15
10	13	13	13
11	15	15	15
12	16	16	16
13	16	16	16
14	24	24	24
15	26	26	26
16	15	15	15
17	17	17	17
18	26	26	26
19	21	26	26
20	21	21	21
Mean ($\bar{x}$)	18.95	19.30	19.40
Standard Error $\widehat{SE}(\bar{x})$	1.13	1.12	1.12

Note that each of the data sets generated as described above yields a different estimate, $\bar{x}$, of the mean MMSE score and a different estimate $\widehat{SE}(\bar{x})$ of the standard error of the mean. If one wanted to make an inference concerning the unknown population mean, $\bar{X}$, taking into consideration the uncertainty in the imputed values, one could obtain from the calculated means and variances, a "within" component representing the estimated variance of the estimated mean conditional on the imputed values, and a "between" component representing the variance of the estimated means over different realizations of the imputation process. One would then combine them to obtain an overall variance estimate. The specific calculations are shown below.

Within variance component:

$$s_w^2 = (1.13^2 + 1.12^2 + 1.12^2)/3 = 1.26$$

Between variance component

$$s_b^2 = \left(1 + \frac{1}{k}\right) \sum_{i=1}^{k} (\bar{x}_i - \bar{x})^2 / (k - 1)$$

where k is the number of realizations ($k = 3$ in this instance), $\bar{x}_i$ is the estimated mean for the ith realization of the imputation, and $\bar{x}$ is the mean of these $\bar{x}_i$. For these data we have

$$\bar{x} = (18.95 + 19.30 + 19.40)/3 = 19.22$$
$$s_b^2 = (4/3) \times 0.0558 = 0.074$$

and the overall variance and standard error of the estimated mean is given by

$$\text{Var}(\bar{x}) = 0.074 + 1.26 = 1.334$$
$$\text{SE}(\bar{x}) \sqrt{1.334} = 1.15$$

Note that in this example, the standard error estimated from the multiple imputation process is just slightly higher than what would have been estimated had any of the three combinations shown above been used by itself. This indicates that there is relatively little variability among the means attributable to the specific values imputed relative to the variability in the means attributable to the sampling variance of the distribution of MMSE scores. □

The discussion above of multiple imputation merely introduces the topic and gives a simple illustration of how it can be used. A more comprehensive discussion would entail familiarity with Bayesian methods of inference and other theoretical concepts that are beyond the scope of this text. The reader interested in pursuing this area is referred to the texts by Rubin [1] and by Little and Rubin [2].

13.7 SUMMARY

In this chapter we discussed problems caused by incomplete data in sample surveys. In particular, we described the effect of nonresponse on estimates observed from sample surveys of households; we discussed the reasons why nonresponse might result; and we suggested several methods for increasing the response rate in such surveys. In one widely used sample design, questionnaires are mailed to sample households and then data are obtained on a subsample of non-respondents by intensive effort. This sample design, if properly executed, results in estimates that are not biased seriously by the nonresponse. Finally, we discussed the problem of missing items in a data file, and we described several imputation methods, including multiple imputation, to convert an incomplete data set into a complete one.

EXERCISES

13.1 In a community containing 200 households, it is desired to conduct a mail survey for purposes of estimating X (the number of persons 18–64 years of age in the community), R_1 (the proportion of employed persons among all persons 18–64 years of age), and R_2 (the average number of work days lost per employed person per year among employed persons 18–64 years old). From a collection of ten households in a nearby similar community, the accompanying data were obtained. How large a sample is needed in order to be virtually certain of estimating X to within 20%, R_1 to within 30%, and R_2 to within 25%?

Household	Persons 18–64 Years	Employed Persons 18–64 Years	Work Days Lost in Past Month
a	4	3	1
b	2	1	1
c	3	2	2
d	1	0	0
e	1	1	2
f	0	0	0
g	2	2	3
h	5	4	2
i	0	0	0
j	2	1	2

Table 13.2 Data that would be Obtained from Mail Survey

Household	Persons 18–64 Years Old	Employed Persons 18–64 Years Old	Work Days Lost in Past Month	Household	Persons 18–64 Years Old	Employed Persons 18–64 Years Old	Work Days Lost in Past Month
1	0	0	0	25	*		
2	2	1	1	26	*		
3	*			27	*		
4	*			28	*		
5	1	1	0	29	2	0	0
6	*			30	3	1	1
7	4	1	0	31	4	3	2
8	1	0	0	32	3	3	6
9	4	0	0	33	3	1	1
10	3	3	5	34	5	1	1
11	*			35	3	2	3
12	0	0	0	36	*		
13	2	1	1	37	4	0	0
14	3	0	0	38	2	2	3
15	4	3	6	39	4	1	1
16	*			40	5	1	1
17	2	0	0	41	5	1	0
18	5	3	2	42	*		
19	2	2	1	43	*		
20	1	0	0	44	3	3	5
21	*			45	3	0	0
22	2	2	1	46	4	0	0
23	0	0	0	47	5	1	0
24	2	1	1	48	2	2	0

Table 13.2 Data that would be Obtained from Mail Survey (*continued*)

Household	Persons 18–64 Years Old	Employed Persons 18–64 Years Old	Work Days Lost in Past Month	Household	Persons 18–64 Years Old	Employed Persons 18–64 Years Old	Work Days Lost in Past Month
49	5	1	0	73	*		
50	5	2	3	74	3	2	1
51	4	0	0	75	*		
52	0	0	0	76	*		
53	0	0	0	77	0	0	0
54	0	0	0	78	2	0	0
55	3	2	1	79	*		
56	4	1	1	80	1	1	1
57	1	1	1	81	3	1	1
58	0	0	0	82	4	2	1
59	0	0	0	83	5	0	0
60	*			84	3	0	0
61	*			85	4	3	1
62	*			86	3	3	1
63	3	3	4	87	5	1	0
64	3	3	1	88	*		
65	2	1	2	89	*		
66	2	2	1	90	1	1	2
67	5	0	0	91	2	2	4
68	*			92	1	0	0
69	2	0	0	93	*		
70	4	0	0	94	2	1	1
71	2	1	1	95	*		
72	1	0	0	96	4	2	1

#			
97	2	2	1
98	4	2	0
99	0	0	0
100	*		
101	1	1	2
102	5	0	0
103	1	0	0
104	2	1	1
105	*		
106	4	1	1
107	1	1	1
108	*		
109	5	1	2
110	3	2	4
111	4	2	1
112	0	0	0
113	*		
114	3	2	3
115	*		
116	4	3	3
117	4	3	0
118	3	2	3
119	0	0	0
120	0	0	0
121	4	3	3
122	1	1	0
123	0	0	0
124	*		
125	*		
126	0	0	0
127	3	1	0
128	5	4	5
129	*		
130	3	1	1
131	3	1	1
132	0	0	0
133	4	1	1
134	4	3	5
135	3	1	2
136	4	3	1
137	1	1	0
138	5	4	6
139	2	2	3
140	4	1	0
141	2	1	2
142	4	1	2
143	3	1	0
144	*		
145	*		
146	3	3	2
147	0	0	0
148	3	0	0
149	1	1	0
150	5	4	4
151	0	0	0
152	5	4	2
153	1	0	0
154	5	5	4
155	*		
156	2	1	0

Table 13.2 Data that would be Obtained from Mail Survey (continued)

Household	Persons 18–64 Years Old	Employed Persons 18–64 Years Old	Work Days Lost in Past Month	Household	Persons 18–64 Years Old	Employed Persons 18–64 Years Old	Work Days Lost in Past Month
157	*		0	179	2	1	1
158	1	0	0	180	1	0	0
159	4	2	2	181	4	2	4
160	4	0	0	182	*		
161	5	2	3	183	3	1	1
162	3	1	1	184	3	2	0
163	3	1	1	185	2	1	1
164	2	1	0	186	4	3	1
165	*			187	4	1	1
166	2	0	0	188	*		
167	4	2	0	189	3	1	1
168	0	0	0	190	*		
169	3	2	3	191	*		
170	*			192	3	2	0
171	0	0	0	193	*		
172	3	1	1	194	*		
173	*			195	2	2	2
174	2	1	1	196	3	2	3
175	*			197	*		
176	*			198	4	3	3
177	*			199	4	2	3
178	4	2	2	200	4	3	3

*Missing information on this household (i.e., nonrespondents). See Table 13.3.

Table 13.3 Actual Values for Missing Data in Table 13.2

Household	Persons 18–64 Years Old	Employed Persons 18–64 Years Old	Work Days Lost in Past Month	Household	Persons 18–64 Years Old	Employed Persons 18–64 Years Old	Work Days Lost in Past Month
3	3	2	2	100	1	0	0
4	3	2	2	105	2	2	1
6	2	1	0	108	1	1	0
11	1	1	1	113	3	3	2
16	2	2	1	115	0	0	0
21	3	2	0	124	2	2	1
25	1	1	0	125	1	1	0
26	2	2	1	129	2	2	2
27	1	1	0	144	1	1	1
28	2	2	2	145	2	2	2
36	1	1	1	155	1	1	1
42	1	1	0	157	2	2	1
43	2	2	1	165	1	1	0
60	3	3	3	170	2	2	2
61	3	2	2	173	2	2	2
62	2	2	1	175	2	2	1
68	1	1	0	176	3	3	2
73	1	1	0	177	2	1	0
75	2	2	2	182	2	2	0
76	1	1	1	188	2	2	2
79	2	2	2	190	3	3	1
88	3	3	1	191	2	1	1
89	1	1	0	193	3	3	1
93	0	0	0	194	3	2	2
95	3	2	0	197	3	2	1

13.2   For the data of Exercise 13.1 assume that 20% of the population would not respond to the questionnaire. Assume further that it costs $1.50 per questionnaire for the initial mailing, $10.00 per questionnaire for the processing of mailed questionnaires, and $60.00 per interview (cost of obtaining the interview and processing the data) for nonrespondents. Determine the proportion of nonrespondents that should be sampled and the total number of initial questionnaires that should be mailed.

13.3   Pick a simple random sample of the required number of households (as calculated in Exercise 13.2), and from the data given in Tables 13.2 and 13.3, using the appropriate sampling of nonrespondents, estimate X, R_1, and R_2.

13.4   Consider the data presented in the example used to illustrate the hot deck method. Impute the missing values for MMSE using the hot deck method as used in that example with the following modification. Assume that the individuals with missing values will in general have lower MMSEs than those who had measured values on this variable. To take this into consideration, use as an imputed value 80% of the value taken from the hot deck method. How does the resulting estimated mean and its standard error compare with that obtained from the hot deck method without this modification?

13.5   Repeat the illustrative example presented in Section 13.6 with the modification discussed in Exercise 13.4. How does the estimated mean and its standard error computed on the basis of multiple imputation compare with that originally obtained?

13.6   Use the hot deck method to impute missing values for the data in Table 13.2. How does the resulting estimated mean and its standard error compare with that which would have been obtained had there been 100% response?

BIBLIOGRAPHY

The following books written in the 1980s deal exclusively with issues relating to nonresponse and statistical analysis with missing data.

1. Rubin, D. B., *Multiple Imputation for Nonresponse in Surveys*, Wiley, New York, 1987.
2. Little, R. J. A., and Rubin, D. B., *Statistical Analysis With Missing Data*, Wiley, New York, 1987.
3. Kalton, G., *Compensating for Missing Survey Data*, Research Report Series, Institute for Social Research, University of Michigan, Ann Arbor, 1983.

Chapter 4 of the recent text by Lehtonen and Pahkinen discusses issues relating to the handling of missing data. It gives an especially comprehensive treatment of reweighting methods for unit nonresponse.

4. Lehtonen, R., and Pahkinen, E. J., *Practical Methods for Design and Analysis of Complex Surveys*, rev. ed., Wiley, Chichester, U.K., 1994.

The following recent reviews and expository articles give overviews of methods used in the handling of missing data due to unit and/or item nonresponse. These reviews are especially useful for their inclusion of references to very recent work on these topics.

5. Dillman, D. A., Call-backs and mail-backs in sample surveys. In *The Encyclopedia of Biostatistics*, Armitage, P. A., and Colton, T., Eds., Wiley, Chichester U.K., 1998.

6. Little, R. J., Biostatistical analysis with missing data. In *The Encyclopedia of Biostatistics*, Armitage, P. A., and Colton, T., Eds., Wiley, Chichester U.K., 1998.

7. Barnard, J., Rubin, D. B., and Schenker, N., Multiple imputation. In *The Encyclopedia of Biostatistics*, Armitage, P. A., and Colton, T., Eds., Wiley, Chichester U.K., 1998.

8. Kviz, F., Nonresponse in sample surveys. In *The Encyclopedia of Biostatistics*, Armitage, P. A., and Colton, T., Eds., Wiley, Chichester U.K., 1998.

9. Sudman, S., Response effects in sample surveys. In *The Encyclopedia of Biostatistics*, Armitage, P. A., and Colton, T., Eds., Wiley, Chichester U.K., 1998.

The two following classic books give excellent discussions of methods of improving response rates, primarily in mail and telephone surveys.

10. Erdos, P., Professional Mail Surveys, McGraw-Hill, New York, 1970.

11. Dillman, D. A., *Mail and Telephone Surveys. The Total Design Method*, Wiley, New York, 1978.

The following publications are reports of substantive studies which have used methods discussed in this chapter to deal with issues of nonresponse and missing values.

12. Mullner, R., Levy, P. S., Byre, C. S., and Matthews, D., Effects of characteristics of the survey instrument on response rates to a mail survey of community hospitals. *Public Health Reports*, **97**: 465, 1982A.

13. National Center for Health Statistics, A Study of the Effect of Renumeration upon Response in the Health and Nutrition Examination Survey, PHS Publication No. 1000, Series 2, No. 67, U.S. Government Printing office, Washington, D.C., 1973.

14. Rich, S., Chomka, E., Hasara, L., Hart, K., Drizd, T., Joo, E., and Levy, P. S., The prevalence of pulmonary hypertension in the U.S. *Chest* 236, 1989.

15. Barr, D., Hershow, R., Levy, P. S., Furner, S., and Handler, A., Assessing prenatal heptatis B screening in Illinois using an inexpensive study design adaptable to other jurisdictions. *American Journal of Public Health*, Jan. 1999.

In January, 1998, a WINDOWS-based PC program entitled SOLAS became available. This software product can imput missing values using several methods including hot deck and multiple imputation. The users manual includes discussion of each of these methods.

16. Statistical Solutions Ltd., *SOLAS for Missing Data 1.0*, Statistical Solutions Ltd., Cork, Ireland, 1998.

CHAPTER 14

Selected Topics in Sample Design and Estimation Methodology

In this chapter we discuss some sampling and estimation techniques that have been developed for special purposes. More specifically, we will first discuss some sampling methods that have been developed for use in health surveys conducted in developing countries, and then examine techniques that have been used in developed countries in order to meet special needs.

14.1 WORLD HEALTH ORGANIZATION EPI SURVEYS: A MODIFICATION OF PPS SAMPLING FOR USE IN DEVELOPING COUNTRIES

The World Health Organization (WHO), through its Expanded Program on Immunization (EPI) aimed to ensure the availability of immunization to all children of the world. As part of that program, it developed methodology for estimating, by use of relatively quick and inexpensive sample surveys, immunization levels of children in areas that would be targeted for special immunization programs if the levels were low. The methodology makes use of a modification of probability proportional to size (PPS) sampling developed originally in the United States [1] and later modified for use in the Smallpox Eradication Program in West Africa [2].

Although it can be adapted to meet other objectives, the major objective of an EPI survey is to estimate the immunization coverage (i.e., the proportion of children having all their required immunizations) in a given target area (this could be a village, town, city, etc.). Over the years, the practice evolved in these surveys of selecting 30 sample clusters and 7 children within each cluster, which would yield a sample size of 210 children. In fact, these surveys became referred to as "30 × 7" surveys.

Although hundreds of these "30 × 7" surveys have been conducted, the rationale for the choice of the sample size is rather unusual. Assuming that 50% of the target population is covered by immunization, a simple random sample of size 96 would be required to be 95% confident of estimating this proportion to within 10 percentage points of the true value. Simple random sampling in the environment in which EPI surveys are conducted, however, is not cost effective, and so some cluster sampling technique would normally be employed. If one assumed a design effect of 2, the required sample size would be doubled, and one would need 192 (2 times 96) individuals in the sample. The developers of the EPI methodology were determined to use 30 clusters. Therefore, a sample of 30 clusters with 7 individuals per cluster would yield slightly more than the desired sample size. This is described in more detail by Lemeshow and Stroh [3].

Clusters in the EPI surveys depend on the particular population being surveyed and are generally villages, cities, towns, or health service districts for which population information is available. At the first stage, a PPS sample of 30 clusters is taken (as described in Chapter 11). At the second stage, however, for budgetary and logistic reasons, the process of selecting the seven individuals differs markedly from traditional cluster sampling. Instead of taking the seven subjects at random from all available subjects, the EPI methodology calls for randomly selecting a starting household (HH), collecting all relevant information on eligible subjects in that HH, and then proceeding to the HH whose front door is physically closest to the HH just visited. This process of visiting next closest HHs and collecting information on *all* eligible individuals in those HHs continues until the required seven subjects are studied.

The particular procedures used for selecting the first HH at random at the second stage of sampling depends on the nature of the cluster. For example, in a rural area, the interviewer might be instructed to go to a centrally located landmark in the cluster (such as a church or market), randomly select a direction in which to walk (i.e., north, south, east, or west) and count the number of households (K) found in that direction from the starting point to the town boundary. A random number between 1 and K would then be selected, which would designate the first HH chosen. As an operating rule, data are collected on all eligible children in the household contributing the seventh child, even if that results in including more than 7 children in a cluster.

The method as described above of selecting children within sample clusters in EPI surveys has been found to be relatively easy to implement in the field. The costs of taking a true random selection at the second stage would be prohibitive for the resources typically allocated to these EPI surveys. In an effort to evaluate the effect on estimates of immunization coverage of this nonrandom selection of individuals within clusters, a computer simulation model was developed [4]. This model compared the results of the EPI selection method to the results obtained by more traditional methods using artificially created populations having specified characteristics. It was found that although the EPI method performed poorly within particular clusters when there was pocketing of nonimmunized individuals, the resulting estimates, over all clusters, tended to be accurate to within 10 percentage points of the true population levels. This was within the goals specified by the EPI Program and may be attributed to the fact that a large number of clusters is selected and biases occurring within clusters tend to average out over the set of 30. Thus, the method appears quite useful when used for the target areas as a whole, but could provide highly unacceptable estimates if used for particular clusters or subgroups.

14.2 QUALITY ASSURANCE SAMPLING

The EPI survey design described in Section 14.1 has the major advantages of simplicity and low cost that make it an attractive option for estimating parameters such as vaccination coverage in countries or regions of interest. The EPI methodology, because it is a cluster survey technique, however, cannot provide information on small population units or health areas. Health program managers need this information to focus supervisory activities, since some health units may be performing less adequately than others in carrying out their specific functions. By identifying the health units that are not achieving their stated objectives (e.g., high immunization coverage), managers can direct their efforts to those areas where the most improvement is necessary. The quality assurance sampling (QAS) procedure has been suggested and is receiving considerable attention as an alternative to EPI sampling for use as a supervisory tool.

QAS methods were originally used in sampling and inspecting a manufactured product where it was necessary to keep labor and other sampling costs to minimal levels. One type of QAS sampling, lot quality assurance sampling (LQAS) is essentially stratified sampling, but the sample sizes are too small to provide what are usually considered acceptably narrow confidence intervals for estimates within a specific stratum (usually called a "batch" or "lot"). Rather, a decision is made about the quality of a particular batch or lot based on the probability that the number of defective items in a sample from it is less than or equal to a specified number. The results of the samples taken from all of the mutually exclusive and exhaustive batches can be combined to provide a precise overall estimate of the average quality of the total product.

The average quality of a product is often continually monitored by a manufacturer to (1) identify where improvement can be made in the manufacturing process, and (2) adjust the sample design as the average quality of the product changes. Generally, a lot is an "operationally useful" unit. For example, in an industrial application, if there were several machines producing the same part, lots could be chosen that are produced by the same machine, particularly if any variation in the parts produced is more likely to be due to machine drift than to operator input. The manufacturer's sampling interval should be short enough to identify any drift in measurements before tolerances are exceeded. For this type of application, it would also be worthwhile to monitor the sequence of measurements for early identification of tendency to drift.

For public health applications, a national manager might define lots as recipients of services from a single operational unit, such as a particular immunization team, over a specified period of time. The amount of time between sampling might be related to intervals between "high incidence" seasons for immunizable diseases, but would probably be related as much to the amount of time and cost associated with the sampling than any other single consideration.

In public health applications, a serious error would be made if the population were judged to be adequately covered ("accept the lot") when, in fact, it was not. In order to control for this possibility, the procedure is set up as a one-sided statistical test. Let d denote the number of persons not vaccinated from our sample of n subjects. Let P denote the true proportion of individuals not vaccinated in the population of size N. It is assumed that N is very large relative to n. (If it happens that N is not large relative to n, then the reader should consult a text such as Brownlee [29, Section 3.15] that demonstrates how the hypergeometric distribution is used to evaluate the LQAS procedure.)

The null hypothesis is

$$H_0: P \geq P_0 \quad \text{(i.e., proportion of unvaccinated children } \geq .50)^*$$

versus

$$H_a: P < P_0 \quad \text{(i.e., proportion of unvaccinated children } < .50)$$

The following four-celled table describes the consequences of the testing procedure.

Consequences of Hypothesis Testing in LQAS Procedure

Actual Population

		Not adequately vaccinated	Adequately vaccinated	
D e c i s i o n	Fail to reject H_0: not adequate coverage	Test recognizes or is sensitive to lack of adequate coverage $1 - \alpha$ Sensitivity	*Provider Risk* β False positive rate	← Reject the lot
	Reject H_0: adequate coverage	*Consumer Risk* α False negative rate	Test recognizes adequate coverage $1 - \beta$ Specificity	← Accept the lot

*The level 50% is chosen here as an example. Actually, any level could have been chosen.

Note that in this table, because the test is set up as one-sided, and because we assume the population is not adequately covered unless we reject H_0, the type I error, that is, accepting the lot when it is defective (false negative), the probability which we can control, is the most serious error. That is, using the example of immunization, if a population (lot) of children is thought to have an acceptable proportion immunized when, in fact, it does not, the larger number of susceptible children in the population increases the risk of transmission of the disease when introduced into the lot. Hence, we consider the "cost" to be high of declaring that the population is adequately vaccinated, when, infact, it is not. On the other hand, the type II error—rejection of an acceptable lot—is judged to be less serious since the result of a false positive decision would be to concentrate program resources on an already adequately vaccinated population.

The fundamental problem in LQAS sampling is not so much simply determining sample size as choosing an appropriate balance between sample size and critical region. The computation of the type II error probability, β, will, in all cases, depend upon what the actual value of P is when it is assumed to be different from P_0. The method of computing probabilities and determining sample sizes can be accomplished by use of the binomial distribution and is described in detail elsewhere [30], [31].

The method of quality assurance sampling described to this point is known as "single sampling," because only one sample is taken to make a decision regarding the disposition of the lot. A modification of the LQAS procedure incorporates a "double sampling" strategy and may be useful under certain field conditions.

A double sampling, or two-stage sampling plan, can be used to lower the sampling costs of a survey. In this scenario, two critical values, d_1^* and d_2^*, where $d_1^* \leq d_2^*$, are designated, and two sample sizes, n_1 and n_2, are specified. At the first stage, n_1 individuals are studied. If the observed number of unvaccinated individuals is less than or equal to d_1^*, we would conclude that the actual proportion unvaccinated in the population is significantly less than P_0. If the observed number of unvaccinated individuals in the first-stage sample of size n_1 is greater than d_2^*, we would conclude that the actual proportion unvaccinated in the population is not significantly less than P_0. If the observed number of unvaccinated individuals in the first stage is greater than d_1^* but less than or equal to d_2^*, we then proceed to the second stage and continue sampling until either $d_2^* + 1$ unvaccinated individuals are observed, indicating a low level of vaccination coverage, or a total of $n_1 + n_2$ individuals have been sampled without exceeding d_2^*, indicating a high level of vaccination coverage.

Rather than thinking of double sampling as a single sampling plan followed by an additional sampling stage, one should realize that the total sample size and critical value of the two stages correspond to the single sampling plan discussed previously, while the first stage represents a preliminary "reduced" sample. Herein lies the source of increased economy offered by the double sampling. When the results are extreme in the first stage, a health planner can make a conclusion based on fewer subjects sampled than if a one-stage sampling plan had been used. Otherwise, the health planner will continue sampling knowing that the maximum number sampled will be equal to the sample size from a one-stage plan. In other words, utilizing a double sampling plan will ensure that the number of people sampled will be less than or equal to that in a one-stage sampling plan.

While double sampling within the context of an LQAS scheme may be able to increase the economy of a health survey under certain conditions, it may be impractical in other situations. For example, if the medical test results cannot be analyzed on the spot, then a double sampling plan may require that a health team return to a community for further sampling if the statistical results are not extreme/conclusive in the first sample. The cost in terms of time and travel may offset the potential gain in economy attained through double sampling. However, if the cost per subject of administering the medical test is high, the health planner may feel that the potential gain from possibly having to carry out only the first stage of the sampling makes double sampling preferable.

LQAS is a stratified sampling technique. Instead of constructing confidence interval estimates of unknown parameters, it reduces the problem to a series of hypothesis tests. It does not, however, provide more information than conventional stratified random sampling because, using the latter technique, confidence intervals could be established for each stratum (or lot) and decisions could be made on values covered by each such interval if sample sizes were large enough to provide useful confidence intervals.

Although the sample sizes in each stratum in an LQAS scheme are typically too small to provide useful confidence intervals for estimates for each stratum, an appropriately designed LQAS scheme may provide a means for continually testing strata and classifying them as "acceptable" or "unacceptable" in terms of a particular outcome. Because LQAS sample sizes are relatively small, there is greater likelihood that sampling can be done more frequently. Perhaps samples could be drawn concurrently with other duties that take staff to the field. Because the rules are simple to follow, the surveyor/classifier needs minimal training. Results for strata can be combined to provide adequate estimates for groups of strata such as districts, regions, or the nation as a whole.

Although confidence intervals will always provide much more information than a simple binary decision, the sample sizes required to obtain any useful level of precision on estimates for relatively small strata may be prohibitive. In such instances, an appropriate QAS scheme may be an alternative worthy of consideration.

14.3 SAMPLE SIZES FOR LONGITUDINAL STUDIES

An important design used in epidemiological studies is the *cohort study*. In such a study, individuals are identified, measured at the time of identification, and sometimes followed over a period of years for determination of outcome variables (e.g., incidence of or mortality from specific diseases of interest). The main objectives in such studies are to examine relationships between these outcome variables and characteristics of the individuals present at the time of the initial identification. Examples of such studies include the Framingham study of cardiovascular disease [32], the physical activities study conducted by Ralph Paffenbarger [33], and the Longitudinal Study of Aging [34].

Such studies often require a large cohort size that is determined on the basis of the hypotheses to be tested concerning relationships between incidence of the outcome variables and the characteristics present at the time the cohort is ascertained. Methods for determining such necessary cohort sizes have been described in the epidemiological literature (e.g., Rothman and Boice [35]). Once the necessary cohort size has been determined, however, it becomes necessary to identify a sufficient number of individuals who satisfy criteria for inclusion in the cohort.

Often identification of cohort members is done by means of a sample survey in which a sample of individuals is selected, and the sample individuals are screened for satisfaction of criteria for inclusion in the cohort. Those satisfying the criteria are then recruited into the cohort for subsequent study. The size of the sample that should be taken for this screening is stated below for two sample designs: simple random sampling of individuals, and simple one-stage cluster sampling.

14.3.1 Simple Random Sampling

In order to have $100(1 - \alpha)\%$ certainty of obtaining at least n^* subjects who meet certain criteria, the approximate number n of subjects required to be sampled is given by

$$n = \left[A + \sqrt{A^2 + \frac{n^*}{P}} \right]^2 \tag{14.1}$$

where

$$A = \frac{|z_\alpha|}{2} \times \sqrt{\frac{1 - P}{P}}$$

z_α = the $100 \times \alpha$ percentile of the normal distribution

P = the proportion of persons in the population who meet the criteria for inclusion in the cohort study (i.e., the penetration of persons eligible to be included in the cohort)

The sample size given in relation (14.1) is based on the population size being much greater than the sample size and on approximation of the normal distribution to the binomial.

Illustrative Example. Suppose that 200 chief executive officers (CEOs) of hospitals are needed for a long-term follow-up study of job mobility. In order to be included in the study, the CEO has to be between 30 and 39 years of age. The method of recruiting these individuals into the study is as follows. A simple random sample is to be taken from a file which contains the names of CEOs from the approximately 6000 community hospitals in the United States. A telephone call is made to each sample CEO and he/she is queried on his/her age. If his/her age is between 30 and 39, then an attempt is made to secure the CEO's participation in the study. It is guessed that approximately 30% of all CEOs are in the target age range. If one wishes to be 95% certain of obtaining at least 200 CEOs (assuming 85% participation among all eligible sample persons), how many CEOs should be sampled?

Using relation (14.1) with $P = .30$, $n^* = 200$, and $z_\alpha = -1.645$, we have

$$A = \frac{1.645}{2} \times \sqrt{\frac{1 - .30}{.30}} = 1.256$$

and

$$n = \left[1.256 + \sqrt{(1.256)^2 + (200/.30)} \right]^2 \approx 735$$

and, allowing for 85% recruitment success, the final n required is given by

$$n = 735/.85 \approx 865.$$

Thus, 865 CEOs would have to be sampled in order to be 95% certain of recruiting at least 200 in the target age group.   □

The formulation described above is for simple random sampling. A sampling design more likely to be used in practice for identification of individuals, however, is cluster sampling, where a household might be a cluster and individuals within each sample household would be screened for eligibility to be recruited into the cohort. The analogous specification of sample size would be to sample a sufficient number, m, of clusters so that, with $100 \times (1 - \alpha)\%$ certainty, the required number n^* of individuals would be identified for recruitment into the cohort. Under this specification, and under a simple one-stage cluster sampling design, relation (14.1) applies with the following modifications.

14.3.2 Simple One-Stage Cluster Sampling

$$m = \left[A + \sqrt{A^2 + \frac{n^*}{\bar{N}}} \right]^2 \tag{14.2}$$

where

$A = |z_\alpha| \times V_N/2$

$V_N = \sigma_N/\bar{N}$

$\sigma_N = \sqrt{\sum_{i=1}^{M}(N_i - \bar{N})^2/M}$

M = the number of clusters in the population

N_i = the number of eligible individuals in cluster i; $i = 1, \ldots, M$

$\bar{N} = \sum_{i=1}^{M} N_i/M$ (the mean number of eligible individuals per cluster)

It should be noted that $\bar{N}$, the mean number of eligible individuals per cluster, is analogous to P, the proportion of eligible individuals in the population in the specification for sample size under simple random sampling.

Illustrative Example.   Suppose that we wish to take a sample of households in a large city and screen every person in the household for the purpose of identifying 500 unmarried women aged 25–39 who are employed full time and have at least one child of school age. Suppose further that there are approximately 30,000 such women in the city; that the city has approximately 300,000 households; and that $\sigma_N \approx \sqrt{\bar{N}}$. How many households would have to be sampled in order to identify with 95% certainty at least 500 women meeting the above criteria?

$\bar{N} = 30,000/300,000 = 0.1$ (mean number of unmarried women per household)

$\sigma_N = \sqrt{0.1} = .316$

$V_N = .316/0.1 = 3.16$

$A = 1.645 \times 3.16/2 = 2.60$

$m = \left[2.60 + \sqrt{(2.60)^2 + (500/.1)} \right]^2 \approx 5382.$

Thus, one would have to sample 5382 households in order to be 95% certain of identifying at least 500 eligible women (assuming 100% participation among the eligible women). □

14.3.3   Cluster Sampling with More Than One Domain

It is often the situation that one wishes to identify n^* individuals in each of several specified domains for future study. For example, one might wish to identify 1500 persons in each of four race–sex categories (white male, black male, white female, black female). If the sample design specified for identification of these individuals is simple one-stage cluster sampling, then the required number of clusters that should be sampled in order to obtain at least n^* individuals in each of these domains is given by

$$m = \max(m_1, \ldots, m_H) \tag{14.3}$$

where

$$m_h = \left[A_h + \sqrt{A_h^2 + \frac{n^*}{\bar{N}_h}} \right]^2, \qquad h = 1, \ldots, H \tag{14.4}$$

A_h and $\bar{N}_h$ are domain-specific analogues of the parameters defined for relation (14.2) and $H = $ the number of domains of interest.

We can assume without loss of generality that $m_1 \leq m_2 \leq \cdots \leq m_H$. Then, with simple one-stage cluster sampling, all domains except domain H would be likely to have as eligible subjects more than the number required to meet the specifications. This is due to the fact that in ordinary single-stage cluster sampling, once a cluster is selected in the sample, there is no further subsampling of individuals. Levy et al. [5], [6] developed a variation of simple one-stage cluster sampling in which the sample clusters are randomized into one of H groups. Those in group 1 can recruit individuals in all of the H domains; those in group 2 can recruit individuals in domains 2 through H but not in domain 1, and so forth, with clusters in group h recruiting only individuals in domain H. This modification of simple one-stage cluster sampling, called *telescopic single-stage cluster sampling*, results in the specifications being satisfied exactly for each domain, and avoids the problem of recruiting too many individuals in most of the domains. This methodology was used successfully in a large survey of elderly persons in Shanghai, China [5], [6].

14.4   ESTIMATION OF PREVALENCE OF DISEASES FROM SCREENING STUDIES

It is often desired to estimate the prevalence of a disease or condition in a population on the basis of a screening test that has less than perfect *sensitivity* and *specificity*, where these two terms have the following meanings:

> *Sensitivity* is defined as the probability that a person having the particular disease or condition will have a positive screening test.

Specificity is the probability that a person *not having* the disease or condition will not have a positive screening test.

The screening test is usually a test that is inexpensive and feasible to use in the field in comparison to a more accurate diagnostic test which, although available, would not be feasible to use in a survey situation. For example, the Mini Mental State Examination (MMSE) consists of a few questions that are used to screen individuals for cognitive impairment that may or may not indicate a dementing illness [6], whereas it would require a complex battery of neurological and psychiatric tests to diagnose dementia to any reasonable degree of accuracy.

The major objectives of screening programs are generally to identify for subsequent intervention individuals having the condition or disease, and the major statistical issues involve the evaluation of the likelihood that an individual screened as positive really has the disease and, analogously, the likelihood that an individual screened as negative really does not have the disease (called, respectively, *predictive value of a positive test* and *predictive value of a negative test*). The epidemiologic literature abounds with discussions of these issues [7], and we will concentrate instead on the problem of estimating the prevalence of the disease from a screening test.

The basic methodology involves taking a sample of n individuals from a population of N individuals and giving the screening test to each of the sample individuals. If k of the n sample individuals are screened as positive, then it was shown by Levy and Kass [8] that the maximum likelihood estimate, $\hat{\pi}$, of the unknown prevalence, π, of persons having the disease is given by

$$\hat{\pi} = \frac{\hat{p} + S_p - 1}{S_e + S_p - 1} \tag{14.5}$$

where $\hat{p} = k/n =$ the proportion having positive tests, $S_e =$ the sensitivity of the test, and $S_p =$ the specificity of the test. One can see from relation (14.5) that, in situations where the sum of the specificity and sensitivity are less than unity or when the sum of the prevalence of the test and its specificity are less than unity, the estimated prevalence $\hat{\pi}$ would be negative. Gastwirth [9] and Lew and Levy [10] proposed modifications of Equation (14.5) which would eliminate the possibility of negative estimates of prevalence. In practice, a screening test having a sensitivity and/or specificity so low that negative estimates of prevalence are likely would have little utility as a screen for the particular disease or condition.

The standard error of the estimated prevalence, $\hat{\pi}$, is given by

$$SE(\hat{\pi}) = \frac{SE(\hat{p})}{(S_e + S_p - 1)} \tag{14.6}$$

where the standard error, $SE(\hat{p})$, of $\hat{p}$ would depend on the particular sample design and estimation procedures used.

   Illustrative Example.   Suppose that a simple random sample of 150 members was taken from the membership of a union representing teachers employed in seven school districts in a large county in Illinois. The seven school districts employed 2560 teachers. All teachers sampled were given a screening test for glaucoma known to have a sensitivity of 96% and a specificity of 89%. Of the 150 teachers tested, 23 were positive. From these data, it is desired to estimate and obtain 95% confidence intervals for the proportion of teachers in the union that have glaucoma. From our knowledge of simple random sampling (Chapter 3), we have

$$\hat{p} = \tfrac{23}{150} = .153$$

and

$$\widehat{SE}(\hat{p}) = \left(\frac{N-n}{N}\right)^{1/2} \left(\frac{\hat{p}(1-\hat{p})}{n-1}\right)^{1/2}$$
$$= \left(\frac{2560-150}{2560}\right)^{1/2} \left(\frac{.153 \times .847}{149}\right)^{1/2}$$
$$= .029$$

and from relations (14.5) and (14.6), we have

$$\hat{\pi} = \frac{.153 + .89 - 1}{.96 + .89 - 1} = \frac{.043}{.85} = .051$$

and

$$\widehat{SE}(\hat{\pi}) = \frac{.029}{.85} = .034.$$

Finally, 95% confidence intervals for π, the unknown prevalence of glaucoma among all teachers in the seven school districts, is given by

$$.051 - 1.96 \times .034 \leq \pi \leq .051 + 1.96 \times .034$$

or

$$0 \leq \pi \leq .118.$$

Note that the lower limit was computed as $-.016$ and set equal to zero, since a negative proportion makes no sense.   □

The methodology presented above assumes that the sensitivity and specificity of the screening test are known. If they are not known, then a double sampling design can be used to estimate the unknown prevalence, π. In this design, a subsample would be taken from those individuals screened as positive and another subsample taken from those screened as negative. Individuals in both samples would be given a more definitive diagnostic examination for the disease or condition, which would be the "gold standard" used to substantiate or repudiate the results of the original screening test. In this type of design, the estimate, $\hat{\pi}$, of prevalence is given by

$$\hat{\pi} = \frac{\dfrac{k_1}{m_1} \times m + \dfrac{k_2}{m_2} \times (n - m)}{n}, \tag{14.7}$$

where

$n =$ the number screened from the population of N elements
$m =$ the number positive for the screening test
$n - m =$ the number negative for the screening test
$m_1 =$ the number sampled from the group of m individuals initially positive for the screening test
$k_1 =$ the number confirmed as positive from the m_1 subjects initially positive and resampled
$m_2 =$ the number sampled from the group of $n - m$ individuals initially negative for the screening test
$k_2 =$ the number of subjects confirmed as positive from the m_2 subjects initially negative and resampled

An estimate of the variance of this estimate (obtained by use of conditional variance and ignoring finite population corrections) is given by

$$\widehat{\mathrm{Var}}(\hat{\pi}) = \left(\frac{k_1}{m_1} - \frac{k_2}{m_2}\right)^2 \times \frac{\dfrac{m}{n}\left(1 - \dfrac{m}{n}\right)}{n} + \left(\frac{m}{n}\right)^2 \frac{\dfrac{k_1}{m_1}\left(1 - \dfrac{k_1}{m_1}\right)}{m_1}$$
$$+ \left(1 - \frac{m}{n}\right)^2 \frac{\dfrac{k_2}{m_2}\left(1 - \dfrac{k_2}{m_2}\right)}{m_2}. \tag{14.8}$$

Illustrative Example. A simple random sample of 120 persons is taken from 423 persons who work in toll booths in the state highway system of a large state. Each sample employee is given a very rapid screening test that assesses hearing deficiency. Of the 120 employees screened in this way, 63 showed evidence of hearing loss. A simple random sample of 30 individuals was taken from the 63 screened positive and these 30 were given a more definitive test for hearing loss. Of these 30, 23 had a confirmed hearing loss. Likewise, a sample of 30 individuals was taken from the 57 initially screened as negative, and 14 of these had hearing loss when given the more definitive test. From Equation (14.7), we have

$$n = 120 \qquad m = 63 \qquad n - m = 57$$
$$m_1 = m_2 = 30 \qquad k_1 = 23 \qquad k_2 = 14$$
$$\hat{\pi} = \frac{\frac{23}{30} \times 63 + \frac{14}{30} \times 57}{120} = .62$$

From relation (14.8), the standard error of $\hat{\pi}$ is estimated by

$$\widehat{SE}(\hat{\pi}) = \left\{ \left(\frac{23}{30} - \frac{14}{30}\right)^2 \frac{.525 \times .475}{120} \right.$$
$$\left. + (.525)^2 \frac{.767 \times .233}{30} + (.475)^2 \frac{.467 \times .533}{30} \right\}^{1/2} = .061$$

Thus, 95% confidence intervals for the proportion π having the disease or condition being screened for is given by

$$.62 - 1.96 \times .061 \leq \pi \leq .62 + 1.96 \times .061$$

or

$$.50 \leq \pi \leq .74 \qquad \qquad \square$$

The above example illustrates the importance of double sampling when the sensitivity and the specificity of the screening test are not known. If the proportion positive at the initial screen had been used, the resulting estimate, $63/120 = .525$, would have been considerably lower than the estimate given in relation (14.7).

It is often of interest in screening studies, not only to estimate the prevalence of the particular disease or condition, but also to estimate the sensitivity and specificity of the particular screening test. This can be done if samples are taken both of those initially screened negative and those initially screened positive. The appropriate estimates, $\hat{S}_e$ and $\hat{S}_p$, of the sensitivity and specificity are given by

$$\hat{S}_e = \frac{m\,\dfrac{k_1}{m_1}}{m\left(\dfrac{k_1}{m_1} - \dfrac{k_2}{m_2}\right) + n\,\dfrac{k_2}{m_2}} \tag{14.9}$$

and

$$\hat{S}_p = \frac{(n - m)\left(1 - \dfrac{k_2}{m_2}\right)}{m\left(\dfrac{k_2}{m_2} - \dfrac{k_1}{m_1}\right) + n\left(1 - \dfrac{k_2}{m_2}\right)} \tag{14.10}$$

14.5 ESTIMATION OF RARE EVENTS: NETWORK SAMPLING

We have shown that modification of a basic simple random sampling plan without alteration of the estimation procedure (e.g., stratified random sampling with proportional allocation) can sometimes lead to estimates that have smaller sampling errors than those obtained through simple random sampling. We have also discussed how a simple random sampling plan using a modified estimation procedure (e.g., ratio estimation) can also lead to estimates with lower sampling errors. In a similar way, in this section, we will show how modification of a counting rule can lead to estimates that have lower sampling errors than what would have been obtained through conventional counting rules.

A counting rule is an algorithm that links enumeration units (or listing units) to elementary units. For example, in a sample survey of households conducted to estimate total births that occur in the population during a specified time period, an obvious counting rule is to allow births to be reported in the household of the parents of the newborn. Such a counting rule links each element (e.g., birth) to one and only one enumeration unit (e.g., household). However, an alternative counting rule allows births to be reported in the household of the grandparents of the newborn as well as in the household of the parents. This counting rule would then allow an element to be linked to more than one listing unit.

A counting rule that allows an element to be linked to only one enumeration unit is called a *conventional counting rule*. A counting rule that allows an element to be linked to more than one enumeration unit is called a *multiplicity counting rule*. Sample designs that use multiplicity counting rules are called *network samples*. Network samples have received considerable attention over the past two decades, especially in the health and behavioral sciences, and especially in situations involving rare events or rare characteristics. Let us investigate this design through the following example.

Illustrative Example. Let us consider a county that has 100 identified primary health care providers. Suppose that we are interested in conducting a sample survey of ten health care providers in order to estimate the total number of persons who were treated for skin cancer during a particular time period. This process would be a simple one if every patient had been treated by one and only one health provider. However, a person with skin cancer may be treated by several providers (e.g., internist, surgeon, radiologist, physical therapist). Thus, in designing the sample survey, we must specify a counting rule that allows us to link the elements (i.e., persons treated for skin cancer) with more than one enumeration unit (i.e., health care providers).

Let us suppose that three persons were treated for skin cancer during the year. Person 1 was treated by four physicians (physicians 1, 2, 3, and 4); person 2 was treated by two physicians (physicians 4 and 5); and person 3 was treated by one physician (physician 6). We then have the network linking health care providers with skin cancer patients that is shown in Figure 14.1. The solid lines in the figure indicate the *first* provider (chronologically) who treated the patient.

If we use a conventional counting rule—such as linking patients with the first provider who treated them—then patients 1 and 2 would be reported by provider 4 and patient 3 would be reported by provider 6; the other 98 providers would report no patients. If we let X_i be the number of patients reported by the ith provider according to this counting rule, then $X_4 = 2$, $X_6 = 1$, and the remaining $X_i = 0$. For a simple random sample of $n = 10$ health care providers, we see that the estimator $x' = (100/10)x$, by enumerating all samples, has the following distribution

x'	**Relative Frequency**
0	.8091
10	.0909
20	.0909
30	.0091

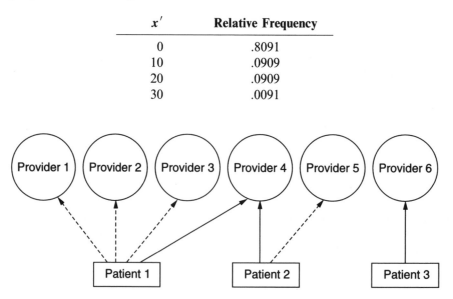

Figure 14.1 Network sample for health care providers and skin cancer patients.

The mean, $E(x')$, of the distribution of x' is equal to 3 (the true population total), and the standard error, $SE(x')$, of x' is equal to 6.681. Notice that in more than 80% of the samples, no patients would be identified and the estimate, x', would be equal to 0. □

Referring to the example above, suppose now that we use a counting rule that allows a patient to be reported by *any* health provider treating the patient. This is a multiplicity rule since it allows a patient to be reported by more than one provider. Since those patients who were treated by more than one provider have a greater chance of being selected than those treated by only one provider, a modified estimation procedure must be used to obtain an unbiased estimator of the total. This is done by defining for each enumeration unit, i, (e.g., health care provider) the following variable, x_i^*, given by

$$x_i^* = \sum_{j=1}^{m} \frac{\delta_{ij}}{s_j}$$

where

m = the total number of elements (patients) identified in the sample

$$\delta_{ij} = \begin{cases} 1 & \text{if the } i\text{th enumeration unit (provider } i) \text{ is linked} \\ & \text{to the } j\text{th element by the counting rule} \\ 0 & \text{otherwise} \end{cases}$$

s_j = the number of enumeration units linked to element j
(called the *multiplicity* of element j)

The s_j represent extra information that must be obtained from the sample enumeration units (if possible) or, in some cases, from some other source, such as the elements themselves. We note that this process of obtaining the multiplicities might add considerably to the cost of the survey.

For simple random samples of health care providers from a population of N such providers, the estimated total, x'_{mult}, is given by

$$x'_{\text{mult}} = \left(\frac{N}{n}\right) x^*$$

where x^* is the sample total of the x_i^*. Let us return to our example.

Illustrative Example. Referring to the previous example, let us use a counting rule that allows a patient to be reported by any health care provider treating the patient. Then, for the sample shown in Figure 14.1, we have

$$s_1 = 4 \qquad s_2 = 2 \qquad s_3 = 1$$

$$x_1^* = \tfrac{1}{4} \qquad x_2^* = \tfrac{1}{4} \qquad x_3^* = \tfrac{1}{4} \qquad x_4^* = \tfrac{1}{4} + \tfrac{1}{2} = \tfrac{3}{4} \qquad x_5^* = \tfrac{1}{2} \qquad x_6^* = 1$$

Table 14.1 gives the distribution of x'_{mult} for simple random samples of $n = 10$ of the $N = 100$ health care providers in this example.

The mean, $E(x'_{mult})$, and the standard error, $SE(x'_{mult})$, as calculated from the distribution shown in Table 14.1 (and using expressions 2.24 given in Box 2.4), are

$$E(x'_{mult}) = 3 = X \quad \text{and} \quad SE(x'_{mult}) = 4.13$$

Thus we see that, for this example, the estimated total, x'_{mult}, is not only an unbiased estimator for the population total X but has in this instance a much smaller standard error than x', the estimated total obtained from the conventional counting rule.   □

The theory of network sampling is discussed in greater detail in articles by Sirken [11], [12] and by Sudman, Sirken and Cowan [13]. It has been shown to be especially useful in estimating the incidence or prevalence of attributes that occur in less than 3% of the population (i.e., "rare events"). For example, it has been used to estimate the number of births and marriages [14] and crime victims [15] occurring in a population during a specified time period, as well as the prevalence of such diseases as cystic fibrosis [12], cancer [16], and diabetes [17]. It has been extended to stratification [12], [18], ratio estimation [19], and cluster sampling [20].

Multiplicity counting rules can improve the reliability of an estimate because they often increase the yield of a sample. For instance, in the example used above, approximately 81% of all samples of size $n = 10$ would yield no patients with skin cancer if a conventional counting rule were used, whereas only about

Table 14.1   Distribution of x'_{mult}

x'_{mult}	Relative Frequency[a]
0.0	.5223
2.5	.1843
5.0	.0807
7.5	.08132
10.0	.08251
12.5	.03076
15.0	.01003
17.5	.00839
20.0	.00192
22.5	.00074
25.0	.00019
27.5	.00001
30.0	.000003

[a]Obtained from combinatorial theory.

52% of all samples would yield no skin cancer patients under the multiplicity rule. Under the multiplicity rule, the network of health providers eligible to report skin cancer patients has tripled from 2 to 6 (see Figure 14.1).

14.6   ESTIMATION OF RARE EVENTS: DUAL SAMPLES

Another strategy that sometimes can be used to estimate the prevalence of rare events or members of rare populations is the use of two independent surveys or a survey in combination with a registration system. Estimation from this type of dual system is as follows. Let N = the unknown number of rare events in the universe, x_1 = the total number of rare events identified in the first survey, x_2 = the total number of rare events identified in the second survey, and x_{12} = the number of rare events identified in both surveys. This can be represented as follows

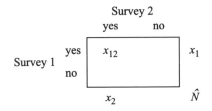

If the two surveys are independent, then the number, x_{12}, of rare events included in both surveys should be approximately equal to $(x_1 x_2 / N)$, and N can be estimated by $\hat{N}$ given by

$$\hat{N} = \frac{x_1 x_2}{x_{12}} \tag{14.9}$$

This estimate was developed originally by Chandra Sekar and Deming [21] who used it to estimate vital events in developing countries. In this use of it, the two sources reporting vital events were a registration system and a sample survey. More recently, Cowan and Malec extended this methodology to more complex situations in which there is a clustering of events that are not captured by either system [22].

Illustrative Example.   Suppose that the vital registration system for a developing country enumerates 20,543 deaths during a given year, and that a sample survey of one in 100 households enumerates 185 deaths, of which 146 match deaths which had been listed in the vital registry.

Using the estimator shown in relation (14.9), we have

$$x_1 = 20{,}543$$
$$x_2 = 100 \times 185 = 18{,}500$$
$$x_{12} = 100 \times 146 = 14{,}600$$
$$\hat{N} = \frac{20{,}543 \times 18{,}500}{14{,}600} \approx 26{,}031$$

Thus, we would estimate that there were 26,031 deaths in that country during that period. □

14.7 ESTIMATION OF CHARACTERISTICS FOR LOCAL AREAS: SYNTHETIC ESTIMATION

The planning of health and social services in the United States is often done on a subnational geographic basis, with areas such as groups of states, individual states, counties, and municipalities serving as the functional "analytic units." For this reason, it is of considerable importance to have valid and reliable estimates of health and social characteristics for these local areas so that planning decisions can be made on the basis of accurate information.

On the other hand, such estimates for local areas are often not easily obtainable. Although estimates of births, deaths, marriages, and divorces can be obtained for local areas through the vital statistics registration system, estimates of morbidity, disability, and utilization of services are often not available on a local basis. The major reason for lack of local area health data lies in the fact that most health data are collected from a system of nationwide surveys conducted by the National Center for Health Statistics (NCHS). This system of health surveys can provide reliable and valid estimates for the United States as a whole and for large geographic subregions (i.e., Northeast, North Central, South, West). Limitations in the sample size and in the design of these surveys, however, make them generally unsuitable for production of accurate estimates for the relatively small areas that often serve as planning units.

The major characteristic of the designs of these nationwide surveys that makes them unsuitable for production of small-area estimates is the way the strata are constructed. For example, in the National Health Interview Survey (NHIS), which is a nationwide household interview survey yielding estimates of morbidity, disability, and utilization of health services, strata consist of one or more counties or Standard Metropolitan Statistical Areas (SMSAs) grouped according to similar demographic characteristics. For example, an NHIS stratum might include three counties: one from Iowa, one from Nebraska, and one from Kansas. Only one of these three would be selected in the sample to represent the entire stratum. Estimates for the United States are obtained by aggregating such stratum estimates over all the strata. However, it is virtually impossible to piece together estimates for such areas as states, cities, or health planning areas, which are generally not combinations of NHIS strata.

One method of using data from nationwide health surveys for purposes of obtaining estimates for small areas that has found some acceptance—mainly because of its simplicity and intuitive appeal—is called *synthetic estimation.* This procedure obtains small-area estimates of characteristics by combining nationwide estimates of the characteristics specific to population groups with estimates of the proportional distribution within the small-area population into these same population groups. The groups are chosen on the basis both of their relevance to the characteristic being estimated and of the availability of small-area population data specific to the group.

More formally, a *synthetic estimate* $\tilde{\bar{x}}_a$ of the mean level $\bar{X}_a$ of characteristic $\mathcal{X}$ for area a is given by

$$\tilde{\bar{x}}_a = \sum_{k=1}^{K} \hat{P}_{ak} \bar{x}_k \qquad (14.10)$$

where, for $k = 1, \ldots, K$, $\bar{x}_k$ is the *estimated nationwide mean level* of characteristic $\mathcal{X}$ for persons in group k obtained from the nationwide survey, and $\hat{P}_{ak}$ is the *estimated proportion* of all persons in area a who are in group k. The $\hat{P}_{ak}$ are estimates of local population proportions generally obtained from a U.S. Census or from local agencies; K represents the total number of population groups chosen for study.

We see that the synthetic estimate $\tilde{\bar{x}}_a$ has some characteristics that are very similar to the estimates developed in the discussion of poststratification in Chapter 6 (although there are also important differences). The similarity to poststratification lies in the fact that both methods combine means specific to groups that are not strata with population proportions appropriate for the groups. The major difference lies in the fact that the group-specific means $\bar{x}_k$ used in constructing a synthetic estimate are themselves constructed from data that in most instances are obtained from individuals outside the small area.

As mentioned earlier, synthetic estimation has found some acceptance because it is a more feasible alternative, in terms of resources and costs, to conducting a survey in the small area for which estimates are desired. Statistical properties of synthetic estimates have been investigated by Gonzalez and Hoza [23] and by Levy and French [24]. They are *biased* estimates, with bias given by

$$B(\tilde{\bar{x}}) = \sum_{k=1}^{K} \hat{P}_{ak} (\bar{X}_k - \bar{X}_{ak}) \qquad (14.11)$$

where for $k = 1, 2, \ldots, K$, $\bar{X}_k$ is the mean level of characteristic $\mathcal{X}$ on the national level for group k, and $\bar{X}_{ak}$ is the mean level of characteristic $\mathcal{X}$ for individuals in area a who are in group k.

An expression for the appropriate variance of a synthetic estimate is given by

$$\text{Var}(\tilde{x}) \approx \sum_{k=1}^{K} P_{ak}^2 \, \text{Var}(\bar{x}_k) + 2 \sum_{k<r} P_{ak} P_{ar} \, \text{Cov}(\bar{x}_k, \bar{x}_r) \tag{14.12}$$

where

$\text{Var}(\bar{x}_k)$ = variance of estimated mean level of $\mathscr{X}$ in group k (nationwide)

$\text{Cov}(\bar{x}_k, \bar{x}_r)$ = covariance between estimated mean levels of characteristic $\mathscr{X}$ in groups k and r (nationwide)

Since synthetic estimates are generally based on large samples, their sampling errors are often quite small, and their accuracy depends largely on the magnitude of their bias. Note that the bias in a synthetic estimate is a weighted average of the differences between the mean for a group on the nationwide level and that for the same group in the small area.

If an unbiased estimate $\bar{x}_a'$ exists for the small area and is independent statistically of the synthetic estimate, then the mean square error of the synthetic estimate can be estimated by the following expression:

$$\widehat{\text{MSE}}(\tilde{x}_a) = (\tilde{x}_a - \bar{x}_a')^2 - \widehat{\text{Var}}(\bar{x}_a') \tag{14.13}$$

where $\widehat{\text{Var}}(\bar{x}_a')$ is an unbiased estimate of the variance of $\bar{x}_a'$. Generally, the variance of the available unbiased estimate, $\bar{x}_a'$, is too unstable for Equation (14.13) to be useful (otherwise $\bar{x}_a'$ might be the estimator of choice rather than the synthetic estimate). However, these estimators of the mean square error of individual synthetic estimates can be averaged over a number of similar expressions among several small areas to arrive at a more stable estimate, which has the interpretation of being the *average mean square error (AMSE)* of a collection of synthetic estimates (e.g., states within the United States).

Illustrative Example. Let us suppose that we are interested in estimating the mean number of days lost from work because of health reasons for a large state and that national estimates shown below exist for each of four race–sex domains, along with the distribution of the population of the state according to these four race–sex groups.

Sex–Race Group	Proportion of State Population in Sex– Race Group (P_{ak}')	National Level Estimate of Work- Loss Days/Person Year ($\bar{x}_k$)
White male	.39	5.2
White female	.43	5.6
All other male	.08	5.9
All other female	.10	6.3

From relation (14.1) the synthetic estimate for the state is given by

$$\tilde{\tilde{x}}_a = .39 \times 5.2 + .43 \times 5.6 + .08 \times 5.9 + .10 \times 6.3 = 5.54 \text{ days/person-year}$$

Suppose that an unbiased estimate exists for the state and is equal to 6.85 with variance estimated at 76.29. Then the estimated mean square error of the synthetic estimate is given by

$$\widehat{\text{MSE}}(\tilde{\tilde{x}}_a) = (6.85 - 5.54)^2 + 76.29 = 78.01$$

and the estimate of its root mean square error would be $\sqrt{78.01} = 8.83$. $\quad\square$

Synthetic estimation is one of several methods of obtaining estimates of the characteristics of small areas. Regression models have been increasingly used. This methodology generally develops from regression equations expressing relationships between an estimate of the outcome variable of interest and a set of indicator variables available for the local areas. These regression equations are then used to provide an improved estimate of the outcome variable of interest for the local area based on the available indicator variables for the local area. A more thorough discussion of this type of methodology and other methods of obtaining small-area estimates can be found in a review by Levy [25].

14.8 EXTRACTION OF SENSITIVE INFORMATION: RANDOMIZED RESPONSE TECHNIQUES

In many sample surveys, information of a sensitive nature must be extracted from individuals selected in the sample. For example, in a study of family planning practices, it might be necessary to ask questions concerning use of drugs, contraceptive practices, or history of abortions. To some individuals, such questions might be threatening or embarrassing. In order to avoid an excess of refusals or misleading responses, a method called *randomized response*, developed originally by Warner [26], has been used with some success in many surveys.

The randomized response technique in its most basic form presents the respondent with two questions: a sensitive question and an innocuous question. The respondent is then given some randomization device such as a bag containing red and white chips and told to select a chip from the bag without letting the interviewer see it. If a red chip is selected, the respondent is instructed to answer "yes" or "no" to the innocuous question. If the white chip is selected, the respondent is to answer "yes" or "no" to the sensitive question. The interviewer then records the respondent's answer without knowing which question is being answered.

The rationale behind this method is that the respondent will be willing to answer the sensitive question if he or she feels that the interviewer does not know whether the response is to the sensitive or to the innocuous question. To illustrate, the respondent might be given the following flash card:

1. Have you ever used cocaine for recreational purposes?
2. Is the last digit in your Social Security number an odd number (1, 3, 5, 7, 9)?

After being told to respond to question 1 if a white chip is chosen and to question 2 if a red chip is chosen, the respondent answers "yes" or "no" without indicating to the interviewer which question is being answered.

If both the composition of the randomization device and the theoretical probability of answering "yes" to the innocuous question are known, an estimate can be obtained of the proportion of individuals in the population who have the attribute specified in the sensitive question from the total proportion of respondents for whom a "yes" response is recorded. This estimate is given by

$$\hat{P}_1 = \frac{p^* - P_2(1 - \theta)}{\theta} \tag{14.14}$$

where $\hat{P}_1$ is the estimated proportion in the population who have the attribute specified by the sensitive question; p^* is the proportion of "yes" responses obtained in the survey; P_2 is the theoretical probability of answering "yes" to the innocuous question; and θ is the probability of answering the sensitive question (e.g., the proportion of red chips in the bag).

Illustrative Example. In the example given above, suppose that the bag contained 75% white chips and that the last digit of an individual's Social Security number is equally likely to end in an odd digit as in an even digit. Then we have θ and P_2 given by

$$\theta = \frac{3}{4} = .75 \quad \text{and} \quad P_2 = \frac{1}{2} = .50$$

Suppose that 40% of all respondents answered "yes." In other words, $p^* = .40$. Then the estimated proportion, $\hat{P}_1$, of persons who use cocaine for recreational purposes is given by

$$\hat{P}_1 = \frac{.40 - .50 \times (1 - .75)}{.75} = .367$$

Thus, we would estimate that 36.7% of all individuals in this population used cocaine for recreational purposes. ☐

Because the responses to the innocuous question in a sense waste information, randomized response techniques generally require larger sample sizes than conventional surveys to meet specified standards of reliability. Also, it is possible to obtain negative estimates by this method.

A more detailed exposition of this method is given in papers by Abernathy et al. [27], and some elaborations of this technique are discussed by I-Cheng et al. [28].

14.9   SUMMARY

In this chapter we discussed some applications of sampling and estimation methods that are relevant to specific problems in the health sciences. One of these methods, a variation of probability proportional to size sampling, was developed for the purpose of determining immunization levels in developing countries. Another method—telescopic sampling—was developed for a survey of dementia in Shanghai, Peoples Republic of China. This technique is useful in situations where it is not feasible to subsample within clusters. Other topics discussed include methods for estimating the prevalence of diseases or conditions from screening tests which have imperfect sensitivity and specificity; estimation of rare events or rare population groups; estimation methods for small areas; and methods of obtaining sensitive information from sample surveys.

EXERCISES

14.1   A simple random sample was taken of 525 workers in a plant employing 3575 workers. All persons sampled were given an electrocardiogram which was read for abnormalities independently by two physicians. Of the 525 sample persons, 25 had abnormalities noted by both physicians; 15 had abnormalities noted by physician A, but not by physician B; 37 had abnormalities noted by physician B only; and the remainder had no abnormalities noted by either physician. Based on these data, what would be the estimated number of abnormalities among the 3575 workers?

14.2   These same persons were screened for diabetes on the basis of a single fasting blood glucose test. The particular screening method has a known sensitivity equal to 80% and a specificity equal to 96%. Based on findings of 14 positive tests, estimate and give 95% confidence intervals for the prevalence of diabetes among these employees.

14.3   These sample persons were also screened for hypertension by use of a standard sphygmomanometer examination and, based on this examination, 63 were positive. Of those screened as positive, 25 were given a more intensive evaluation for hypertension, and 21 were confirmed as being hypertensive. A sample of 50 persons was taken from those originally screened as negative, and 8 of these were found on the more intensive evaluation to be hypertensive. Based on these findings, what is the estimated prevalence of hypertension in this population? Give 95% confidence intervals for this estimated proportion.

14.4   From the data presented in the previous exercise, estimate the sensitivity and the specificity of the sphygmomanometer examination used in the screening for hypertension.

14.5   A simple random sample was taken of 300 households in a community containing 3562 households. Respondents from each household were queried on whether there had been a burglary during the past year in either that house or any other house on the block segment containing that house. The following six (6) burglaries were reported:

Burglary	Number of Households Eligible to Report the Burglary
1	3
2	2
3	7
4	6
5	8
6	2

Based on these findings, estimate the number of burglaries that occurred in that community over the past year.

BIBLIOGRAPHY

The following publications discuss the methodology used in the EPI Surveys.

1. Serfling, R. E., and Sherman, I. L., *Attribute Sampling Methods*, Publication No. 1230, U.S. Department of Health and Human Services, Public Health Service, Washington, D.C., 1975.

2. Henderson, R. H., et al., Assessment of vaccination coverage, vaccination scar rates, and smallpox scarring in five areas of West Africa, *Bulletin of the World Health Organization*, **48**: 183, 1973.

3. Lemeshow, S., and Stroh, G., Jr., *Sampling Techniques for Evaluating Health Parameters in Developing Countries*, National Academy Press, Washington, D.C., 1988.

4. Lemeshow, S., et al., A computer simulation of the EPI survey strategy, *International Journal of Epidemiology*, **14**: 473, 1985.

The following publications discuss the Shanghai Survey of Alzheimer's Disease and Dementia and single-stage cluster sampling with a telescopic respondent rule.

5. Levy, P. S., Yu, E. S. H., Liu, W. T., Zhang, M. Y., Wang, Z. Y., Wong, S., and Katzman, R., Single stage cluster sampling with a telescopic respondent rule: A variation motivated by a survey of dementia in elderly residents of Shanghai. *Statistics in Medicine*, **8**, 1537, 1989.

6. Levy, P. S., Yu, E. S. H., Liu, W. T., Zhang, M., Wang, Z., Wong, S., and Katzman, R., Variation on single stage cluster sampling used in a survey of elderly people in Shanghai. *International Journal of Epidemiology*, **17**: 931, 1988.

The following publications discuss estimation of prevalence from screening tests.

7. Weiss, N. S., *Clinical Epidemiology: The Study of Outcome of Disease*, Oxford University Press, New York, 1986.

8. Levy, P. S., and Kass, E. H., A three population model for sequential screening for Bacteriuria. *American Journal of Epidemiology*, **91**: 148, 1970.

9. Gastwirth, J., The statistical precision of medical screening procedures: Application to polygraph and AIDS antibodies test data. *Statistical Science*, **2**: 213, 1987.

10. Lew, R. A., and Levy, P. S., Estimation of prevalence on the basis of screening tests. *Statistics in Medicine*, **8**: 1225, 1989.

The following publications deal with network sampling.

11. Sirken, M. G., Household surveys with multiplicity. *Journal of the American Statistical Association*, **65**: 257, 1970.

12. Sirken, M. G., Stratified sample surveys with multiplicity. *Journal of the American Statistical Association*, **67**: 224, 1972.

13. Sudman, S., Sirken, M. G., and Cowan, C.D., *Science* 240, 991–996, 1988.

14. Nathan, G., Schmelz, U. O., and Kenvin, J., *Multiplicity Study of Marriages and Births in Israel*, Vital and Health Statistics, Series 2, No. 70, National Center for Health Statistics, Rockville, MD, 1977.

15. Czaja, R., Blair, J., Using network sampling for rare populations: An application to local crime victimization surveys. American Statistical Association, Proceedings of the Survey Research Section, 38–43, 1988.

16. Czaja, R., Snowden, C., and Cassady, R., Reporting bias and sampling errors in a survey of a rare population using multiplicity counting rules. *Journal of the American Statistical Association*, **81**: 411, 1986.

17. Sirken, M. G., Inderfurth, G. P., Burnham, C. E., and Danchik, K. M., Household sample survey of diabetes: design effects of counting rules. *Proceedings of the American Statistical Association, Social Statistics Section*, 659, 1975.

18. Levy, P. S., Optimum allocation in stratified random network sampling for estimating the prevalence of attributes in rare populations. *Journal of the American Statistical Association*, **72**: 758, 1978.

19. Sirken, M. G., and Levy, P. S., Multiplicity estimation of proportions based on ratios of random variables. *Journal of the American Statistical Association*, **69**: 68, 1974.

20. Levy, P. S., Simple cluster sampling with multiplicity. *Proceedings of the American Statistical Association, Social Statistics Section*, 963, 1977.

The following publications develop methodology for estimation of events from dual systems.

21. Chandra Sekar, C., and Deming, W. E., On a method of estimating birth and death rates and the extent of registration. *Journal of the American Statistical Association*, **44**: 101, 1949.

22. Cowan, C. D., and Malec, D., Capture-recapture models when both sources have clustered observations. *Journal of the American Statistical Association*, **81**: 347, 1986.

The following publications discuss methodology for obtaining estimates for small areas.

23. Gonzalez, M. E., and Hoza, C., Small area estimation with applications to unemployment and housing estimates. *Journal of the American Statistical Association*, **73**: 7, 1978.

24. Levy, P. S., and French, D., *Synthetic Estimation of State Health Characteristics Based on the Health Interview Survey*, Vital and Health Statistics, Series 2, No. 75, DHEW publication No. (PHS) 78-1349, U.S. Government Printing Office, Washington, D.C., 1977.

25. Levy, P. S., Small-area estimation—Synthetic and other procedures, 1968–1978, *Proceedings of the Workshop on Synthetic Estimates for Small Areas*, National Institute of Drug Abuse, Research Monography 24. U.S. Government Printing Office, Washington, D.C., 1979.

The following publications discuss randomized response methodology.

26. Warner, S. L., Randomized response: A survey technique for eliminating evasive answer bias. *Journal of the American Statistical Association*, **60**: 63, 1975.

27. Abernathy, J. R., Greenberg, B. G., and Horvitz, D. G., Estimates of induced abortion in urban North Carolina. *Demography*, **7**: 19, 1970.

28. I-Cheng, C., Chow, L. P., and Rider, R. V., The randomized response technique as used in the Taiwan outcome of pregnancy study. *Studies in Family Planning (A Publication of the Population Council)*, **3**: 265, 1972.

The following publications deal with issues related to acceptance sampling.

29. Brownlee, K. A., *Statistical Theory and Methodology in Science and Engineering*, 2nd ed., Wiley, New York, 1965.

30. Lemeshow, S., and Stroh, G., Jr., *Sampling Techniques for Evaluating Health Parameters in Developing Countries*, National Academy Press, Washington, D.C., 1988.

31. Lemeshow, S., Hosmer, D., Klar, J., and Lwanga, S., *Adequacy of Sample Size in Health Studies*, Wiley, New York, 1990.

The following publications deal with issues related to cohort studies described in Section 14.3.

32. Kannel, W. B., An epidemiological study of cardiovascular disease. In: *Fifth Conference on Cerebral Vascular Diseases*, R. G. Sickert and J. P. Whisnat, eds., Grune and Stratton, New York and London, 1966.

33. Paffenbarger, R. L., Physical activity, all-cause mortality, and longevity of college alumni. *New England Journal of Medicine*, **314**: 605, 1986.

34. Kovar, M. G., Fitti, J. E., and Chyba, M. M., The longitudinal study of aging: 1984–1990. *Vital and Health Statistics*, **1**: 28, 1992.

35. Rothman, K. J., and Boice, J. D., *Epidemiologic Analysis with a Programmable Calculator*. Epidemiology Resources, Inc., Boston, 1982.

The following expository articles on topics discussed in this chapter have appeared recently in the Encyclopedia of Biostatistics.

36. Cohen, S., Small area estimation. In *The Encyclopedia of Biostatistics*, Armitage, P. A., and Colton, T., Eds., Wiley, Chichester, U.K., 1998.

37. Franklin, L., Randomized response techniques in sample surveys. In *The Encyclopedia of Biostatistics*, Armitage, P. A., and Colton, T., Eds., Wiley, Chichester, U.K., 1998.

38. Krotki, K., Sampling in developing countries. In *The Encyclopedia of Biostatistics*, Armitage, P. A., and Colton, T., Eds., Wiley, Chichester, U.K., 1998.

39. Sirken, M., Network sampling. In *The Encyclopedia of Biostatistics*, Armitage, P. A., and Colton, T., Eds., Wiley, Chichester, U.K., 1998.

CHAPTER 15

Telephone Sampling

Robert J. Casady and James M. Lepkowski

15.1 OVERVIEW

The use of the telephone for survey data collection requires the selection of samples of telephone numbers to identify sampling units for interviewing. The basic sampling techniques employed to make these selections are the same as those used for many other sample design problems. There are, however, several unique features of the frames used for telephone sample selection that have stimulated the development of sample designs specific to telephone surveys.

The available frames vary from one country to the next and from one type of unit (e.g., household vs. establishment) to the next. We limit the discussion here to frames and sampling designs for telephone households in the United States. Frames and designs in other countries or for units other than households will have similar features to those described here. As one might expect, however, specific aspects of designs for other countries or for other units would be somewhat modified to improve efficiency and other properties of survey operation.

Telephone household sampling must begin with a careful review of the features of the frames available. Sample selection methods have been developed to address the particular features of each frame. We discuss the frames and basic designs employed for them in the remainder of this section. In Section 15.2 we examine in more detail the properties of alternative designs, contrasting the relative efficiencies of several designs to provide guidance on selection of a suitable design for a given problem. Estimation for the principal telephone sampling methods is addressed in Section 15.3. The chapter concludes in Section 15.4 with a comparison of designs based on cost, variance, implementation, and bias considerations.

15.1.1 The Telephone Household Population

One of the principal reasons that telephone surveys were first used in household surveys was to reduce the costs of data collection. Telephone contact is substantially less expensive than face-to-face contact, and often much more convenient for both the researcher and the respondent. Telephones were used for household surveys as early as the 1930s in the United States and, even then, it was recognized that these surveys were limited to a subset of all households. The method gained popularity among commercial survey organizations in the 1960s as the proportion of households with telephones increased.

Despite the recognition that telephone surveys were limited to telephone households, telephone survey results were, and still are, often presented as though they apply to the entire population of all households. This practice rests on an assumption that there are no differences between households with and without telephones for the kind of characteristics being studied. While this assumption may be correct, it is important that, to the extent possible, it be tested. The test of differences may be limited to characteristics that are only mildly correlated with those being measured in a survey. For example, because age and gender are related to attitudes, investigators in a survey of economic attitudes may be satisfied that the residents of telephone and nontelephone households have similar age and gender distributions.

Approximately 5% of U.S. households do not have a telephone, and the percentage of persons who live in households without a telephone is approximately 4%. While this overall rate of noncoverage is small, and may be reassuring to some investigators, noncoverage varies substantially by a number of characteristics that may be related to variables being measured in a survey. For example, nontelephone households tend to have younger and more mobile persons. They tend to be located in higher proportions in rural areas of the South region of the United States, and in central cities. Noncoverage rates can rise to 15% or higher for some subpopulations, a level that is considered unacceptable to those who must produce estimates for many small subgroups of the U.S. population from the survey data.

The characteristics of nontelephone households have been examined in several reviews (see, for example, Thornberry and Massey [16]). Nontelephone households tend to have higher rates of unemployment, have higher rates of smokers, and experience higher rates of crime victimization. Thus, telephone surveys could produce biased estimates of employment, health, or social characteristics.

Some investigators have attempted to adjust telephone samples of households through standard survey weighting procedures. Noncoverage in surveys is often adjusted through the use of poststratification weights. In the case of telephone samples, these adjustments may indeed compensate partially for noncoverage bias. The use of poststratification, or population control adjustments, for this purpose is discussed later.

15.1.2 Telephone Systems

In the United States, telephone numbers are grouped into geographical areas. U.S. telephone numbers consist of three parts: a three-digit area code, a three-digit prefix (or central office code), and a four-digit suffix. The area code and prefix are established as part of an international system that extends across the United States, Canada, Mexico, and the Caribbean. These numbers are not, of course, assigned at random across the entire geographic area covered by the phone system. Area codes are assigned to specific geographic regions that in the United States do not, for the most part, cross state boundaries. However, area codes do not otherwise correspond to political boundaries such as counties, cities, or other minor civil divisions. Until recently (due to area code "overlays"), there has been a one-to-one correspondence between an area code and a geographic area.

Prefixes within area codes are not generally geographically defined. Further, the same prefix may be used across many different area codes. Within an area code, prefixes are grouped into geographic areas called exchanges. Exchanges (or places, in the more generic terminology of the telephone system) are geographic areas defined for the purposes of providing and maintaining phone service. For example, the Detroit exchange within the 313 area code is a geographic area roughly approximating the city of Detroit and a few surrounding areas. The Detroit exchange is assigned to more than 125 different prefixes.

Households and businesses requesting telephone service within the geographic area defined as the Detroit exchange must be assigned a telephone number whose prefix is one of those serviced by the exchange. No other exchange within the same area code can use the prefixes assigned to the Detroit exchange.

Within the Detroit exchange, there is little further geographic differentiation with respect to prefixes. A household located anywhere within the exchange may be assigned a telephone number from any prefix available in the exchange. Some exchanges with large numbers of prefixes will be divided into wire centers responsible for a subdivision of the area covered by the exchange. Thus, in these exchanges, there is a small degree of geographic grouping of prefixes within the exchange. But this type of geographic differentiation of prefixes within an exchange is the exception and not the rule.

The majority of the exchanges in the United States have a small number of telephone numbers assigned. As a result, most exchanges are assigned only a single prefix. Until the recent past, exchanges have been areas designated by public service commissions within which companies were able to obtain exclusive rights to provide phone service. Service requirements are such that the land area covered by an exchange is limited. Yet population density for a given exchange can vary enormously. Thus, some exchanges have very few customers, and enough numbers are available in a single prefix to assign to all customers. Other exchanges have large numbers of customers, and multiple prefixes are assigned to the exchange.

Suffixes are grouped in sets of 10,000. They are typically assigned by local telephone service personnel based on existing assignment patterns. There does not appear to be any standard system to assign new customer requests for household telephone numbers within a prefix.

Empirical investigations have uncovered patterns of assignment of suffixes within prefixes, at least when the entire system is examined. In exchanges with multiple prefixes and large numbers of customers, prefixes and suffixes appear to be assigned haphazardly. There is no obvious clustering of assigned telephone numbers within banks of numbers. But in exchanges with a single prefix and a small number of customers, suffixes have historically been assigned in clusters to reduce the cost of assignment. Older electro-mechanical switching equipment allowed smaller companies to assign all numbers in a single "1000-bank" of consecutive numbers, numbers that all began with the same first digit of the four-digit suffix. A company covering a small population would only have to purchase a single or limited number of banks of 1000 to have an adequate number of telephone numbers for its customers. Telephone numbers in the more numerous single-prefix exchanges are thus clustered, at the 1000 bank level. Empirical investigation has revealed that this "clustering" of assigned numbers increases as the size of a bank decreases. For example, the clustering is more intensive for banks defined by the first two digits of a suffix, or a "100 bank." Several telephone sampling methods described subsequently take advantage of this clustered assignment of numbers to improve the efficiency of identifying telephone numbers assigned to residential units.

15.1.3 Sampling Frames

There are four types of frame problems that arise in telephone sampling. Listings on the frame that are not elements of the population are referred to as *blanks*, while elements in the population for which there is no corresponding listing are referred to as *noncovered* elements. Listings on the frame which yield multiple elements in the population are referred to as *clusters*, while elements in the population which have two or more listings on the frame are referred to as *duplicate listings*.

Each of these deficiencies can lead to bias in survey estimates, or inefficiency in survey operations. Sampling statisticians have developed selection procedures that reduce or eliminate bias due to these deficiencies. They also have been instrumental in finding selection procedures that reduce the inefficiencies.

Three principal frames are used for telephone sampling: telephone numbers, directories, and commercial lists. The frame of telephone numbers can be created through two primary sources. Each combines a list of area code and prefix combinations with randomly generated suffixes. The area code-prefix combinations can be obtained for local studies from examination of local telephone directories, which generally contain up-to-date lists of prefixes within the exchanges covered by the directory. For surveys covering larger geographic areas, area code-prefix combinations can be obtained in the United States from a commercial firm, Bell Core Research, Inc., (BCR).

The BCR frame is updated monthly and contains all area code and prefix combinations for the United States, as well as for Canada, Mexico, and the Caribbean. The BCR frame affords virtually complete coverage of telephone households, but it suffers from a substantial number of blank listings. In fact, less than 25% of the generated numbers are assigned to residential units, so, it is operationally inefficient to use a scheme of a randomly generated suffix appended to an area code and prefix selected from the BCR frame. Other methods based on the BCR frame (discussed below) have been developed to take advantage of the inherent clustering of residential numbers in 1000 banks to decrease the proportion of blanks generated from the frame.

There is another disadvantage of the BCR frame, as well as the other two frames. Households with more than one telephone number used for residential purposes are represented on the frame multiple times. Probability sampling methods require that the number of telephone numbers in a household be acquired and used to develop a compensatory weight for estimation.

The second frame, directories, has been widely used as a frame for local studies. Directories provide a list of telephone numbers that is inexpensive to acquire for a local area. Simple list sampling methods (e.g., systematic sampling) can be used to select samples quickly, although not necessarily easily. Directory frames are difficult to assemble for wider geographic areas since there are more than 5000 directories published across the United States each year. Their popularity as a sampling frame is due to cost and convenience and to the lower proportion of blank listings in the directory frame compared to the telephone number frame: approximately 10–15% of listings in a residential directory in the United States are no longer residential.

On the other hand, directory frames suffer from substantial noncoverage of the telephone household population because of unlisted numbers and changes in telephone status of households. The percentage of telephone households that do not appear in U.S. directories exceeds 35%, varying from low percentages (10%) in suburban and rural areas to more than 60% in some urban locations. Survey designers cannot accept these high proportions of unlisted or out-of-date listings, and choose to use random digit dialing methods or other schemes that afford higher coverage.

Further, directories have higher levels of duplicate listings than the BCR frame because subscribers can purchase additional listings. For example, a married couple at the same address with different surnames may, for a small fee, choose to appear in the directory under both names. The duplicate listing increases the chance of their telephone household being selected, which must, from a probability sampling point of view, be compensated for through a weight for the household.

The third type of frame is assembled by commercial firms in electronic files based on directories collected from across the country. Directory entries (name, address, and phone number) are either keyed or added to the file when an electronic format is available. Lists based on commercial directories are supplemented by other lists, the largest of which is automobile registrations obtained from approximately 30 states that release such data publicly. The combined file is subjected to processing to assign a ZIP code to each entry for the purposes of mailing. Several firms have taken advantage of the availability of telephone numbers in such files to create national telephone directories and to draw and sell samples of telephone numbers from them. The commercial frames suffer from a small proportion of blank listings (approximately 10–15%, the same as for directories), the failure to cover unlisted numbers, and duplicate listings.

15.2 TELEPHONE SAMPLE DESIGNS

Sampling statisticians have developed sampling methods that attempt to take advantage of the strengths of each of these three frames. The methods are often classified as one of three types: simple list frame sampling methods suitable for directories, random digit dialing methods based on the telephone number frame, and list-assisted methods based on directories or commercial lists, generating samples that include unlisted numbers as well. We do not discuss the sampling methods as applied to directories here; they are essentially applications of methods already discussed in previous chapters of this text. We instead examine the random digit dialing and list-assisted methods, since they are novel applications of methods described elsewhere in this text.

15.2.1 Sample Designs Using the BCR Frame

The simplest and most direct approach to utilizing the BCR frame is, as described previously, to randomly select telephone numbers from the frame, call the selected numbers, and conduct an interview when a household is reached. Numbers are selected and called until the desired sample size, say n, of in-scope households is attained. As noted earlier, only about 25% of the sample telephone numbers will be assigned to households, so, the number of numbers required, say n', will be considerably larger than n. The expected number of required numbers is n/p, where p is the proportion of telephone numbers assigned to residential households. Thus, in order to account for ineligible listings, the sample of telephone numbers from the BCR frame must be approximately four times as large as the desired sample of n telephone households.

In general, the determination of the status of a telephone number is a costly matter, especially for telephone numbers not assigned to households. Frequently, a number must be dialed several times in order to determine its status. Since procedures must be specified for each type of dialing outcome, the use of the BCR (or any list with a high proportion of blank listings) will greatly increase the administrative and operational costs of telephone survey operations (see Lepkowski [10]).

It will be useful for comparing various designs to summarize the operational costs of the use of each frame. The costs of using the BCR frame can be summarized in a simple cost model as follows. Let C_0 be the cost of determining the status of a number not assigned to an in-scope household (i.e., a household that has a telephone); C_1 denote the cost of determining the status of a number assigned to an in-scope household; and C_2 denote the cost of conducting the survey interview. The total cost of a survey based on the BCR frame is then given by $C = n(C_1 + C_2) + (n' - n)C_0$. Incorporating the proportion of telephone numbers that are in-scope, the expected total cost of a simple random digit dialing survey is given by $E(C) = n((C_1 + C_2) + C_0(1 - p)/p)$. For p in the neighborhood of .25, the component of expected cost due to unproductive calls [i.e., $nC_0(1 - p)/p$] will be a substantial proportion of total expected cost C. The telephone designs described in the following sections were all motivated by a desire to reduce the proportion of cost due to unproductive calls.

15.2.1.1 The Mitofsky–Waksberg Design

The two-stage random digit design proposed by Mitofsky [11] and more fully developed by Waksberg [18] has been so widely employed in telephone surveys that it has become nearly synonymous with random digit dialing telephone surveys. The method capitalizes on the fact that telephone numbers assigned to residential households tend to be clustered in banks of consecutive telephone numbers. While only 25% of the numbers in the BCR frame are assigned to households overall, among banks of 100 consecutive numbers where there is at least one number assigned to a household, over 60% of the numbers are assigned to residential households. Clearly, if the 100-banks with one or more residential numbers could be identified, and if sampling were restricted to those banks, then the proportion of unproductive calls could be substantially reduced, and overall operational costs would be reduced.

The Mitofsky–Waksberg technique starts by grouping the numbers in the BCR frame into banks of 100 consecutive numbers using the area code, the three-digit prefix and the first two digits of the suffix to specify a *bank* (or *100-bank*). In the first stage, 100-banks are selected at random with replacement, a telephone number within the bank is selected at random, and the number is dialed. If the selected number is found to be residential, the bank is retained for second-stage sampling. The process is continued until a specified sample of m 100-banks is attained. Within each retained 100-bank, telephone numbers are selected at random without replacement, until a total of k residential numbers (including the original number used to retain the 100-bank) have been identified. Residential status of a telephone number can only be determined by calling it.

Thus, the Mitofsky–Waksberg technique utilizes a two-stage design, where 100-banks are selected with probability proportional to number of residential telephone numbers in the first stage, and a fixed-size sample of residential households is selected in the second stage. Thus, the sample of $n = mk$ residential households is selected with equal (but unknown) probability. The efficiency of the Mitofsky–Waksberg technique derives from the fact that the eligible telephone numbers are concentrated in a relatively small proportion of the 100-banks.

For the purpose of determining the cost of using this alternative sample design for the BCR frame, we let t be the proportion of 100-banks with no eligible numbers. Then the total expected number of numbers across the first and second stages is $n(1 - t(k - 1)/k)/p$ and the expected total operational cost is

$$E(C) = n((C_1 + C_2) + C_0(1 - p - t(k - 1)/k)/p)$$

Clearly, both the expected number of calls and the expected cost decrease as k increases. Nationally, t is in the neighborhood of .65, so even modest values of k can lead to substantial cost savings.

Although the Mitofsky–Waksberg technique offers an elegant method to improve telephone survey efficiency, there are practical problems. The most obvious is that some 100-banks may have fewer than the requisite k eligible households, in which case all numbers in the bank will, of necessity, be called. Then compensatory weighting will be required. A second problem is that it is not always possible to accurately determine the eligibility status of a selected number. In the first stage, this may lead to the incorrect inclusion or exclusion of 100-banks. In the second stage, some numbers may still be unresolved at the end of the survey period, so that fewer than k eligible households are identified for the bank. Finally, a more subtle problem is intrabank correlation, a topic which will be discussed in more detail in Section 15.3, when estimation is examined.

15.2.1.2 The Potthoff Design

A design suggested by Potthoff [12] is similar to the Mitofsky–Waksberg design, except that eligibility is extended to a broader class of telephone numbers. Rather than determining eligibility of a 100-bank based on whether a telephone number is assigned to a residence, Potthoff proposed defining eligibility in terms of the status of the number after it was dialed. He termed numbers that were eligible under a variety of outcomes as *auspicious numbers*. Typically, the auspicious numbers include not only the residential household numbers, but also numbers that ring without answer and have an unknown residential status after dialing. This broader definition reduces the amount of screening needed for the first stage and the amount of replacement required at the second stage. Potthoff [12], [13] also proposed that $c \geq 2$ numbers be selected per 100-bank in the first stage. Sampling in the second stage then depends on the number of auspicious numbers observed in the first stage. The details of the Potthoff method will not be discussed in detail in this text.

The Potthoff sampling design yields an equal probability sample of eligible numbers. Replacement is required for only a small number of selected prefix areas and it reduces ambiguities about the status of numbers dialed at the first stage. Also, as c, the number of numbers selected per 100-bank in the first stage, increases, the chances of obtaining a bank that will be exhausted in the second stage are reduced. Implementation of the Potthoff design requires knowledge about the proportion of auspicious numbers that are actually eligible numbers in order to determine the appropriate sample size. The administrative structure is more complex and the training requirements for operational staff are increased for this procedure relative to the Mitofsky–Waksberg design.

15.2.2 Sample Designs Utilizing Published Residential Telephone Numbers

As described above, 85 to 90% of the telephone numbers on commercial lists are connected to residential households. A straightforward systematic selection (random selection is only feasible if the list is numbered sequentially) of numbers from such a list would be much more efficient than the designs used for sampling from the BCR list. Unfortunately, the typical directory-based list only includes about 70% of the residential telephone households due to datedness of the listed and unlisted numbers. Comparisons of telephone households with and without published numbers indicates that substantial bias may result if households without published numbers are omitted from the sampling frame (Brunner and Brunner [2]). The designs discussed in this section attempt to capitalize on the efficiency inherent in directory-based sampling while extending the coverage of the design to include the entire residential telephone population.

15.2.2.1 Plus Digit Dialing
Plus digit dialing is a directory-assisted procedure in which a sample of telephone numbers is selected from the directory and one is added to the suffix of the number. For instance, in plus one dialing the integer "one" is added to the suffix of each number selected from the directory. Thus, if the number selected were 734-936-0021, the one plus replacement would be 734-936-0022. The resulting sample of telephone numbers generally includes both listed and unlisted numbers; in addition, it yields a higher proportion of productive numbers than does the simple random digit dialing design.

Unfortunately this procedure has a number of operational and theoretical problems. Empirical investigations of the method have shown that there is considerable bias in selection of residential households in one plus dialing. In addition, the numbers in the target population have unequal and unknown probabilities of selection. In fact, some of the unlisted numbers may have a zero probability of selection unless the unlisted numbers are evenly mixed among the listed numbers. Generalizations of this design in which the last d

digits (two or more) are replaced by a randomly generated d digit number have been suggested.

A closely related design, based on half-open intervals of telephone numbers, was suggested by Frankel and Frankel [5]. In numeric-order directories, a cluster is defined to consist of a listed telephone number together with all numbers up to, but not including, the next listed number. A sample of clusters is selected from the directory by simply selecting a simple random sample of telephone numbers from the directory. All numbers within a selected cluster are then dialed. This method achieves known, nonzero, probabilities of selection for all telephone households. However, the potentially large variation in cluster size can introduce formidable operational problems. Sample size could vary substantially from a target level. Furthermore, this method is subject to estimation difficulties, as cluster and sample size are both random variables.

15.2.2.2   Two-Stage Sampling

A two-stage sampling design utilizing a directory list was proposed by Sudman [15]. This procedure, which was originally suggested by Stock [14], uses 1000-banks of telephone numbers (which are identified by the first six digits of the 10-digit telephone number) as the first-stage sampling unit. The selection of 1000-banks is similar to first-stage selection in the Mitofsky–Waksberg method except that the directory of listed numbers is used to select the first-stage sample. Thus, the probability of selection in the first stage is proportional to the number of listed numbers in the 1000-bank. In the second-stage, numbers are selected until a predetermined fixed number of listed numbers are selected. Interviews are attempted for households with both listed and unlisted numbers. It should be noted that unlisted numbers in 1000-banks with no listed numbers have zero probability of selection, but the proportion of telephone households in such 1000-banks is small, and in most cases this is not a serious problem. Of more concern is the fact that the determination of listed status depends on a respondent self-report, which can be in error. A "reverse telephone number order directory," available in many metropolitan areas, can eliminate this source of error.

Unlike the Mitofsky–Waksberg method, the Sudman procedure will produce unequal-size clusters of telephone households (although it produces equal-sized clusters of listed telephone households). The variation in cluster size is usually not very large. Also, the potential for exhausted clusters exists, but with 1000 numbers instead of 100 numbers in a bank as in the Mitofsky-Waksberg method, this is of minor concern.

15.2.3   Designs Using the BCR Frame and Published Telephone Numbers

It should be noted that the designs discussed in Section 15.2.1 require only the BCR frame, while those discussed in Section 15.2.2 require only a published list of residential telephone numbers. The designs discussed in this section require both. The basic idea behind these designs is to directly unite the desirable coverage properties of the BCR frame with the relatively high sampling efficiency of a frame of listed telephone numbers.

15.2.3.1 Dual-Frame Designs

A random digit dialing sample of n_B telephone households is selected from the BCR frame, and simultaneously a sample of n_D telephone households is selected from the directory list frame. Letting n'_B and n'_D be the respective number of numbers required to achieve the desired sample sizes, the cost of the dual-frame design is given by

$$C = (n_B + n_D)(C_1 + C_2) + C_0(n'_B + n'_D - n_B - n_D)$$

The expected cost of a dual-frame survey is given by

$$E(C) = n(C_1 + C_2 + C_0(\lambda(1 - p_B)/p_B + (1 - \lambda)(1 - p_D)/p_D))$$

where $n = n_B + n_D$ is the total sample size, $\lambda = n_B/n$ is the proportion of the total sample allocated to the BCR frame, p_B is the proportion of telephone numbers in the BCR frame assigned to residential households, and p_D is the proportion of telephone numbers in the directory frame assigned to residential households. Since p_B is in the neighborhood of .25, and p_D is usually about .85, the expected cost (for a fixed total sample size n) will decrease as λ decreases.

There are several possible ways to combine the data from the two frames for estimation. In general, dual-frame estimators are more complicated than the estimators for the previously discussed designs. Groves and Lepkowski [6] provide a detailed discussion of the issue of dual-frame estimation and the problem of sample allocation to the two frames so as to attain minimum cost for a specified variance.

In order to implement dual-frame methodology, the directory status (i.e., listed or unlisted) of each residential household from the BCR sample must be known. In order to avoid using potentially unreliable respondent reports regarding their listing status, numbers selected from the BCR frame can be matched to the directory list at the time of sample selection. If the directory frame contains addresses for the listed numbers, then it is possible to send advance letters for the purpose of improving response rates. In general, the dual-frame design requires a somewhat more sophisticated administrative operation. Costs are increased by the need to match the BCR sample to the directory frame to determine which numbers were eligible for selection in both frames, the mailing of advance letters, and by the use of a more complicated estimator. The benefits of a higher response rate more than offset the costs of advance letters.

15.2.3.2 Directory-Based Stratification

The directory list may be used for the purpose of stratifying the BCR frame so as to improve sampling efficiency from the BCR frame. In a typical application, the directory list is used to identify all 100-banks in the BCR frame with one or more directory-listed telephone numbers. The BCR frame is then partitioned into two strata: one stratum contains all telephone numbers in 100-banks with one or more listed numbers, and the other stratum contains all other numbers. The first stratum is referred to as the high-density stratum, while the second is referred to as the residual stratum. Simple random digit dialing samples are then selected from each stratum, with a much larger sample selected from the high-density stratum since it contains nearly all of the residential telephone numbers.

The stratified design attempts to use the same clustered feature of the telephone number frame as the Mitofsky–Waksberg design. Telephone numbers for residential households, both listed and unlisted, tend to be clustered within 100-banks. If banks containing such telephone numbers can be identified and sampled at a higher rate, then sampling efficiency can be greatly improved. Casady and Lepkowski [3] found that at the national level the proportion of the telephone numbers in the BCR frame assigned to the high-density stratum would be approximately .38, and that it would contain more than 97% of the numbers assigned to residential households. They showed that the proportion of numbers in the high-density stratum assigned to households is approximately .55, while the proportion of numbers assigned to households in the residual stratum is only about .02.

Assuming a random digital dialing sample of n_1 telephone households is selected from the high-density stratum, and a sample of n_2 telephone households is selected from the residual stratum, then the cost for the stratified design is given by

$$C = (n_1 + n_2)(C_1 + C_2) + C_0(n_1' + n_2' - n_1 - n_2)$$

where n_1' and n_2' are the respective number of numbers required to achieve the desired sample sizes. The expected cost of the stratified sample is

$$E(C) = n(C_1 + C_2 + C_0(\gamma(1 - p_1)/p_1 + (1 - \gamma)(1 - p_2)/p_2))$$

where n is the total sample size, $\gamma = n_1/n$ is the proportion of the total sample allocated to the high-density stratum, p_1 is the proportion of telephone numbers in the high-density stratum assigned to residential households, and p_2 is the proportion of telephone numbers in the residual stratum assigned to residential households. Since p_1 is approximately .55, and p_2 is usually about .02, the expected cost (for a fixed total sample size n) will decrease as γ increases. The allocation of the sample to the strata to minimize cost for a fixed variance (or minimize variance for a fixed cost) is discussed in detail in Casady and Lepkowski [3].

The probability of selection is known, positive, and equal within strata, so the estimation of population totals is straightforward. The estimation of a population mean at the stratum level is also straigthtforward, but the estimation of the overall population mean requires that the total residential telephone population be estimated for each stratum and a ratio estimator be used to estimate the population mean. A more detailed discussion of estimated means and variances is given in Section 15.3.

Under the relatively simple cost model given above, this design compares favorably with the Mitofsky–Waksberg design. In practice, directory-based stratification with simple random digit dialing sampling within strata has proven to have an advantage with respect to implementation and administration. There are two costs associated with this design that are not included in the simple model: the cost of the commercial list itself, and the cost of stratifying the BCR frame. The cost of the commercial list will vary by vendor, but for any large-scale, continuing survey operation, this should be a relatively minor cost component. Both of these costs are fixed and can be amortized over multiple studies to greatly reduce the impact on any single study.

15.2.3.3 Directory-Based Truncation

A special case of the stratified method discussed in the last section allocates no sample to the residual stratum; that is, the BCR frame is truncated by removing the residual stratum. The greatly increased hit rate, together with the other advantages of the directory-based stratification design, make this an extremely attractive approach. The obvious disadvantage is that not all of the target population is covered when the frame is truncated. In the example given above, approximately 2% of the telephone households will not be covered. However, empirical evidence indicates (Brick et al. [1]; Connor and Heeringa [4]) that for many variables the out-of-scope population is very similar to the target population, and very little bias results from truncation. As previously noted, approximately 5% of the U.S. household population is not included in the telephone population, and any additional bias due to truncation of the BCR frame is probably minimal.

15.3 ESTIMATION

The probability features of these designs must be taken into account in the computation of estimates from the samples. The basic principles of such estimation are described briefly here for means (and by implication, for proportions, as well) and their sampling variances. In addition, poststratification, or population control adjustment, is in some cases applied to telephone survey data in order to attempt to adjust the telephone household sample to the distribution of all households.

15.3.1 Estimating Means

For the simple random digit dialing design, let $\bar{y}_{RDD}$ be the simple mean of the n observations of the household variable $\mathcal{Y}$. Similarly, let $\bar{y}_{MW}$ be the simple mean of the mk observations under the Mitofsky–Waksberg design. Both $\bar{y}_{\mathrm{RDD}}$ and $\bar{y}_{MW}$ are design unbiased for the population mean $\bar{Y}$; furthermore,

$$\mathrm{var}(\bar{y}_{\mathrm{RDD}}) = \frac{\sigma^2}{n} \quad \text{and} \quad \mathrm{var}(\bar{y}_{MW}) \cong \frac{\sigma^2}{mk}(1 + \rho(k-1))$$

where σ^2 is the population variance and ρ is the intra-100-bank correlation for the variable $\mathcal{Y}$.

The estimation of the population mean for the directory-based stratified designs is somewhat more complicated. Sampling within stratum is random digit dialing, so $\bar{y}_h$ (the simple mean of the n_h observations from the h^n stratum) is unbiased for the stratum mean $\bar{Y}_h$. It follows that

$$y_t' = \sum_{h=1}^{H} N_h \left(\frac{n_h}{n_h'}\right) \bar{y}_h$$

is approximately unbiased for the population aggregate of the y values for telephone households and

$$N_t' = \sum_{h=1}^{H} N_h \left(\frac{n_h}{n_h'}\right)$$

is approximately unbiased for the total number of telephone households, say N_t. Thus, the ratio estimator, $\bar{y}_{\mathrm{strat}} = (y_t'/N_t')$, is approximately unbiased for the population mean and

$$\mathrm{var}(\bar{y}_{\mathrm{strat}}) \cong \sum_{h=1}^{H} \frac{z_h^2 \sigma_h^2 (1 + (1 - p_h)\lambda_h)}{n_h}$$

where p_h is the proportion of telephone numbers in the hth stratum assigned to residential households, z_h is the proportion of the telephone household population included in the hth stratum, and $\lambda_h = (\bar{Y}_h - \bar{Y})^2/\sigma_h^2$.

Several other statistical issues should be kept in mind when utilizing telephone designs:

1. In general, ratio estimators are required for estimating subclass means, in which case the relatively simple variance expressions above are not applicable.
2. These designs yield samples of households not persons. If persons are selected within households, then additional weighting and more complex estimators are required.

3. In order to have unbiased estimators, the weights of households with multiple telephones must be adjusted to account for their larger probability of selection.

4. The estimators above are based on the use of random digit dialing to achieve fixed sample size. This requires that the status of all numbers selected be determined, which, in turn, requires careful recordkeeping and close supervision. Because fixed sample sizes are required for each retained 100-bank, the Mitofsky–Waksberg method is more complex, and thus the need for tight control is even more important.

15.3.2   Estimating Sampling Variance

For the purpose of estimating $\text{Var}(\bar{y}_{rdd})$, let y_i be the value of the variable $\mathcal{Y}$ for the ith household selected. An unbiased estimator for $\text{Var}(\bar{y}_{rdd})$ is given by

$$\widehat{\text{Var}}(\bar{y}_{rdd}) = \frac{\hat{\sigma}^2}{n} \quad \text{where} \quad \hat{\sigma}^2 = \frac{\sum_{i=1}^{n}(y_i - \bar{y}_{rdd})^2}{n-1}$$

For the Mitofsky–Waksberg sampling we let y_{ij} be the value of the variable $\mathcal{Y}$ for the jth selected household in the ith retained 100-bank. An unbiased estimator for $\text{Var}(\bar{y}_{mw})$ is given by

$$\widehat{\text{Var}}(\bar{y}_{mw}) = \frac{1}{m} \frac{\sum_{i=1}^{m}(\bar{y}_i - \bar{y}_{mw})^2}{m-1}$$

where

$$\bar{y}_i = \frac{\sum_{j=1}^{k} y_{ij}}{k}$$

For the stratified design we let y_{hi} be the value of the variable $\mathcal{Y}$ for the ith household selected in the hth stratum. Applying the linearization technique to the ratio estimator $\bar{y}_{strat}$ yields the variance estimator

$$\widehat{\text{Var}}(\bar{y}_{strat}) = \sum_{h=1}^{H} \frac{\hat{z}_h^2 \hat{\sigma}_h^2 (1 + (1 - \hat{p}_h)\hat{\lambda}_h)}{n_h}$$

where

$$\hat{p}_h = \frac{n_h}{n_h'} \qquad \hat{z}_h = \frac{N_h \hat{p}_h}{N_t'} \qquad \hat{\sigma}_h^2 = \frac{\sum_{i=1}^{n_h} (y_{hi} - \bar{y}_h)^2}{n_h - 1} \qquad \hat{\lambda}_h = (\bar{y}_h - \bar{y}_{\text{strat}})^2 / \hat{\sigma}_h^2.$$

Although results are not given in detail, the linearization technique can also be used to derive estimators for the variance of the ratio estimators required for subclass means.

15.3.3 Poststratification

In traditional sampling theory, poststratification arises when the variables to be used to create strata are not available at the time of selection. That is, one may be interested in partitioning the population into G poststrata using variables collected during the survey. As under proportionally allocated stratified sampling, improvements in precision are possible with suitable modification to variance estimation. Poststratification requires that for each sample element the poststrata be known and that poststratum weights, say W_g, are available for each poststratum. The poststratum weights must come from an outside source such as a census, census projections, or administrative records. For example, poststrata based on age and gender may be created for the respondents if suitable population counts or proportions W_g can be found for age and gender groups in the population.

In telephone sampling, poststratification often adjusts not to the population residing in telephone households, but rather to the population residing in all households. This form of poststratification is applied in order to obtain estimates that have, in a certain sense, been adjusted to the distribution of the population in all households and not just telephone households.

The steps in poststratification may be summarized as follows:

1. Sort the sample into G poststrata based on some observed characteristic(s).
2. Obtain sample weights W_g for the population, typically from an outside source such as a larger survey, a census, census projections, or administrative records.
3. Compute the means $\bar{y}_g$ for the characteristic of interest separately for each poststratum and compute the overall mean $\bar{y}_{ps} = \sum_{g=1}^{G} W_g \bar{y}_g$.
4. For variance estimates, use

$$\widehat{\text{Var}}(\bar{y}_{ps}) \cong \frac{1}{n} \left[\sum_{g=1}^{G} W_g s_g^2 + \sum_{g=1}^{G} W_g (1 - W_g) \frac{s_g^2}{N_g} \right]$$

or alternatively

$$\widehat{\text{Var}}(\bar{y}_{ps}) \cong \frac{1}{n} \sum_{g=1}^{G} W_g s_g^2 \left[1 + \frac{1 - W_g}{N_g} \right]$$

where, s_g^2 is an estimate of the within poststratum element variance, and N_g is the population size for poststratum g. The form of the estimate s_g^2 will depend on the sample design.

In almost all practical situations the poststratified estimate, $\bar{y}_{ps}$, will have smaller variances than the estimated mean without the poststratification.

Poststratification is also often referred to as *population control adjustment*. Poststratified weights are developed for each element. Weighted estimates computed using the poststratified weights are "adjusted" to the outside distribution represented by the W_g. In the case of the random digit dialing design the effects of this adjustment can be seen more clearly if we re-express the poststratified estimate of the mean as follows. Let r denote the number of respondents in the sample and r_g denote the number of respondents in the gth poststratum. In addition, let y_{gi} denote the value of the characteristic $\mathscr{Y}$ for the ith respondent in the gth poststratrum. Then the poststratified mean can be written in terms of element weights, w_{gi}, as follows:

$$\bar{y}_{ps} = \sum_{g=1}^{G} W_g \bar{y}_g = \frac{\sum_{g=1}^{G} N_g \bar{y}_g}{N} = \frac{\sum_{g=1}^{G} \left(\frac{r}{N}\right) \left(\frac{N_g}{r_g}\right) \sum_{i=1}^{r_g} y_{gi}}{\sum_{g=1}^{G} \left(\frac{r}{N}\right) N_g}$$

$$= \frac{\sum_{g=1}^{G} \sum_{i=1}^{r_g} w_{gi} y_{gi}}{\sum_{g=1}^{G} \frac{N_g/N}{1/r}} = \frac{\sum_{g=1}^{G} \sum_{i=1}^{r_g} w_{gi} y_{gi}}{\sum_{g=1}^{G} \sum_{i=1}^{r_g} \left(\frac{1}{r_g}\right) \frac{N_g/N}{1/r}} = \frac{\sum_{g=1}^{G} \sum_{i=1}^{r_g} w_{gi} y_{gi}}{\sum_{g=1}^{G} \sum_{i=1}^{r_g} w_{gi}}$$

That is, the weight, w_{gi}, is the ratio of the proportion in the population in the gth poststratum to the proportion in the sample in the gth poststratum: $w_{gi} = (N_g/N)/(r_g/r)$. Thus, poststratification of a telephone household sample of respondents to a distribution based on all households provides a simultaneous adjustment for nonresponse and noncoverage of the households without telephones.

There are several features of poststratification for telephone samples that are important to observe. Typically, the W_g are census or other related data for all households, not just telephone households. Second, while the poststratification adjustment may be viewed as an adjustment for both nonresponse and noncoverage, it is often applied in practice after some form of nonresponse compensation through weighting. Third, it may not be possible to obtain population weights, W_g, across a full cross-classification of characteristics for the population, but marginal distributions may be available. Raking ratio adjustment procedures (see Kalton and Kasprzyk [7]) can be used to generate a complete distribution of the cross-classification based on the marginal distributions. For example, population weights may be available for age and education, but not their cross-classification. Raking ratio estimation can be used to generate the cross-classification based on a "main effects" model for age and education. The raked cross-classification weights for the population are then applied to the respondent distribution to generate element level weights as indicated above.

15.4 COMPARISON OF DESIGNS

15.4.1 Cost-Variance Trade-offs

The cost function in Section 15.2.1.2, and the sampling variance of an estimated mean in Section 15.3.1, determine the size of the within 100-bank sample size k that minimizes the expected cost of a fixed sampling variance (or minimizes the variance for a fixed cost) for the Mitofsky–Waksberg design. An explicit expression for the optimal value of k can be found in Waksberg [18]. Similarly, the cost function in Section 15.2.3.2, and the variance of the estimated mean in Section 15.3.1, determine the sample allocation across strata that will minimize expected cost for a fixed variance (or minimize the variance for a fixed cost) for directory-based stratification. Explicit expressions for sample allocation can be found in Casady and Lepkowski [3].

Using generally accepted values of cost factors and population parameters for the simple cost models and the variance expressions cited above, Casady and Lepkowski concluded that both the Mitofsky–Waksberg design and directory-based stratification offer considerable improvement over the simple RDD design. They also concluded that, on the basis of the simple cost model alone, there was little difference in efficiency between the two approaches. However, if the possibility of additional bias could be tolerated, then the truncated design was by far the most efficient.

15.4.2 Implementation Considerations

There are a host of features of the telephone system that affect the implementation of the designs described in the last section. We discuss several of the more important ones briefly in this subsection.

The identification of the residential status of each telephone number generated in random digit dialing or list-assisted samples is not always an easy process. Numbers that are answered must be checked for residential use, and those used for mixed residential and business purposes suitably classified (usually any residential use is sufficient to classify a number as residential). Some numbers are readily identified as nonresidential because they are not in service, and a recording clearly indicates that status. Many numbers that are not in service are not connected to a recording to indicate their status, but are connected to a "ringing machine." Thus, interviewers screening telephone numbers to determine residential status cannot distinguish residential numbers where no one is at home from numbers not currently in service.

This latter problem is an important consideration in implementation of some designs. It is difficult to manage the ring-without-answer numbers in two-stage random digit dialing designs that require the replacement of non-residential numbers, particularly in time-limited survey data collection periods. Many survey organizations treat ring-without-answer numbers that have been called at varying times of day and days of the week as nonresidential. If the nonresidential classification is made late in the study period, the replacement number has a relatively short period during which it can be called. Replacements often do not get the same variation in time of day and day of week calling that original numbers received. Survey organizations prefer sampling procedures that give them a fixed sample of telephone numbers rather than one that may generate new telephone numbers late in the survey period.

At the end of the study period, ring-without-answer numbers that have been called repeatedly must be classified as residential or not in order to close out the study. If a number has been called at a variety of times and days, it may be arbitrarily classified as nonresidential. It thus does not count against the response rate for the survey because it has been classified as nonsample. On the other hand, ring-without-answer numbers that have not been called enough times are typically classified as residential and nonresponding, leading to a conservative calculation of the response rate.

In order to overcome these difficulties, and to reduce the costs of screening telephone numbers for residential status, automated screening systems have been developed to identify, at a minimum, telephone numbers that are connected to recordings indicating whether they are in service. The typical "not-in-service" recording is preceded by a "tri-tone," which occurs without any ringing. Proprietary hardware and software has been developed which dials telephone numbers and detects the tri-tone recording. Numbers with a tri-tone recording are dropped from further sampling. Numbers without the tri-tone will often experience a "ring splash," in which the telephone will ring momentarily while the hardware disconnects the call.

Surveys that are statewide or national in scope have geographic boundaries for the population that correspond to area code boundaries. Sample numbers generated within the sample area codes will be assigned to residences within the target geographic area. Many surveys target geographically defined populations whose boundaries do not match area code and exchange boundaries. In these cases, one may redefine the population, limiting it to that residing in specified exchanges, or one may select a sample from a set of exchanges that covers the entire geographic area but includes areas outside of the target. Telephone numbers must then be screened not only for residential status but also for location of residence, based on respondent self-report. The classification of ring-without-answer numbers is even more problematic in these screening surveys.

Identification of duplicates in each of the frames also typically involves a respondent self-report. Responding households are asked if they have more than one telephone number assigned to the household, and, if so, the number of such numbers assigned. This self-reported number of telephone numbers through which a household may be reached is subsequently used to generate a weight for estimation. Many survey organizations also check for wrong connections and operator-incorrect dialing. Incorrectly dialed numbers are discarded, as are wrong connections, in order to avoid further complications in the weighting process for duplicate listings of a household.

Social science and health surveys also frequently select a single eligible person in a household for more interviewing. For example, on a survey involving marital satisfaction, one adult will be selected in order to avoid contamination of responses among adults who converse about the content of the survey between interviews. Respondent selection must be done at an early stage in the interview. The procedure for objective respondent selection described by Kish [8] has been widely used in telephone surveys for this purpose, but it leads to an undesirable consequence–increased nonresponse rate. Households are reluctant to participate in a survey when the first questions are designed to obtain a roster of eligible persons living in the household. Alternative methods include a procedure described by Troldahl and Carter [17] and the nearest birthday method (see Lavrakas [9], for a description). This latter procedure has been shown to be biased in selection, but it continues to be used because it is easy to apply and avoids concerns about increased nonresponse rates associated with the Kish within-household selection procedure.

Finally, answering machines and cellular telephones are posing increasing problems for telephone sampling operations. Answering machines do allow, for the most part, ready identification of residential units. Messages can be left asking that the household call a toll-free number, and calling of households with answering machines can be scheduled at a variety of times of day and days of week to try to reach the household at a time when a person will answer the phone. Cellular telephones pose a different problem. Are such telephone numbers residential or business? Further, the subscriber may incur a charge when they receive calls. Cellular telephone numbers are not, for the most part, located in separate prefixes, but are mixed in the same prefixes as other numbers. This distribution makes identification difficult. Yet cellular phones may be more readily answered than telephones at a residence. In addition, a well-trained interviewer can make arrangements to call a household at another number, reducing the cost to the telephone subscriber.

15.4.3 Choice Among Alternative Designs

As indicated previously, the choice among alternative designs is largely based on a consideration of cost and error properties of each design. Three basic cost factors are typically considered: the cost of generating the sample of telephone numbers, the cost of screening the sample, and the "convenience" of working with the sampling procedure in implementation (a cost consideration that is often difficult to quantify). On the error side, there are two principal concerns, coverage of the telephone household population and sampling variance.

If we examine three chief competitors on these characteristics, we can see why organizations are today making particular choices among alternative designs. For example, it is inexpensive to generate telephone numbers in the Mitofsky–Waksberg two-stage random digit dialing sample design. Screening is efficient in the second stage since more than 60% of the telephone numbers are residential. The Mitofsky–Waksberg design presents a number of difficulties in implementation, including replacement of nonresidential numbers and exhausted clusters. These can be substantial inconveniences for some survey operations, and alternative methods that avoid these problems have substantial attraction. On the error side, the Mitofsky–Waksberg design does provide complete coverage of the telephone household population. Sampling variances are larger than for element sample designs because of the cluster sample selection and increases in variance due to within-100-bank homogeneity among sample elements. That is, design effects for Mitofsky–Waksberg samples are greater than one.

The stratified design has a somewhat different set of characteristics. The sample generation costs can be high. The list stratum sample can be purchased from a commercial sampling firm at a reasonably low cost per sample number, but the unlisted stratum sample requires further stratification of numbers and two-stage RDD samples drawn from each unlisted stratum. Screening costs are also higher than for the Mitofsky–Waksberg design, since approximately 50% of the sample telephone numbers in the listed stratum are residential, and a very low percent are residential in the unlisted stratum. Given that different sampling methods are used across strata, sample selection is less convenient for the stratified design than the Mitofsky–Waksberg design. However, the stratified design does eliminate the need to replace numbers and exhausted clusters. The stratified design does cover the entire telephone household population. Sampling variances will be smaller for the stratified design than the Mitofsky–Waksberg design because element sampling has smaller variances, and some improvements in precision due to stratification can be expected.

The truncated design has the disadvantage relative to the Mitofsky–Waksberg and stratified designs of noncoverage of telephone households in 100-banks with no listed numbers. The level of noncoverage is low and empirical investigations have shown that the difference for many characteristics between the covered and noncovered populations is small. Samples drawn using the truncated design are inexpensive when obtained from commercial sampling firms. The screening costs of the truncated design are intermediate to those of the Mitofsky–Waksberg and the stratified designs since approximately 55% of the generated telephone numbers will be residential. The truncated design is the most convenient among the three designs considered here since no replacement numbers are needed, the sample is drawn only from the listed stratum, and no two-stage sampling is needed from the unlisted stratum. The sampling variances of estimates should be the smallest for the truncated design since it is a stratified element sample with no cluster sampling.

The sampling practitioner is thus faced with a choice between designs that provide complete coverage but a number of inconveniences in selection and a design with less than complete coverage but a number of conveniences in selection. Given the empirical evidence on the size of the bias due to the non-coverage of telephone households in 100-banks without listed numbers, current practice favors the latter truncated design. That is, practitioners are choosing truncated sampling methods for telephone surveys based on a classic, although informal, cost–error trade-off.

15.5   SUMMARY

In this chapter we develop methods suitable for sampling telephone households using telephone number and telephone directory-based frames. Two-stage random digit dialing procedures as developed by Mitofsky and elaborated by Waksberg are widely used. Current alternative approaches have, relative to this procedure, coverage and cost deficiencies. These deficiencies are addressed through telephone sample designs which use listed number information to improve the cost efficiency of random digit dialing. The telephone number frame is divided into a stratum for which listed number information is available at the 100-bank level and one for which no such information is available. The efficiencies of various sampling schemes for this stratified design are compared to simple random digit dialing and the Mitofsky–Waksberg technique. Modest gains in efficiency of these alternative designs relative to the Mitofsky–Waksberg technique can be demonstrated for nearly all such designs. We also discuss briefly the use of poststratification to make inferences from the telephone household population to a broader population, and operational issues that arise in the implementation of telephone sampling methods.

EXERCISES

15.1   A telephone survey with a desired $n = 1600$ completed interviews is to be conducted in a large metropolitan area. The expected working residential rate in the area is 35%. One adult aged 21 or older is to be selected from each household (expected household eligibility 95%) and a response rate of 70% is expected. A two-stage Mitofsky–Waksberg random digit dialing sample design is proposed.

a. If we fix the cluster size at $b = 8$ residential numbers, how many primary numbers should be generated and how many clusters obtained?

b. If we expect a secondary working rate of 65%, how many numbers will be generated in the second stage?

c. Several problems are anticipated during interviewing. Describe in a single sentence whether these numbers would be classified "sample/nonsample" and how you would recommend handling each:

    1. A wrong connection.

    2. A household is contacted and an appointment is made for a later time. When redialed at appointment time, the number is out of service.

    3. The dialed number is used by a small accounting business in a home, but it is also used for personal calls.

    4. At the end of the study, there are a small number of numbers that are ringing without answer after from 1 to 20 calls.

15.2 A telephone sample is selected in an exchange. One hundred (100) consecutive telephone numbers in a 100-bank selected in the first stage of a Mitofsky–Waksberg design are placed in random order. Suppose that for one of the selected banks the first 40 numbers in the randomized list have been called, and the following results known for each:

(1) 936-0071	Interview	(21) 936-0026	Interview
(2) 936-0053	Business	(22) 936-0049	Business
(3) 936-0046	Busy (6 calls)	(23) 936-0084	Disconnected
(4) 936-0084	Not assigned	(24) 936-0003	Ring, no answer
(5) 936-0089	Not assigned	(25) 936-0094	Disconnected
(6) 936-0079	Business	(26) 936-0019	Business
(7) 936-0050	Refusal	(27) 936-0031	Interview
(8) 936-0024	Interview	(28) 936-0056	Refusal
(9) 936-0021	Wrong connection	(29) 936-0016	Ring, no answer
(10) 936-0001	Disconnected	(30) 936-0093	Not assigned
(11) 936-0038	Interview	(31) 936-0087	Ring, no answer
(12) 936-0090	Pay phone	(32) 936-0049	Business
(13) 936-0048	Hang up (5)	(33) 936-0010	Noise
(14) 936-0045	Ring, no answer (15)	(34) 936-0093	Not assigned
(15) 936-0014	Ring, no answer (11)	(35) 936-0095	Not assigned
(16) 936-0002	Hospital page	(36) 936-0022	Business
(17) 936-0017	Refusal	(37) 936-0011	Interview
(18) 936-0030	Answer machine	(38) 936-0075	Refusal
(19) 936-0096	Not assigned	(39) 936-0037	Not assigned
(20) 936-0044	Number changed to 747-1101	(40) 936-0012	Not assigned

For each of the following types of results, state whether at the end of the study, if you obtained these results, you would classify it as residential or nonresidential:

a. Disconnected

b. Not in service

c. RNA (Ring No Answer) for 11 or more calls

d. Wrong connection (on 2 dialings)

e. Answering machine

f. Telephone number changed

g. Hang up/RNA for many calls

15.3 Consider the following design features for a stratified telephone sample design

Stratum	Description	W_h	C_h
1	Listed 100-bank	0.35	$0.75
2	Unlisted 100-bank, listed prefix, unlisted 1000-bank	0.24	7.30
3	Remainder	0.41	1.45

a. Develop an optimal allocation for a three-stratum design with screening costs no more than $1250. Assume the element variances across the strata are approximately the same. Give the weights for elements in each of the strata needed to compensate for the unequal probabilities of selection.

b. Suppose that the decision is made to drop stratum 2 because of the expense of screening numbers there (i.e., use a truncated frame design). Now what optimal allocation would be used? And what would be the element weights needed to compensate for unequal probabilities of selection?

BIBLIOGRAPHY

1. Brick, J. M., Waksberg, J., Kulp, D., and Starer, A., Bias in list assisted telephone samples. *Public Opinion Quarterly*, 59(2): 218–235, 1995.

2. Brunner, J. A., and Brunner, G. A., Are voluntarily unlisted telephone subscribers really different? *Journal of Marketing Research*, 8: 121–124, 1971.

3. Casady, R. J., and Lepkowski, J. M., Stratified telephone sampling designs. *Survey Methodology*, 19(1): 103–113, 1993.

4. Connor, J., and Heeringa, S., Evaluation of two cost-efficient RDD designs. Paper Presented at the Annual Meeting of the American Association for Public Opinion Research, St. Petersburg, FL, 1992.

5. Frankel, M. R., and Frankel, L., Some recent developments in sample survey design. *Journal of Marketing Research*, 14: 280–293, 1977.

6. Groves, R. M., and Lepkowski, J. M., Dual frame mixed mode survey designs. *Journal of Official Statistics*, 1(3): 263–286, 1985.

7. Kalton, G., and Kasprzyk, D., The treatment of missing survey data. *Survey Methodology*, 12: 1–16, 1988.

8. Kish, L., *Survey Sampling*, Wiley, New York, 1965.

9. Lavrakas, P. J., *Telephone Survey Methods: Sampling, Selection, and Supervision*. Sage Publications, Newbury Park, Calif., 1987.

10. Lepkowski, J. M., Telephone sampling methods in the United States. In *Telephone Survey Methodology*, Groves, R. M., Biemer, P. P., Lyberg, L. E., Massey, J. T., Nicholls, W. L., II, and Waksberg, J., Eds., Wiley, New York, 1988.

11. Mitofsky, W., Sampling of Telephone Households. Unpublished CBS News memorandum, 1970.

12. Potthoff, R. F., Some generalizations of the Mitofsky–Waksberg techniques for random digit dialing. *Journal of the American Statistical Association*, 82(298): 409–418, 1987.

13. Potthoff, R. F., Generalizations of the Mitofsky–Waksberg technique for random digit dialing: Some added topics. *Proceedings of the Section on Survey Research Methods*, American Statistical Association, 615–620, 1987.

14. Stock, J. S., How to improve samples based on telephone listings. *Journal of Marketing Research*, 2(3): 50–51, 1962.

15. Sudman, S., The uses of telephone directories for survey sampling. *Journal of Marketing Research*, 10(2): 204–207, 1973.

16. Thornberry, O. T., and Massey, J. T., Trends in U.S. telephone coverage across time and subgroups. In *Telephone Survey Methodology*, Groves, R. M., Biemer, P. P., Lyberg, L. E., Massey, J. T., Nichols, W. L., II, and Waksberg, J., Eds., Wiley, New York, 1988.

17. Troldahl, V. C., and Carter, R. E., Jr., Random selection of respondents within households in phone surveys. *Journal of Marketing Research*, 1(2): 71–76, 1964.

18. Waksberg, J., Sampling methods for random digit dialing. *Journal of the American Statistical Association*, 19(1): 103–113, 1978.

The following review was written for the Encyclopedia of Biostatistics *and contains, in a different format, much of the material that is in this chapter.*

19. Casady, R. J., and Lepkowski, J. M., Telephone sampling. In *The Encyclopedia of Biostatistics*, Armitage, P. A., and Colton, T., Eds., Wiley, Chichester, U.K., 1998.

CHAPTER 16

Strategies for Design-Based Analysis of Sample Survey Data

Researchers typically design sample surveys to provide valid and reliable estimates of population parameters such as means, totals, and proportions, but increasingly are also interested in evaluating interrelationships among variables. More often than not, widely available statistical software packages have been used to analyze such data, particularly when multivariable modeling has been involved in the analysis. Unfortunately, such software generally does not take into consideration many of the design features of the particular sample survey undergoing analysis. In this book we have been focusing on use in analysis of survey data of SUDAAN and STATA because, unlike many other statistical packages currently available, they have the capability to analyze survey data in such a way that the relevant design features are taken into consideration. As we have indicated earlier, our use of these two products reflects our own familiarity with them and should not be interpreted as an endorsement over others having similar capabilities that are currently available, or those that may become available in the future. The strategies outlined in this chapter and throughout this book are based on sampling theory and should be independent of and transferable to any software product that purports to perform *design-based* analysis of sample survey data as defined below.

Design-based analysis of sample survey data is analysis which takes into consideration the features involved in the sample design. These features often include, among others, stratification, clustering, sampling fractions large enough to benefit from use of finite population corrections, and sampling weights. Analysis that is not design-based, that is, that does not take into consideration design features such as those listed above, will be referred to as *model-based analysis*. Our use of this latter term is broader than that often used in the literature in that we include under model-based analysis, analysis that has been done under no explicitly stated model but that seems to assume independent random sampling from an infinite population ("classic" assumptions).

481

We have indicated in previous sections that when design features of a survey are ignored in the analysis, the potential exists for the results to be incorrect. In this chapter we will illustrate how the relevant design features are identified, and then appropriately incorporated into the analysis of sample survey data. We will also show how failure to incorporate these features can result in incorrect estimates and invalid inferences.

16.1 STEPS REQUIRED FOR PERFORMING A DESIGN-BASED ANALYSIS

The following steps are required in order to perform a design-based analysis.

1. Identify the following elements of the sample design:
   Stratification
   Clustering variables used
   Population sizes required for determination of finite population corrections
2. On the basis of the above information, determine the sampling weight for each sample subject.
3. Determine for each sample record a final sampling weight that takes into consideration any nonresponse and poststratification adjustments that are desired.
4. Ensure that all stratification, clustering, and population size data required for an appropriate design-based analysis are identified on each sample record.
5. Determine the procedure and the set of commands for performing the required analysis for the particular software package that will be used.
6. Run the analysis and carefully interpret findings.

Illustrative Example. Let us consider a state consisting of 5 regions and containing 57 nursing homes, as shown in Table 16.1. Suppose that we take a stratified random sample of two nursing homes within each region and, within each nursing home, take a sample of five admissions for determining the total number of patients admitted in 1997 to nursing homes in the five-region area whose source of payment is Medicaid. The resulting data are shown in Table 16.2 and the variables shown in this table are described below:

REGION identifies the region
NURSHOME identifies the sample nursing home
PATIENT identifies the sample patient
MEDICAID equals "1" if the sample patient is on Medicaid; "0" otherwise
RGNHOMES is the total number of nursing homes in the region

Table 16.1 Number of Nursing Homes in Five Regions in a State

Region	Number of Nursing Homes in Region	Total Admissions Among Nursing Homes in Region During 1997
1	12	1245
2	20	3887
3	11	583
4	8	400
5	6	2376

NHADMISS is the total number of admissions to the nursing home during 1997

We will go through the six steps listed above to obtain a design-based estimate of the total number of patients admitted to nursing homes in 1997 whose source of payment is Medicaid.

1. This is a two-stage stratified cluster sample with nursing homes chosen by simple random sampling without replacement at the first stage within each stratum, and patients chosen by simple random sampling within each selected nursing home. The stratification variable is REGION; the clustering variable is NURSHOME; the variable, RGNHOMES, is the number of nursing homes within each region and is the variable used to compute the finite population correction for the first stage of sampling; the variable NHADMISS is the total number of patients admitted during 1997 to each sample nursing home and serves as the variable used for computing the finite population correction at the second stage of sampling.

2. The sampling weight for each sample record is obtained as follows:

   Let M_h = the number of nursing homes in region h

   Then the probability, f_{1h}, of any nursing home being selected in the sample is given by

   $$f_{1h} = \frac{2}{M_h}$$

   Let N_{hi} = the number of 1997 admissions to nursing home i within stratum h

   Then the second stage sampling fraction, f_{2hi}, is given by

   $$f_{2hi} = \frac{5}{N_{hi}}$$

Table 16.2 Resulting Data from Sample of Nursing Homes

REGION	NURSHOME	PATIENT	MEDICAID	RGNHOMES	NHADMISS
1	1	1	1	12	123
1	1	2	1	12	123
1	1	3	1	12	123
1	1	4	0	12	123
1	1	5	1	12	123
1	2	1	0	12	89
1	2	2	0	12	89
1	2	3	1	12	89
1	2	4	0	12	89
1	2	5	0	12	89
2	1	1	1	20	231
2	1	2	0	20	231
2	1	3	1	20	231
2	1	4	0	20	231
2	1	5	1	20	231
2	2	1	0	20	187
2	2	2	0	20	187
2	2	3	0	20	187
2	2	4	1	20	187
2	2	5	0	20	187
3	1	1	1	11	43
3	1	2	1	11	43
3	1	3	1	11	43
3	1	4	0	11	43
3	1	5	1	11	43
3	2	1	1	11	49
3	2	2	1	11	49
3	2	3	1	11	49
3	2	4	1	11	49
3	2	5	0	11	49
4	1	1	0	8	56
4	1	2	1	8	56
4	1	3	1	8	56
4	1	4	0	8	56
4	1	5	0	8	56
4	2	1	0	8	38
4	2	2	0	8	38
4	2	3	0	8	38
4	2	4	0	8	38
4	2	5	1	8	38
5	1	1	1	6	359
5	1	2	0	6	359
5	1	3	1	6	359
5	1	4	1	6	359
5	1	5	0	6	359

Table 16.2   Resulting Data from Sample of Nursing Homes (*continued*)

REGION	NURSHOME	PATIENT	MEDICAID	RGNHOMES	NHADMISS
5	2	1	0	6	460
5	2	2	1	6	460
5	2	3	0	6	460
5	2	4	1	6	460
5	2	5	0	6	460

Thus, the overall probability of a patient being included in the sample is given by

$$f_{hi} = \frac{2}{M_h} \times \frac{5}{N_{hi}}$$

and the sampling weight, w_{hi}, is given by

$$w_{hi} = \frac{M_h N_{hi}}{10} \tag{16.1}$$

3. In this illustrative example, we are assuming that there is complete response and that there is no plan for poststratification.
4. Examination of Table 16.2 indicates that the stratification, clustering, and finite population correction variables are present for each sample record. While not shown explicitly in Table 16.2, we have constructed for each sample record, a variable, *WEIGHT*, given by equation (16.1).
5. We will use SUDAAN for this illustrative example since STATA does not make use of finite population corrections for cluster sample designs. The appropriate commands in SUDAAN are shown below:

```
PROC DESCRIPT DATA = "A:CH16ILLI" FILETYPE = SAS DESIGN = WOR
DEFF TOTALS;
NEST REGION NURSHOME;
TOTCNT RGNHOMES NHADMISS;
VAR MEDICAID;
WEIGHT WEIGHT;
SETENV COLWIDTH = 15;
SETENV DECWIDTH = 4;
```

The first command line indicates the appropriate SUDAAN procedure for estimating a total, locates the appropriate data set, indicates that it is a SAS data file, specifies the appropriate sample design (the WOR design is appropriate when finite population corrections are required).

The second command line or "nest" statement indicates the stratification and cluster variables (unless otherwise specified, the first variable indicated in the nest statement is interpreted as a stratification variable).

The third line or "totcnt" statement indicates the population variables needed to compute finite population corrections at each stage of sampling.

The fourth command line specifies the variable(s) for which estimates are to be made.

The fifth line indicates the sampling weight variable.

The last two lines give specifications for output.

6. The resulting output is shown below:

| Number of observations read: | 50 | | Weighted count: | 8791 |
| Deonominator degrees of freedom: | 5 | | | |

Variance Estimation Method: Taylor Series (WOR)
by: Variable, One.

Variable		One
		– –
MEDICAID	Sample Size	50.0000
	Weighted Size	8791.0000
	Total	4180.2000
	SE Total	1112.7529
	Mean	0.4755
	SE Mean	0.1052
	DEFF Mean #4	2.1748
	DEFF Total #4	3.1479

The findings shown above estimate that 4180 patients were admitted to nursing homes in this state during 1997 having Medicaid as the source of payment. The standard error of this estimated total is 1113, and the design effect for the total is 3.15, which implies a high amount of clustering for this variable.   □

16.2   ANALYSIS ISSUES FOR "TYPICAL" SAMPLE SURVEYS

All sample surveys incorporate some, but not necessarily all, of the design features listed above, and some have designs that are considerably more complex. It is useful at this point to describe a "typical" sample survey. The type of design that we will portray here is typical of the vast majority of real-life survey situations. Of course, more complex situations exist, especially in the large ongoing survey programs that are maintained by nations. Often, however, even these can be simplified, for analysis purposes, to resemble the typical situation we will describe here, and results will often be close to what would have been correct if the full survey design parameters could have been specified.

We now consider a survey whose design is very similar to that of the survey discussed in Section 16.1, but with larger sample size, some additional complications not considered earlier, and a much more complex analytic agenda. More specifically, the design of this survey is such that all population elements are grouped into one of L mutually exclusive and exhaustive strata. Within the hth stratum, the population is divided into M_h clusters [termed primary sampling units (PSUs)] and m_h of these are selected for inclusion in the sample. Within each sample cluster, a second stage of sampling is performed and n_{hi} enumeration units are selected. Each unit selected from a particular PSU is assigned a *sampling weight*, as discussed earlier. This weight may be thought of as the number of units in the population that this unit represents and, in this example, is determined by the stratum and the PSU in which this unit resides. Again, it is computed as the reciprocal of the probability that the unit is included in the sample. When population sizes are known, they may be incorporated into the analysis in the form of *finite population corrections*.

Illustrative Example. To illustrate these concepts we consider the analysis of data collected as part of the PAQUID (Personnes Agees Quid) study, a stratified cluster sample of elderly French citizens [1], [2]. Noninstitutionalized residents who were 65 years of age and over on December 31, 1987, and who lived in two administrative areas, or "departments," in the South-West of France: Gironde (10,000 km^2, 1,127,546 inhabitants) and Dordogne (9060 km^2, 377,356 inhabitants), were included. A total of 3777 community residents were selected for the purpose of identifying baseline and lifetime factors that might be related to cognitive loss, dementia, and Alzheimer's disease. Baseline data were collected in 1988–1989 and subjects have since been studied periodically up to the present time.

The departments of Gironde and Dordogne are comprised of 543 and 555 smaller areas called *parishes*, respectively. To select the study subjects, the parishes within each department were placed on the basis of population size, into one of four groups:

Group 1: parishes with $> 50,000$ inhabitants

Group 2: parishes with between 10,000 and 49,999 inhabitants

Group 3: parishes with between 2000 and 9999 inhabitants

Group 4: parishes with fewer than 2000 inhabitants

Within each group, parishes were selected with probability proportional to the size of the parish. There were no parishes with $> 50,000$ inhabitants in

Dordorgne. In total, 37 parishes were selected from Gironde and 38 were selected from Dordogne.

Within each selected parish, subjects were selected at random from the electoral lists of each parish, stratified by age and sex. Selected subjects were asked to provide written agreement to participate in the study. This resulted in a total study population of 3777 subjects: 2792 from Gironde, and 985 from Dordogne.

All study subjects were contacted by telephone or (when possible) by mail to request their permission to participate in the study. Those agreeing to participate (68.5%) were interviewed by a trained psychologist in their homes to obtain baseline data. A structured questionnaire was administered to each participant. Subjects were revisited at regular intervals to screen for development of cognitive dysfunction and dementia.

Clearly, this is not a simple random sample, but instead is a sample survey that incorporates many of the features outlined previously. In the subsequent discussion we will employ the following notation:

- h refers to one of 7 strata (defined by department and group)
- M_h is the number of clusters (or parishes) making up the hth stratum, $h = 1, \ldots, 7$
- m_h is the number of clusters selected from the hth stratum, $h = 1, \ldots, 7$
- i refers to the parish number within the stratum
- N_{hi} is the number of individuals 65 and older living in the ith sampled parish within stratum h (based on census data)
- N_h is the number of individuals 65 and older living in stratum h (based on census data)
- n_{hi} is the number of individuals actually studied in parish i within stratum h

Table 16.3 presents a summary of the selection process.

We can consider that we have 7 strata and that samples were selected within each stratum. In Gironde there were only 3 parishes with populations $> 50,000$ (stratum 1), and each of these parishes was selected. In Dordogne there were only 2 parishes with population between 10,000 and 49,999 (stratum 3), and both of these were selected. For these two strata, since $m_h = M_h$, the probability of selecting a particular unit is (n_{hi}/N_{hi}), so for these two strata the sampling weight is $1/(n_{hi}/N_{hi}) = N_{hi}/n_{hi}$. For the other five strata, the approximate probability of selecting a particular unit is equal to the product of the approximate probability of selecting the parish using a probability proportional to size (PPS) sampling design, $m_h \times (N_{hi}/N_h)$ (see proof of this at the end of the chapter), times the probability of selecting the individual in the selected parish, n_{hi}/N_{hi}. That is, the probability of selecting an individual in these five strata is

Table 16.3 Selection of Sample Subjects from Departments of Gironde and Dordogne

Department	Group	Stratum	M_h	m_h	$\sum_{i=1}^{m_h} N_{hi}$	$\sum_{i=1}^{m_h} n_{hi}$
Gironde	1	1	3	3	49,786	1,231
Gironde	2	2	14	4	35,253	473
Dordogne	2	3	2	2	11,764	71
Gironde	3	4	73	10	37,024	361
Dordogne	3	5	26	13	17,687	311
Gironde	4	6	453	20	44,980	727
Dordogne	4	7	527	23	46,250	603
Total			1,098	75	242,744	3,777

$$\left(m_h \times \frac{N_{hi}}{N_h}\right) \times \left(\frac{n_{hi}}{N_{hi}}\right) = \frac{m_h n_{hi}}{N_h}.$$

It follows that the sampling weight in these strata is $(N_h/(m_h n_{hi}))$.

Although these weights, as intended, are correct in the sense of portraying the number of persons in the population each study subject represents, the sum of the weights within specified age/sex subgroups may not correctly sum to the know population sizes within these subgroups. To remedy this situation, a poststratification adjustment is needed which modifies the initial weight in such a way that the sum of the weights over all sampled individuals in each of the age–sex subgroups is identical to the known population sizes within each of those subgroups. The subgroups are:

Males, ages 65–74	Females, ages 65–74
Males, ages 75–84	Females, ages 75–84
Males, ages 85+	Females, ages 85+

For example, in Gironde stratum 1 there were 10,105 males between the ages of 65 and 74 on the voting lists. This represented 20.3% of all subjects on the voting list from that stratum. In the sample, however, there were 284 males between the ages of 65 and 74, representing 23.07% of the sample from that stratum. Therefore, we may adjust each weight by multiplying by the ratio $.203/.2307 = .88$. If we call these adjustment factors c_{hijk}, where h denotes the stratum, i denotes the PSU, j denotes the subgroup, and k denotes the individual, then the final statistical weights, w_{hijk}, may be expressed as

$$w_{hijk} = \left(\frac{N_h}{m_h n_{hi}}\right) \times c_{hijk} \qquad \square$$

The above discussion demonstrates that the PAQUID study may be characterized as a stratified multistage design where, at the first stage of sampling, parishes (or PSUs) are selected from the strata and, at the second stage, subjects are selected at random from the electoral lists within the selected parish. Until recently, as stated in earlier chapters, analyzing survey data of this type was relatively difficult because most statistical software packages assume the data have been selected by simple random sampling. This assumption can give rise to errors in estimation and inference when analyzing sample survey data not resulting from a simple random sampling design. Such programs may produce biased point estimates and may grossly underestimate the standard errors of these estimates. As mentioned repeatedly in previous chapters of this book, programs such as SUDAAN and STATA make it possible to analyze sample survey data appropriately.

We use the sample survey capabilities of STATA to analyze these data. To do this, we simply specify that there are seven strata and, within them, the PSUs are parishes. We also provide the statistical weights, w_{hijk}, computed following the process described above.

Survey design parameters are specified to STATA using *svyset* commands. In this example, the variables that contain information on stratum, sampling weight, and primary sampling unit are named: STRATUM, WEIGHT, and PSU, respectively. These specifications are saved as part of the data set and are invoked each time a survey analysis is run:

```
.svyset strata STRATUM
.syvset pweight WEIGHT
.svyset psu PSU
```

The objective of this analysis is to estimate the 3-year incidence of dementia among those individuals who were *not* demented at the time of the initial survey examination. For this reason, we consider only those subjects free of dementia at the time of initial observation ($n = 2273$). As a first analysis, consider the calculation of the proportion of these subjects having scores on the Mini-Mental State Examination (MMSE) less than or equal to 21. The MMSE is a short test that screens for cognitive impairment, and can range between 0 and 30, with low scores indicating increased likelihood of dementia. Letting the variable mmse01 indicate a score ≤ 21 on the MMSE, we see that ignoring the survey design results in the following estimate of the proportion and associated confidence interval:

Variable	Obs	Mean	Std. Err.	[95% Conf. Interval]	
mmse01	2242	.0816236	.0057836	.0702818	.0929653

To account for the survey design parameters, we issue the following command to STATA:

.syvmean mmse01

and obtain the following results:

Survey mean estimation

pweight:	finalwt	Number of obs	=	2242
Strata:	newstrat	Number of strata	=	7
PSU:	parish	Number of PSUs	=	75
		Population size	=	146863.41

Mean	Estimate	Std. Err.	[95% Conf Interval]		Deff
mmse01	.082957	.0079147	.0671634	.0987506	1.845315

Note that while the point estimates are quite comparable (approximately 8% having MMSE scores less than or equal to 21), the standard error of the estimated proportion based on the survey design is .0079 as compared to .0058, the estimated standard error ignoring the survey design parameters. The *design effect* (indicated in the STATA output as "Deff") is the ratio of the variance of the estimated parameter taking into consideration the survey design parameters over the variance of the estimated parameter assuming simple random sampling. In this case,

$$\text{Deff} = \frac{.0079^2}{.0058^2} = 1.85$$

While the point estimates may be comparable in the two analyses, the standard errors of the means are considerably larger in the design-based analysis. This is as expected for estimates of the sample proportion. Clearly, ignoring the sample survey design parameters results in an underestimate of the sample variance by 85%, and in confidence intervals that are far too narrow.

Typically, design effects for estimated means, totals, and proportions are considerably greater than unity. The design effect can be thought of as a measure of the inflation in variance that is due to homogeneity within clusters. The design effect can be expressed as $1 + \delta_y(\bar{n} - 1)$, where δ_y is the *intracluster correlation coefficient* (i.e., *intraclass correlation coefficient*) and $\bar{n}$ is the average number of units sampled per cluster. As stated earlier, the intracluster correlation coefficient can range from small negative values (when the data within clusters are highly heterogeneous) to unity (when the data within clusters are very homogeneous). Only in very rare instances when the data are highly heterogeneous within clusters will the design effect be less than unity.

An important objective of this study was to investigate whether a relationship exists between consumption of wine and occurrence of dementia, and if so, to estimate the strength of that relationship. Specifically, the outcome of interest in this study was whether the subject had dementia at the time of the 3-year follow-up, and the primary risk factor under consideration was wine consumption as grouped into the following categories:

$$\text{wine} = \begin{cases} 0 & \text{no wine consumption} \\ 1 & \text{up to } 1/4 \text{ liter/day} \\ 2 & \text{more than } 1/4 \text{ liter/day} \end{cases}$$

In this analysis, the dependent variable is presence or absence of dementia, and is based on a battery of neuropsychiatric tests considerably more sophisticated than the MMSE. The cross-tabulation of dementia status at 3 years of follow-up (as determined by this battery of tests) versus wine consumption without consideration of survey design is presented in Table 16.4.

Table 16.5 illustrates that the same odds ratios and confidence intervals can be obtained through the use of a logistic regression model under the assumption of simple random sampling.

Using the features of the survey design, a logistic regression is run with DEMENTIA as the dependent variable and two indicator variables for wine consumption (WINE_1 and WINE_2) as the independent variables. This is accomplished in STATA with the following command:

```
.svylogit DEMENTIA WINE_1 WINE_2, or
```

Table 16.4   Association of Wine Consumption vs. Incident Dementia (Model-Based Analysis)

Wine Consumption	Incident Dementia				Odds Ratio (OR)*	95% CI
	Yes		No			
	n	%	*n*	%		
None	48	4.9	923	95.1	1.000	
≤1/4 liter/day	47	5.1	875	94.9	1.033	.684–1.561
>1/4 liter/day	4	1.1	376	98.9	.205	.073– .571
Total	99		2,174			

*Compared to none as referent group.

This gives rise to the following output:

```
Survey logistic regression

pweight:    WEIGHT                      Number of obs      =          2273
Strata:     STRATUM                     Number of strata   =             7
PSU:        PSU                         Number of PSUs     =            75
                                        Population size    =     148779.94
                                        F(    2,   67)      =          5.99
                                        Prob > F           =        0.0041
```

DEMENTIA	Odds Ratio	Std. Err.	t	P > |t|	[95% Conf. Interval]	
WINE_1	1.040389	.2807133	0.147	0.884	.6072504	1.7824760
WINE_2	.1691458	.0885213	-3.395	0.001	.0595280	.4806197

Table 16.6 presents this analysis in a format similar to the one presented in Table 16.5.

The odds ratios are similar between the two analyses but the protective effect of wine appears 18% greater in the analysis that correctly accounted for the sampling design. It is interesting to note that it is moderate or heavy, not mild wine consumption, that appears to have a protective effect for dementia. In addition, the design effects for the regression coefficients are not as dramatic as was the case for means or proportions. In some cases, the design effects were actually less than 1. Interestingly, design effects for regression coefficients can be approximated by $1 + (\bar{n} - 1)\delta_x\delta_y$. Because this expression depends on the product of the intracluster correlation coefficients for both the independent and dependent variables, both of which are by definition less than or equal to 1, the magnitude of the effect is smaller than or equal to that seen for means, totals, or proportions. Furthermore, it is important to note that δ_x and δ_y are not necessarily in the same direction. It is possible for data within

Table 16.5 Logistic Regression Analysis of Wine Consumption and Incident Dementia Assuming Simple Random Sampling (Model-Based Analysis)

Wine Consumption	Odds Ratio	Standard Error of Odds Ratio	95% Confidence Intervals
None	1.000	—	—
≤ 1/4 liter/day	1.033	.217	[.684, 1.56]
> 1/4 liter/day	.205	.107	[.073, .571]

Table 16.6   Logistic Regression Analysis of Wine Consumption and Incident Dementia Incorporating Sample Survey Parameters (Design-Based Analysis)

Wine Consumption	Odds Ratio	Standard Error of Odds Ratio	95% Confidence Intervals
None	1.000	—	—
≤ 1/4 liter/day	1.040	.281	[.607, 1.782]
> 1/4 liter/day	.169	.089	[.060, .481]

clusters to be heterogeneous with respect to one variable and homogeneous with respect to the other variable. In this case, the product of the intracluster correlation coefficients would be negative and the resulting design effect would be smaller than 1.

Recently survey organizations such as the National Center for Health Statistics and the U.S. Bureau of the Census have distributed data from the National Health and Nutrition Examination Survey (NHANES III) and the National Health Interview Survey (NHIS) to interested investigators via CD-ROM. Confronted by the richness of such databases and the historic relative lack of availability of suitable software to appropriately account for the survey design, researchers have simply ignored the complexities of the survey and analyzed the data as if they resulted from a simple random sample. The availability of modern programs such as STATA and SUDAAN provides data analysts with the new analytical capabilities needed to perform appropriate analyses.

16.3   SUMMARY

In this chapter, we present a 6-step procedure for performing design-based analysis of data from sample surveys that one should be able to use with any software package that can perform such analysis. We illustrate this procedure using a relatively simple two-stage stratified cluster sample design. Using an example that has a more complex sample design, we then illustrate how failure to use a design-based analysis can lead to misleading conclusions.

TECHNICAL   APPENDIX

Proof that the probability of selecting a particular PSU, i, under PPS sampling is given by the following

$$P\{i \in \text{sample}\} = \frac{N_i}{N} m$$

where

N_i = Number of enumeration units in PSU i
N = Total number of enumeration units in population
m = Total number of PSUs in sample

Proof. Assume sampling of PSUs is with replacement:

$$P\{\text{PSU } i \notin \text{sample}\} = \left(1 - \frac{N_i}{N}\right)^m \approx 1 - m\,\frac{N_i}{N}$$

(first term binomial theorem expansion)

Thus,

$$P\{\text{PSU } i \in \text{sample}\} = 1 - P\{\text{PSU } i \notin \text{sample}\} = \frac{N_i}{N}\,m$$

BIBLIOGRAPHY

The following articles describe the design and basic findings of the PAQUID Study:
1. Lemeshow, S., Letenneur, L., Dartigues, J. F., Lafont, S., Orgogozo, J. M., and Commenges, D., An illustration of analysis taking into account complex survey considerations: The association between wine consumption and dementia in the PAQUID study. *American Journal of Epidemiology*, 148(3): 298–306, 1998.
2. Barberger-Gateau, P., Dartigues, J. F., Commenges, D., Gagnon, M., Letenneur, L., Canet, C., Miquel, J. L., Nejjari, C., Tessier, J. F., Berr, C., Dealberto, M. J., Decamps, A., Alpérovitch, A., and Salamon, R., Paquid: An interdisciplinary epidemiologic study of cerebral and functional aging. *Annals of Gerontology*, 383–392, 1992.
3. Letenneur, L., Commenges, D., Dartigues, J. F., and Barberger-Gateau, P. Incidence of dementia and Alzheimer's disease in elderly community residents of South-Western France. *International Journal of Epidemiology*, 23: 1256–1261, 1994.

The following article furnishes another example of the problems that result from ignoring design features in the analysis of data from sample surveys.
4. Brogan D., Software Packages for Analysis of Sample Survey Data, Misuse of Standard Packages. In *Encyclopedia of Biostatistics*, Armitage, P. A., and Colton, T., Eds., Wiley, Chichester, U.K., 1998.

Also many of the references cited in Chapter 12 deal with general issues in analysis of data from complex sample surveys.

Appendix

Table A.1 Random Number Table

Line/Col.	(1)	(2)	(3)	(4)	(5)	(6)	(7)	(8)	(9)	(10)	(11)	(12)	(13)	(14)
1	10480	05011	01536	02011	81647	91646	69179	14194	62590	36207	20969	99570	91291	90700
2	22368	46573	25595	85393	30995	89198	27982	53402	93965	34095	52666	19174	39615	99505
3	24130	48390	22527	97265	76393	64809	15179	24830	49340	32081	30680	19655	63348	58629
4	42167	93093	06243	61680	07856	16376	39440	53537	71341	57004	00849	74917	97758	16379
5	37570	39975	81837	16656	06121	91782	60468	81305	49684	60072	14110	06927	01263	54613
6	77921	06907	11008	42751	27756	53498	18602	70659	90655	15053	21916	81825	44394	42880
7	99562	72905	56420	69994	98872	31016	71194	18738	44013	48840	63213	21069	10634	12952
8	96301	91977	05463	07972	18876	20922	94595	56869	69014	60045	18425	84903	42508	32307
9	89579	14342	63661	10281	17453	18103	57740	84378	25331	12568	58678	44947	05585	56941
10	85475	36857	53342	53988	53060	59533	38867	62300	08158	17983	16439	11458	18593	64952
11	28918	69578	88231	33276	70997	79936	56865	05859	90106	31595	01547	85590	91610	78188
12	63553	40961	48235	03427	49626	69445	18663	72695	52180	20847	12234	90511	33703	90322
13	09429	93969	52636	92737	88974	33488	36320	17617	30015	08272	84115	27156	30613	74952
14	10365	61129	87529	85689	48237	52267	67689	93394	01511	26358	85104	20285	29975	89868
15	07119	97336	71048	08178	77233	13916	47564	81056	97735	85977	29372	74461	28551	90707
16	51085	12765	51821	51259	77452	16308	60756	92144	49442	53900	70960	63990	75601	40719
17	02368	21382	52404	60269	89368	19885	55322	44819	01188	65255	64835	44919	05944	55157
18	01011	54092	33362	94904	31273	04146	18594	29852	71685	85030	51132	01915	92747	64951
19	52162	53916	46369	58586	23216	14513	83149	98736	23495	64350	94738	17752	35156	35749
20	07056	97628	33787	09998	42698	06691	76988	13602	51851	46104	88916	19509	25625	58104
21	48663	91245	85828	14346	09172	30163	90229	04734	59193	22178	30421	61666	99904	32812
22	54164	58492	22421	74103	47070	25306	76468	26384	58151	06646	21524	15227	96909	44592
23	32639	32363	05597	24200	13363	38005	04342	28728	35806	06912	17012	64161	18296	22851
24	29334	27001	87637	87308	58731	00256	45834	15398	46557	41135	10306	07684	36188	18510
25	02488	33062	28834	07351	19731	92420	60952	61280	50001	67658	32586	86679	50720	94953

26	81525	72295	04839	96423	24878	82651	66566	14778	76797	14780	13300	87074	79666	95725
27	29676	20591	68086	26432	46901	20849	89768	81536	86645	12659	92259	57102	80428	25280
28	00742	57392	39064	66432	84673	40027	32832	61362	98947	96067	64760	64584	96096	98253
29	05366	04213	25669	26422	44407	44048	37937	63904	45766	66134	75470	66520	34693	90449
30	91921	26418	64117	94305	26766	25940	39972	22209	71500	64568	91402	42416	07844	69618
31	00582	04711	87917	77341	42206	35126	74087	99547	81817	42607	43808	76655	62028	76630
32	00725	69884	69797	56170	86324	88072	76222	36086	84637	93161	76038	65855	77919	88006
33	69011	65795	95876	55293	18988	27354	26575	08625	40801	59920	29841	80150	12777	48501
34	25976	57948	29888	88604	67917	48708	18912	82271	65424	69774	33611	54262	85963	03547
35	09763	83473	73577	12908	30883	18317	28290	35797	05998	41688	34952	37888	38917	88050
36	91567	42595	27958	30134	04024	86385	29880	99730	55536	84855	29088	09250	79656	73211
37	17955	56349	90999	49127	20044	59931	06115	20542	18059	02008	73708	83517	36103	42791
38	46503	18584	18845	49618	02304	51038	20655	58727	28168	15475	56942	53389	20562	87338
39	92157	89634	94824	78171	84610	82834	09922	25417	44137	48413	25555	21246	35509	20468
40	14577	62765	35605	81263	39667	47358	56873	56307	61607	49518	89656	20103	77490	18062
41	98427	07523	33362	64270	01638	92477	66969	98420	04880	45585	46565	04102	46880	45709
42	34914	63976	88720	82765	34476	17032	87589	40836	32427	70002	70663	88863	77775	69348
43	70060	28277	39475	46473	23219	53416	94970	25832	69975	94884	19661	72828	00102	66794
44	53976	54914	06990	67245	68350	82948	11398	42878	80287	88267	47363	46634	06541	97809
45	76072	29515	40980	07391	58745	25774	22987	80059	39911	96189	41151	15222	60697	59583
46	90725	52210	83974	29992	65831	38857	50490	83765	55657	14361	31720	57375	56228	41546
47	64364	67412	33339	31926	14883	24413	59744	92351	97473	89286	35931	04110	23726	51900
48	08962	00358	31662	25388	61642	34072	81249	35648	56891	69352	48373	45578	78547	81788
49	95012	68379	93526	70765	10592	04542	76463	54328	02349	17247	28865	14777	62730	92277
50	15664	10493	20492	38301	91132	21999	59516	81652	27195	48223	46751	22923	32261	85653

Table A.1 Random Number Table (continued)

Line/Col.	(1)	(2)	(3)	(4)	(5)	(6)	(7)	(8)	(9)	(10)	(11)	(12)	(13)	(14)
51	16408	81899	04153	53381	79401	21438	83035	92350	36693	31238	59649	91754	72772	02338
52	18629	81953	05520	91962	04739	13092	97662	24822	94730	06496	35090	04822	86774	98289
53	73115	35101	47498	87637	99016	71060	88824	71013	18735	20286	23153	72924	35165	43040
54	57491	16703	23167	49323	45012	33132	12544	41035	80780	45393	44812	12515	98931	91202
55	30405	83946	23792	14422	15059	45799	22716	19792	09983	74353	68668	30429	70735	25499
56	16631	35006	85900	98275	32388	52390	16815	69293	82732	38480	73817	32523	41961	44437
57	96773	20206	42559	78985	05300	22164	24369	54224	35083	19687	11052	91491	60383	19746
58	38935	64202	14349	82674	66523	44133	00697	35552	35970	19124	63318	29686	03387	59846
59	31624	76384	17403	53363	44167	64486	64758	75366	76554	31601	12614	33072	60332	92325
60	78919	19474	23632	27889	47914	02584	37680	20801	72152	39339	34806	08930	85001	87820
61	03931	33309	57047	74211	63445	17361	62825	39908	05607	91284	68833	25570	38818	46920
62	74426	33278	43972	10119	89917	15665	52872	73823	73144	86662	88970	74492	51805	99378
63	09066	00903	20795	95452	92648	45454	69552	88815	16553	51125	79375	97596	16296	66092
64	42238	12426	87025	14267	20979	04508	64535	31355	86064	29472	47689	05974	52468	16834
65	16153	08002	26504	41744	81959	65642	74240	56302	00033	67107	77510	70625	28725	34191
66	21457	40742	29820	96783	29400	21840	15035	34537	33310	06116	95240	15957	16572	06004
67	21581	57802	02050	89728	17937	37621	47075	42080	97403	48626	68995	43805	33386	21597
68	55612	78095	83197	33732	05810	24813	86902	60397	16489	03264	88525	42786	05269	92532
69	44657	66999	99324	51281	84463	60563	79312	93454	68876	25471	93911	25650	12682	73572
70	91340	84979	46949	81973	37949	61023	43997	15263	80644	43992	89203	71795	99533	50501
71	91227	21199	31935	27022	84067	05462	35216	14486	29891	68607	41867	14951	91696	85065
72	50001	38140	66321	19924	72163	09538	12151	06878	91903	18749	34405	56087	82790	70925
73	65390	05224	72958	28609	81406	39147	25549	48542	42627	45233	57202	94617	23772	07896
74	27504	96131	83944	41575	10573	03619	64482	73923	36152	05184	94142	25299	84387	34925
75	37169	94851	39117	89632	00959	16487	65536	49071	39782	17095	02330	74301	00275	48280

76	11508	70225	51111	38351	19444	66499	71945	05422	13442	78675	84031	66938	93654	59894
77	37449	30362	06694	54690	04052	53115	62757	95348	78662	11163	81651	50245	34971	52924
78	46515	70331	85922	38329	57015	15765	97161	17869	45349	61796	66345	81073	49106	79860
79	30986	81223	42416	58353	21532	30502	32305	86482	05174	07901	54339	58861	74818	46942
80	63798	64995	46583	09785	44160	78128	83991	42865	92520	83531	80377	35909	81250	54238
81	82486	84846	99254	67632	43218	50076	21361	64816	51202	88124	41870	52689	51275	83556
82	21885	32906	92431	09060	64297	51674	64126	62570	26123	05155	59194	52799	28225	85762
83	60336	98782	07408	53458	13564	59089	26445	29789	85205	41001	12535	12133	14645	23541
84	43937	46891	24010	25560	86355	33941	25786	54990	71899	15475	95434	98227	21824	19535
85	97656	63175	89303	16275	07100	92063	21942	18611	47348	20203	18534	03862	78095	50136
86	03299	01221	05418	38982	55758	92237	26759	86367	21216	98442	08303	56613	91511	75928
87	79626	06486	03574	17668	07785	76020	79924	25651	83325	88428	85076	72811	22717	50585
88	85636	68335	47539	03129	65651	11977	02510	26113	99447	68645	34327	15152	55230	93448
89	18039	14367	61337	06177	12143	46609	32989	74014	64708	00533	35398	58408	13261	47908
90	08362	15656	60627	36478	65648	16764	53412	09013	07832	41574	17639	82163	60859	75567
91	79556	29068	04142	16268	15387	12856	66227	38358	22478	73373	88732	09443	82558	05250
92	92608	82674	27072	32534	17075	27698	98204	63863	11951	34648	88022	56148	34925	57031
93	23982	25835	40055	67006	12293	02753	14827	23235	35071	99704	37543	11601	35503	85171
94	09915	96306	05908	97901	28395	14186	00821	80703	70426	75647	76310	88717	37890	40129
95	59037	33300	26695	62247	69927	76123	50842	43834	86654	70959	79725	93872	28117	19233
96	42488	78077	69882	61657	34136	79180	97526	43092	04098	73571	80799	76536	71255	64239
97	46764	86273	63003	93017	31204	36692	40202	35275	57306	55543	53203	18098	47625	88684
98	03237	45430	55417	63282	90816	17349	88298	90183	36600	78406	06216	95787	42579	90730
99	86591	81482	52667	61582	14972	90053	89534	76036	49199	43716	97548	04379	46370	28672
100	38534	01715	94964	87288	65680	43772	39560	12918	80537	62738	19636	51132	25739	56947

Abridged from *Handbook of Tables for Probability and Statistics*, 2nd ed., edited by William H. Beyer (Cleveland: The Chemical Rubber Company 1968.) Reproduced by permission of the publishers, CRC Press, Boca Raton, Fla.

Table A.2   Selected Percentiles of Standard Normal Distribution

Percentile	z
0.5	−2.576
1.0	−2.327
2.5	−1.960
5.0	−1.645
10.0	−1.282
20.0	−0.842
25.0	−0.674
30.0	−0.524
40.0	−0.253
50.0	0.000
60.0	0.253
70.0	0.524
75.0	0.674
80.0	0.842
90.0	1.282
95.0	1.645
97.5	1.960
99.0	2.327
99.5	2.576

Answers to Selected Exercises

CHAPTER 1

1.1 A

1.2 D

1.3 B

1.4 B

1.5 C

1.6 A

CHAPTER 2

2.1a $\bar{X} = 370, \sigma_x = 277.2$

2.1b $\binom{5}{2} = 10$

2.1c

Sample	Sample Hospitals	$\bar{x}$	$(\bar{x} - E(\bar{x}))^2$
1	A, B	190	32,400
2	A, C	505	18,225
3	A, D	335	1,225
4	A, E	135	55,225
5	B, C	535	27,225
6	B, D	365	25
7	B, E	165	42,025
8	C, D	680	96,100
9	C, E	480	12,100
10	D, E	310	3,600

2.1d $E(\bar{x}) = \frac{1}{10}[190 + 505 + \cdots + 480 + 310] = 370 = \bar{X}$
$\text{Var}(\bar{x}) = 228{,}150/10 = 28{,}815$

2.1e $\text{SE}(\bar{x}) = \sqrt{28{,}815} = 169.75 < \sigma_x = 277.2$

2.1f $\binom{5}{4} = 5$

Sample	Sample Hospitals	$\bar{x}$	$(\bar{x} - E(\bar{x}))^2$
1	A, B, C, D	435.0	4,225.00
2	A, B, C, E	335.0	1,225.00
3	A, B, D, E	250.0	14,400.00
4	A, C, D, E	407.5	1,406.25
5	B, C, D, E	422.5	2,756.25

2.1g $E(\bar{x}) = \frac{1}{5}[435 + 355 + \cdots + 422.5] = 370 = \bar{X}$

2.1h $\text{Var}(\bar{x}) = 24{,}012.5/5 = 4802.5 < 28{,}815 = \text{Var}(\bar{x})$ for $n = 2$

2.3c

Sample	$\bar{x}$	Sample	$\bar{x}$
1, 2	0.80	3, 7	2.00
1, 3	2.00	3, 8	1.80
1, 4	1.286	3, 9	1.75
1, 5	1.00	4, 5	1.50
1, 6	0.33	4, 6	1.33
1, 7	0.50	4, 7	1.286
1, 8	0.60	4, 8	1.25
1, 9	0.25	4, 9	1.14
2, 3	2.00	5, 6	1.00
2, 4	1.375	5, 7	1.00
2, 5	1.167	5, 8	1.00
2, 6	0.75	5, 9	0.80
2, 7	0.80	6, 7	0.33
2, 8	0.833	6, 8	0.50
2, 9	0.60	6, 9	0.00
3, 4	2.14	7, 8	0.60
3, 5	2.20	7, 9	0.25
3, 6	2.33	8, 9	0.40

2.3d $E(\bar{x}) = \dfrac{\Sigma \bar{x}}{T} = \dfrac{38.897}{36} = 1.08$

$\bar{X} = \frac{26}{23} = 1.13$

2.3e $\text{Var}(\bar{x}) = \dfrac{13.82}{36} = .384, \ \text{SE}(\bar{x}) = \sqrt{.384} = .6198$

2.5

Sample	$\bar{x}$
1, 2	235.5
1, 3	418.5
1, 4	653.5
2, 3	309.0
2, 4	544.0

(Note: 3, 4 not possible)

2.5a $E(\bar{x}) = \dfrac{235.5 + \cdots + 544.0}{5} = 432.1$

$\bar{X} = 481.25$

$\text{Var}(\bar{x}) = \frac{1}{5}[(235.5 - 432.1)^2 + \cdots + (544 - 432.1)^2] = 23,105.9$

$\text{SE}(\bar{x}) = 152.01$

$$\text{MSE}(\bar{x}) = 23{,}105.9 + (482.25 - 432.1)^2 = 25{,}521.62$$

2.5b No, $E(\bar{x}) \neq \bar{X}$

2.5c No, 1 and 2 have 60% chance; 3 and 4 have 40% chance

2.7 $p = \dfrac{103 \times .1 + 123 \times 0 + \cdots + 180 \times .1}{1489} = .040$

2.9 1-C
2-F
3-E
4-B
5-A
6-D

CHAPTER 3

3.1

Random Numbers						$\bar{x}$	s_x
10	22	24	09	07	02	5.83	9.22
01	07	02	05	25	09	4.00	4.94
15	06	14	12	21	20	4.17	3.60
04	01	25	22	06	11	1.50	2.35
05	22	04	25	02	16	1.83	2.99
07	10	03	08	09	14	6.50	8.85
24	07	12	06	18	17	4.17	4.79
23	09	13	19	24	18	7.33	14.72
16	20	18	13	19	04	7.83	14.51
14	06	25	20	18	15	2.00	3.35

95% confidence intervals for $\bar{X}$: $\bar{x} \pm 1.96 \left(\dfrac{s_x}{\sqrt{n}}\right)\left(\dfrac{N-n}{N}\right)^{1/2}$

where $N = 25;\, n = 6$

(0, 12.26)
(0.55, 7.45)
(1.66, 6.68)

(0, 3.14)
(0, 3.92)
(0.33, 12.67)
(0.83, 7.51)
(0, 17.60)
(0, 17.96)
(0, 4.34)

Note, $\bar{X} = 5.08$, and 7 of the 10 confidence intervals shown above overlap $\bar{X}$

3.3 $p_y = 11/40 = 0.275$

95% confidence intervals for P_y: $p_y \pm \left(\frac{p_y(1-p_y)}{n-1}\right)^{1/2} \sqrt{\frac{N-n}{N}} =$
(.137, .413)

3.5 $p_y = 12/40 = .30$
95% confidence intervals for P_y: (.1586, .4414)

3.7

Household	No. of Persons	Visits Per Person	Total No. of Visits
1	3	4.0	12
2	6	4.5	27
3	2	8.0	16
4	5	3.4	17
5	2	0.5	1
6	3	7.0	21
7	4	8.5	34
8	2	6.0	12
9	6	4.0	24
10	4	7.5	30
Total			194

$\bar{x} = 194/10 = 19.4$, $N = 3000$, $n = 10$, $\varepsilon = .10$

$s_x = 9.845$, $\hat{\sigma}_x = s_x\sqrt{\frac{N-1}{N}} = 9.84$

$\hat{V}_x^2 = \frac{9.84^2}{19.4^2} = .2575$

$n \geq \frac{9(3000)(.2575)}{9(.2575) + (2999)(.10)^2} = 215.17$

Therefore, choose $n = 216$

3.9 $N = 50,000, \varepsilon = .15, z = 1.96$

a. $P_y = .10$ (low end)

$$n \geq \frac{(1.96)^2(50,000)(.1)(.9)}{(1.96)^2(.1)(.9) + (49,999)(.15)^2(.10)^2} = 1490.85$$

Therefore choose $n = 1491$

b. $P_y = .20$ (high end)

$$n \geq \frac{(1.96)^2(50,000)(.2)(.8)}{(1.96)^2(.2)(.8) + (49,999)(.15)^2(.20)^2} = 673.76$$

Therefore, choose $n = 674$

3.11 $E(x_i) = 1500(.05) = 75, \sigma_x = 300(.05) = 15, \hat{V}_x = 15/75 = .20$
$N = 20, n = 5$

$$n \geq \frac{(1.96)^2(20)(.20)^2}{(1.96)^2(.2)^2 + (19)(.2)^2} = 3.36 < 5$$

Thus, 5 is adequate

CHAPTER 4

4.1a $N/k = 120/3 = 40 = n$
Sample includes #26 and #29
$p_y = 2/40 = .05$

4.1b 95% confidence intervals for P_y: $(0, .106)$

4.1c (1) $p_y = 1/40 = .025$
(2) $p_y = 2/40 = .05$
(3) $p_y = 1/40 = .025$
$E(p_y) = (1/3) \times (.025 + .05 + .025) = .0333$
$\text{Var}(p_y) = [n/(n-1)]P_y(1 - P_y) = .000139$
$\widehat{\text{Var}}(p_y) = .000812 > \text{Var}(p_y) = .000139$

4.1d $p_y = 4/120 = 1/30 = .0333$

$$\text{Var}(p_y) = \frac{P_y(1 - P_y)}{n}\left(\frac{N - n}{N - 1}\right) = .00054 > .000139$$

4.3a $p_y = .04167$, $\widehat{\text{Var}}(p_y) = .001389$, $0 \le P_y \le .115$

4.3b $\widehat{\text{Var}}(p_y) = .001389$ (repeated systematic)
$\text{Var}(p_y) = .000278$ (systematic 1 in 5)

4.5a $\bar{x} = 2.33$, $s^2 = 4.0$, $1.383 \le \bar{X} \le 3.277$

4.7 No, there appears to be a periodicity every 7 visits

4.9 All are true except d

CHAPTER 5

5.1a $\widehat{\text{Var}}(\hat{p}) = [(10{,}000 - 1000)/10{,}000][0.35(1 - .035)/999] = .000030428$
$\widehat{\text{SE}}(\hat{p}) = .005516$

5.1b Stratification would likely be better because of large differences among strata with respect to the proportion testing positive.

5.3 $p_{y,\text{str}} = .0599 = 5.99\%$

5.5a

Elements	x'	Elements	x'
1, 2	108,000	2, 6	57,000
1, 3	96,600	3, 4	240,600
1, 4	276,000	3, 5	75,600
1, 5	111,000	3, 6	45,600
1, 6	81,000	4, 5	255,000
2, 3	72,600	4, 6	225,000
2, 4	252,000	5, 6	60,000
2, 5	87,000		

$$E(x') = 2{,}043{,}000/15 = 136{,}200$$

5.5b $\text{Var}(x') = \sum_{i=1}^{15}[x' - E(x')]^2/15 = 6{,}821{,}520{,}001$

$\text{SE}(x') = 82{,}592.49$

5.5c

Sample	$x_1' = 5\bar{x}_1$	$x_2' = \bar{x}_2$	$x_{str}' = x_1' + x_2'$
(1, 4)	110,000	70,000	180,000
(2, 4)	70,000	70,000	140,000
(3, 4)	51,000	70,000	121,000
(5, 4)	75,000	70,000	145,000
(6, 4)	25,000	70,000	95,000

$E(x_{str}') = 136,200$
$SE(x_{str}') = 28,067.06$

5.5d x_{str}' has lower variance than estimated total x' from simple random sampling

5.7a Number of samples $= \binom{12}{10} \times \binom{20}{10} \times \binom{24}{10} = 23,915,351,690,000$

5.7b $\bar{x} = (12x_1 + 20x_2 + 24x_3)/56$

5.7c $\binom{56}{30} = 6,646,448,384,000,000$

5.9 $p_{y,str} = [12 \times .5 + 20 \times .3 + 24 \times .1]/56 = 0.257$

$$SE(p_{y,str}) = \left\{ \frac{1}{N^2} \sum_{h=1}^{L} N_h^2 \left(\frac{P_{hy}(1 - P_{hy})}{n_h - 1} \right) \left(\frac{N_h - n_h}{N_h} \right) \right\}^{1/2} = .05265$$

CHAPTER 6

6.1a $x_{hi} = \begin{cases} 1 & \text{if sample person } i \text{ in stratum } h \text{ has 1 or more teeth missing} \\ 0 & \text{otherwise} \end{cases}$

$$x_{str}' = \sum_{h=1}^{L} (N_h/n_h) \sum_{i=1}^{n_h} x_{hi}$$

6.1b $n_1 = (300/1500) \times 100 = 20$
$n_2 = (500/1500) \times 100 = 33.33 \approx 33$
$n_3 = (100/1500) \times 100 = 6.67 \approx 7$
$n_4 = (600/1500) \times 100 = 40$

6.1c $n_1 = \dfrac{300 \times 5}{(300 \times 5) + (500 \times 3) + (100 \times 3) + (600 \times 2)} \times 100$

$= 33.33 \approx 33$

$n_2 = \dfrac{500 \times 3}{(300 \times 5) + (500 \times 3) + (100 \times 3) + (600 \times 2)} \times 100$

$= 33.33 \approx 33$

$n_3 = \dfrac{100 \times 3}{(300 \times 5) + (500 \times 3) + (100 \times 3) + (600 \times 2)} \times 100$

$= 6.67 \approx 7$

$n_4 = \dfrac{600 \times 2}{(300 \times 5) + (500 \times 3) + (100 \times 3) + (600 \times 2)} \times 100$

$= 26.67 \approx 27$

6.1d $n_1 = \dfrac{300 \times 15}{(300 \times 15) + (500 \times 15) + (100 \times 10) + (600 \times 10)} \times 100$

$= 23.68 \approx 24$

$n_2 = \dfrac{500 \times 15}{(300 \times 15) + (500 \times 15) + (100 \times 10) + (600 \times 10)} \times 100$

$= 39.47 \approx 39$

$n_3 = \dfrac{100 \times 10}{(300 \times 15) + (500 \times 15) + (100 \times 10) + (600 \times 10)} \times 100$

$= 5.26 \approx 5$

$n_4 = \dfrac{600 \times 10}{(300 \times 15) + (500 \times 15) + (100 \times 10) + (600 \times 10)} \times 100$

$= 31.57 \approx 32$

6.1e One strategy would be to take the mean of the two allocations, that is,

$n_1 = (33 + 24)/2 = 28.5 \approx 29$

$n_2 = (33 + 39)/2 = 36$

$n_3 = (7 + 5)/2 = 6$

$n_4 = (27 + 32)/2 = 29.5 \approx 29$

6.1f $\bar{x} = (300 \times 15 + 500 \times 7 + 100 \times 15 + 600 \times 8)/1500 = 9.53$

$$\sigma_{bx}^2 = [300(15 - 9.53)^2 + 500(7 - 9.53)^2 + 100(15 - 19.53)^2$$
$$+ 600(8 - 9.53)^2]/1500$$
$$= 11.049$$
$$\sigma_{wx}^2 = [300 \times 5^2 + 500 \times 3^2 + 100 \times 3^2 + 600 \times 2^2]/1500 = 10.2$$
$$\sigma_x^2 = \sigma_{bx}^2 + \sigma_{wx}^2 = 11.049 + 10.2 = 21.249$$

6.1g Yes, $\sigma_{wx}^2 < \sigma_x^2$

6.3 $C = \$10,000$
$C_1 = \$10 + .25 \times \$50 = \$22.50, N_1 = 10,000$
$C_2 = \$10 + .15 \times \$50 = \$17.50, N_2 = 20,000$
$C_3 = \$10 + .10 \times \$50 = \$15.00, N_3 = 5000$

$$n_1 = \frac{10,000/\sqrt{22.50}}{10,000 \times \sqrt{22.50} + 20,000 \times \sqrt{17.50} + 5000 \times \sqrt{15.00}} \times 10,000$$

$$= 140.11 \approx 140$$

$$n_2 = \frac{20,000/\sqrt{17.50}}{10,000 \times \sqrt{22.50} + 20,000 \times \sqrt{17.50} + 5000 \times \sqrt{15.00}} \times 10,000$$

$$= 317.74 \approx 318$$

$$n_3 = \frac{5,000/\sqrt{15.00}}{10,000 \times \sqrt{22.50} + 20,000 \times \sqrt{17.50} + 5000 \times \sqrt{15.00}} \times 10,000$$

$$= 85.8 \approx 86$$

6.5 $N = 150,000,000, z = 1.96, \varepsilon = .05, P = .15$
From relation (6.23),

$$n = \frac{Nz_{1-(\alpha/2)}^2(\sigma_{wx}^2/\bar{X}^2)}{z_{1-(\alpha/2)}^2(\sigma_{wx}^2/\bar{X}^2) + N\varepsilon^2}$$

$\sigma_{wx}^2 = .15 \times .85, \bar{X} - .15$, which yields $n = 8707.63$ or
$8707.63/65,000 = 0.13$ per ZIP code. Thus, 1 household per ZIP code
would more than meet specifications.

6.9 $N_1 = 8345, N_2 = 5286, N_3 = 6300$
$C_1 = C_2 = \$30, C_3 = \$40$
$\sigma_{1x}^2 = P_1(1 - P_1) \approx P_1$
$\sigma_{2x}^2 = (P_1/2)(1 - P_1/2) \approx P_1/2$
$\sigma_{3x}^2 = (P_1/3)(1 - P_1/3) \approx P_1/3$
(under the assumption that the proportion, P_1, is small)

From relation (6.19),

$$n_1 = \frac{8345\sqrt{P_1}/\sqrt{30}}{8345\sqrt{P_1}\sqrt{30} + 5286\sqrt{P_1/2}\sqrt{30} + 6300\sqrt{P_1/3}\sqrt{40}} \times \$25{,}000$$

$$= 427.08 \approx 427$$

$$n_2 = \frac{5286\sqrt{P_1/2}/\sqrt{30}}{8345\sqrt{P_1}\sqrt{30} + 5286\sqrt{P_1/2}\sqrt{30} + 6300\sqrt{P_1/3}\sqrt{40}} \times \$25{,}000$$

$$= 191.29 \approx 191$$

$$n_3 = \frac{6300\sqrt{P_1/3}/\sqrt{40}}{8345\sqrt{P_1}\sqrt{30} + 5286\sqrt{P_1/2}\sqrt{30} + 6300\sqrt{P_1/3}\sqrt{40}} \times \$25{,}000$$

$$= 161.29 \approx 161$$

6.9a $N_1 = 14{,}770$, $N_2 = 230$, $n_1 = 175$, $n_2 = 230$

$p_1 = 12/175$, $p_2 = 203/230$

$\hat{p} = [14{,}770(12/175) + 230(203/230)]/15{,}000 = .0811$

6.9b $\widehat{SE}(\hat{p}) = \dfrac{1}{15{,}000}\left(14{,}770^2 \dfrac{(12/175)(163/175)}{174} \dfrac{(14{,}770 - 175)}{14{,}770}\right.$

$$\left. + 230^2 \frac{(203/230)(27/230)}{229} \frac{(230 - 230)}{230}\right)^{1/2} = .0188$$

95% confidence intervals for P

$.0443 \le P \le .1179$

CHAPTER 7

7.1 $\bar{x} = 54.38$, $\bar{y} = 438.30$, $s_x = 20.97$, $s_y = 67.62$

$\rho_{xy} = .208$, $N = 234{,}785$, $\varepsilon = .05$, $z = 1.96$

Ignoring the fpc, we have

$$\hat{V}_x^2 = .149, \ \hat{V}_x = .386, \ \hat{V}_y^2 = .024, \ \hat{V}_y = .154$$

and from Equation (7.13), we have

$$n = 227.7 \approx 228$$

7.3 $n = 3^2 \times .149/(.1)^2 = 134$

7.5 From the pilot study:

$$n = 10, \bar{x} = 1.7, \bar{y} = 2.4, s_x = 2.06, s_y = 2.32$$

$\hat{V}_y = 0.9663, \hat{V}_x = 1.2103, \hat{\rho}_{xy} = 0.21$
$\hat{V}_y / \hat{V}_x = .798 > 0.42 = 2\hat{\rho}_{xy}$

Therefore, simple inflation estimate would be better.

7.7 From Equation (7.13), $n = 605.8 \approx 606$ for $\alpha = .05$ and $\varepsilon = .1$

CHAPTER 8

8.1b Cluster sampling

8.3 Chapters as PSUs, pages as secondary units, lines as listing units, words as elementary units

CHAPTER 9

9.1 $x'_{clu} = 280, \hat{\sigma}_{1x} = 3.16, \widehat{SE}(x'_{clu}) = 52.8$
$176.47 \leq X \leq 383.53$
$r_{clu} = .019, \hat{\sigma}_{1y} = 57.81, \widehat{SE}(\bar{x}_{clu}) = 1.76, \widehat{SE}(\bar{y}_{clu}) = 32.21$
$\widehat{SE}(r_{clu}) = .0023, .0144 \leq R \leq .0236$

9.3a Clusters are hospitals, listing units are patient medical records, elementary units are patients

9.3b $x'_{clu} = 7293, \bar{x}_{clu} = 221, \hat{\sigma}_{1x} = 143.94$
$\widehat{SE}(x'_{clu}) = 1273.46, 4797.02 \leq X \leq 9788.98$

9.3c $y'_{clu} = 99, \bar{y}_{clu} = 3, \hat{\sigma}_{1y} = 2.63$
$\widehat{SE}(y'_{clu}) = 23.27, 53.40 \leq Y \leq 144.61$

9.3d $r_{clu} = .0136, \widehat{SE}(\bar{y}_{clu}) = .7051$
$\widehat{SE}(\bar{x}_{clu}) = 38.59, \widehat{SE}(r_{clu}) = .0033$
$.0071 \leq R \leq .0201$

9.5 $x'_{clu} = \sum_{h=1}^{6} \frac{N_h}{n_h} x_h = (200/2)16 + (200/2)38 + (175/2)31 + (200/2)38$

$$+(150/2)24 + (200/2)4$$
$$= 14{,}112.5 \approx 14{,}113$$

Let σ^2_{1hx} = Variance among listing units in District h; $h = 1, \ldots, 6$

$\widehat{\text{Var}}(x'_{clu}) = \sum_{h=1}^{6} (M_h^2/m_h)\sigma^2_{1hx}\left(\frac{M_h - m_h}{M_h - 1}\right)$

$$= (200^2/2)(2)(198/199) + (200^2/2)(98)(198/199)$$
$$+(175^2/2)(24.5)(173/174) + (200^2/2)(162)(198/199)$$
$$+(150^2/2)(18)(148/149) + (200^2/2)(8)(198/199)$$
$$= 5{,}947{,}005.44$$

$\widehat{\text{SE}}(x'_{clu}) = 2438.6$

95% confidence interval for the number of edentulous; 9333 to 18892

Use combined ratio estimate [Equations (7.18) and (7.19)] to estimate and obtain 95% confidence intervals for the proportion of persons over 30 years of age who are edentulous.

$$y'_{clu} = \sum_{h=1}^{6} \frac{N_h}{n_h} y_h = (200/2)63 + (200/2)72 + (175/2)109$$

$$+ (200/2)54 + (150/2)67 + (200/2)37$$
$$= 37{,}162.5 \approx 37{,}163$$

$\widehat{\text{Var}}(y'_{clu}) = \sum_{h=1}^{6} (M_h^2/m_h)\sigma^2_{1hy}\left(\frac{M_h - m_h}{M_h - 1}\right)$

$$= (200^2/2)(24.5)(198/199) + (200^2/2)(98)(198/199)$$
$$+ (175^2/2)(84.5)(173/174) + (200^2/2)(288)(198/199)$$
$$+ (150^2/2)(312.5)(148/149) + (200^2/2)(84.5)(198/199)$$
$$= 14{,}628{,}751.5$$

$r_{clu} = x'_{clu}/y'_{clu} = 14{,}112.5/37{,}162.5 = 0.3798$

Since there are only 2 clusters sampled per stratum, the within stratum correlation between the number of persons over 30 years of age and the number edentulous cannot be estimated (it requires at least 3 clusters). We can, however, estimate this correlation over all strata (12 sample clusters) and assume that it applies for each stratum. This gives us

$$\hat{\rho}_{hxy} = .66 \quad (\text{for } h = 1, \ldots, 6).$$

Equation (7.19) can now be used to obtain the variance of r_{clu} and subsequent confidence intervals.

9.7   Let x_i = number of quadrants requiring surgery for the ith patient

$\hat{\sigma}_x^2 = (367/368)(1.496)^2 = 2.23$ from sample of 7 patients

$\bar{x}_{clu} = 1.714$

$$m = \frac{(1.96)^2 368(2.23/1.714^2)}{(1.96)^2(2.23/1.714^2) + 367(.15)^2} = 96.04 \approx 97 \text{ persons}$$

CHAPTER 10

10.1 $M = 75, m = 8, \bar{N} = 20, \bar{n} = 4$

10.1a   Let $C = C_1'm + C_2'm\bar{n}$. We let $C_1' = \$20 =$ cost associated with selection of each selected community area and $C_2' = \$30 =$ cost associated with selection of the individual pharmacy. Note: $C_1' =$ cost of compiling a list of all the community areas and the pharmacies in the m selected communities, and $C_2' =$ the cost associated with mailing questionnaires to the selected pharmacies (say \$10.00/pharmacy) plus coding and processing of the returned questionnaires (say \$20.00/pharmacy). Then $C = 20m + 30m\bar{n}$.

10.1b   With $m = 8$ and $\bar{n} = 4, C = 20 \times 8 + 30 \times 8 \times 4 = \$1120$

With $m = 16$ and $\bar{n} = 2, C = 20 \times 16 + 30 \times 16 \times 2 = \$1280$

10.1c $\bar{n} = \sqrt{\dfrac{20}{30} \dfrac{1 - .35}{.35}} = 1.11 \approx 1$

$\bar{n} = 1, m = 6, n = m\bar{n} = 6$

$SE(\bar{\bar{x}}_{clu}) = (1.50/\sqrt{6})[1 + .35(1 - 1)]^{1/2} = .612$

$V(\bar{\bar{x}}_{clu}) = .612/10.00 = .0612$

10.3 Let $n^* = 400$ and $\bar{\bar{x}}_{srs} =$ the mean under simple random sampling

$$SE(\bar{\bar{x}}_{srs}) = \sigma_x/\sqrt{400}$$

For cluster sampling, $\bar{n} = 4$ and $\delta_x = .6$

$SE(\bar{\bar{x}}_{clu}) = (\sigma_x/\sqrt{4m})[1 + .6 \times (4 - 1)]^{1/2} = \sigma_x/\sqrt{400} = SE(\bar{\bar{x}}_{srs})$

$\dfrac{2.8}{4m} = \dfrac{1}{400}$ or $m = 280$

10.5a $x'_{clu} = 14,685, \hat{\sigma}_{1y} = 1057.9, \widehat{SE}(x'_{clu}) = 7052.7$

$$861.9 \leq X \leq 25,508.2$$

10.5b $y'_{clu} = 100, \hat{\sigma}_{1y} = 6.708, \widehat{SE}(y'_{clu}) = 44.72$

$$12.35 \leq Y \leq 187.65$$

10.5c $\bar{x}_{clu} = 1468.5, \widehat{SE}(\bar{x}_{clu}) = 705.27$
$86.18 \leq \bar{X} \leq 2850.8, \bar{y}_{clu} = 10, \widehat{SE}(\bar{y}_{clu}) = 4.472$
$1.23 \leq \bar{Y} \leq 18.77$

10.5d $\bar{\bar{x}}_{clu} = 244.75, \widehat{SE}(\bar{\bar{x}}_{clu}) = 117.545$
$14.36 \leq \bar{\bar{X}} \leq 475.14, \bar{\bar{y}}_{clu} = 1.67, \widehat{SE}(\bar{\bar{y}}_{clu}) = .7453$
$.21 \leq \bar{\bar{Y}} \leq 3.13$

10.5e $r_{clu} = .0068, \widehat{SE}(r_{clu}) = .0002$
$.0064 \leq R \leq .0072$

10.7 $\bar{n} = .727 \approx 1.00$

10.9 From pilot study, $\bar{X} = .60, \sigma_{1x}^2 = 1.84, \bar{\bar{X}} = .06$

$$\sigma_{2x}^2 = \sum_{i=1}^{20} 10\bar{X}_i(1 - \bar{X}_i)/200 = .0076$$
$$\sigma_x^2 = (.06)(1 - .06) = .0564$$
$$\delta_x = [(1.84)/10) - .0564]/[9(.0564)] = .2514$$
$$C_1 = 1, C_2 = 15$$
$$\bar{n} = \left(\frac{1}{15} \times \frac{1 - .2514}{.2514}\right)^{1/2} = .446 \text{ so that optimal } \bar{n} = 1$$

10.11 $N = 39, Y = 7844, M = 20, m = 6$
(The trick is to weight the sample cluster totals by the number of non-trauma hospitals in the county.)

$$x'_{clu} = (20/6)[(2 \times 14) + (4 \times 10) + (3 \times 6) + (4 \times 0) + (1 \times 1)$$
$$+ (3 \times 24)]$$
$$= 530$$
$$y'_{clu} = (20/6)[(2 \times 310) + (4 \times 223) + (3 \times 350) + (4 \times 143)$$
$$+ (1 \times 64) + (3 \times 367)]$$
$$= 14{,}330$$
$$x''_{clu} = \frac{Y}{y'} x' = \frac{7844}{14{,}330} 530 = 290.11 \approx 290$$

10.13 Required $m = 25$

10.15

Optimum Cluster Sizes			
Variable	$N_i = 6$	$N_i = 9$	$N_i = 18$
Bed-days ($\mathfrak{X}$)	3.33	2.52	4.74
Hospital discharges ($\mathfrak{Y}$)	2.03	1.84	1.73
Mean	2.68	2.18	3.24

CHAPTER 11

11.1a Health Center 8 is sampled twice

11.1b $y'_{ppswr} = \dfrac{22{,}965}{40} (12 + 6) = 10{,}334.25$

11.3 Counties and Hospitals Sampled:

County 6-Hospital 1

County 19-Hospital 1

County 19-Hospital 1

County 28-Hospital 1

County 31-Hospital 3

CHAPTER 12

12.1 From linearization:

$$\text{Var}(\bar{z}) = (\bar{z}^2/n)[\hat{V}_x^2 + \hat{V}_y^2 + 2\hat{\rho}_{xy}\hat{V}_x\hat{V}_y]\left(\frac{N-n}{N-1}\right)$$

12.3 $n = 48, M = 6, \bar{n} = 8$

$$s_{bx}^2 = [8/(6-1)] \sum_{i=1}^{6} (p_i - \bar{p})^2 = 1.871$$

$$s_{wx}^2 = \sum_{i=1}^{6} 8p_i(1-p_i)/(6 \times (8-1)) = .0625$$

$$\frac{s_{bx}^2}{s_{wx}^2} = \frac{1.871}{.0625} = 29.94 \quad \text{(highly significant } F \text{ statistic with 5 and 42 df)}$$

$$\delta_x = (29.94 - 1)/(29.94 - 1 + 8) = .78$$

CHAPTER 13

13.1 $N = 200, \bar{x} = 2, s_x = 1.633, \bar{y} = 1.400, s_y = 1.350$
$\bar{z} = 1.300 \times 12 = 15.60, s_z = 12.54$
$\rho_{xy} = .958$
$\rho_{xz} = .514, \rho_{yz} = .606$

$$m_x = 85.7 \approx 86$$
$$m_{r1} = 8.4 \approx 9$$
$$m_{r2} = 63.18 \approx 64$$

CHAPTER 14

14.1 From Equation (14.9)

$$\hat{n} = (62 \times 40)/25 = 99.2$$
$$\hat{N} = (3575/525) \times 99.2 = 675.6 \approx 676$$

14.3
$$\hat{\pi} = \frac{\frac{21}{25} \times 63 + \frac{8}{50} \times 462}{525} = .2516$$

$$\text{Var}(\hat{\pi}) = \left(\frac{21}{25} - \frac{8}{50}\right)^2 \left(\frac{63}{525}\right)\left(1 - \frac{63}{525}\right) + \left(\frac{63}{525}\right)^2 \left(\frac{\frac{21}{25}(1 - \frac{21}{25})}{25}\right)$$

$$+ \left(1 - \frac{63}{525}\right)^2 \left(\frac{\frac{8}{50}(1 - \frac{8}{50})}{50}\right)$$

$$= .0510$$
$$\text{SE}(\hat{\pi}) = .2258$$

95% confidence interval for π: (0, .6032)

CHAPTER 15

15.1a   301 clusters and $(301/.35) = 860$ primary stage numbers

15.1b $(301 \times 8)/(.65) = 3705$ second stage numbers

15.1c   (i) If wrong connection called second time to verify, non-sample

       (ii) Sample

       (iii) Sample

       (iv) If number called more than some arbitrary minimum number of times (e.g., 7) at varying times of day and days of week, non-sample. Otherwise, sample.

15.3a   Stratum I: 349; Stratum II: 77; Stratum III: 294. Total cost $1250.15

15.3b   Stratum I: 633; Stratum II: 534. Total cost $1249.05.

Index

521

WILEY SERIES IN PROBABILITY AND STATISTICS
ESTABLISHED BY WALTER A. SHEWHART AND SAMUEL S. WILKS

Editors
Vic Barnett, Noel A. C. Cressie, Nicholas I. Fisher,
Iain M. Johnstone, J. B. Kadane, David G. Kendall, David W. Scott,
Bernard W. Silverman, Adrian F. M. Smith, Jozef L. Teugels;
Ralph A. Bradley, Emeritus, J. Stuart Hunter, Emeritus

Probability and Statistics Section

*Now available in a lower priced paperback edition in the Wiley Classics Library.

*Now available in a lower priced paperback edition in the Wiley Classics Library.

*Now available in a lower priced paperback edition in the Wiley Classics Library.

*Now available in a lower priced paperback edition in the Wiley Classics Library.

*Now available in a lower priced paperback edition in the Wiley Classics Library.

Texts and References Section

AGRESTI · An Introduction to Categorical Data Analysis

ANDERSON · An Introduction to Multivariate Statistical Analysis, *Second Edition*

ANDERSON and LOYNES · The Teaching of Practical Statistics

ARMITAGE and COLTON · Encyclopedia of Biostatistics: Volumes 1 to 6 with Index

BARTOSZYNSKI and NIEWIADOMSKA-BUGAJ · Probability and Statistical Inference

BERRY, CHALONER, and GEWEKE · Bayesian Analysis in Statistics and Econometrics: Essays in Honor of Arnold Zellner

BHATTACHARYA and JOHNSON · Statistical Concepts and Methods

BILLINGSLEY · Probability and Measure, *Second Edition*

BOX · R. A. Fisher, the Life of a Scientist

BOX, HUNTER, and HUNTER · Statistics for Experimenters: An Introduction to Design, Data Analysis, and Model Building

BOX and LUCEÑO · Statistical Control by Monitoring and Feedback Adjustment

BROWN and HOLLANDER · Statistics: A Biomedical Introduction

CHATTERJEE and PRICE · Regression Analysis by Example, *Second Edition*

COOK and WEISBERG · An Introduction to Regression Graphics

COX · A Handbook of Introductory Statistical Methods

DILLON and GOLDSTEIN · Multivariate Analysis: Methods and Applications

DODGE and ROMIG · Sampling Inspection Tables, *Second Edition*

DRAPER and SMITH · Applied Regression Analysis, *Third Edition*

DUDEWICZ and MISHRA · Modern Mathematical Statistics

DUNN · Basic Statistics: A Primer for the Biomedical Sciences, *Second Edition*

FISHER and VAN BELLE · Biostatistics: A Methodology for the Health Sciences

FREEMAN and SMITH · Aspects of Uncertainty: A Tribute to D. V. Lindley

GROSS and HARRIS · Fundamentals of Queueing Theory, *Third Edition*

HALD · A History of Probability and Statistics and their Applications Before 1750

HALD · A History of Mathematical Statistics from 1750 to 1930

HELLER · MACSYMA for Statisticians

HOEL · Introduction to Mathematical Statistics, *Fifth Edition*

HOLLANDER and WOLFE · Nonparametric Statistical Methods, *Second Edition*

JOHNSON and BALAKRISHNAN · Advances in the Theory and Practice of Statistics: A Volume in Honor of Samuel Kotz

JOHNSON and KOTZ (editors) · Leading Personalities in Statistical Sciences: From the Seventeenth Century to the Present

JUDGE, GRIFFITHS, HILL, LÜTKEPOHL, and LEE · The Theory and Practice of Econometrics, *Second Edition*

KHURI · Advanced Calculus with Applications in Statistics

KOTZ and JOHNSON (editors) · Encyclopedia of Statistical Sciences: Volumes 1 to 9 wtih Index

KOTZ and JOHNSON (editors) · Encyclopedia of Statistical Sciences: Supplement Volume

KOTZ, REED, and BANKS (editors) · Encyclopedia of Statistical Sciences: Update Volume 1

KOTZ, REED, and BANKS (editors) · Encyclopedia of Statistical Sciences: Update Volume 2

LAMPERTI · Probability: A Survey of the Mathematical Theory, *Second Edition*

LARSON · Introduction to Probability Theory and Statistical Inference, *Third Edition*

LE · Applied Categorical Data Analysis

LE · Applied Survival Analysis

MALLOWS · Design, Data, and Analysis by Some Friends of Cuthbert Daniel

MARDIA · The Art of Statistical Science: A Tribute to G. S. Watson

MASON, GUNST, and HESS · Statistical Design and Analysis of Experiments with Applications to Engineering and Science

*Now available in a lower priced paperback edition in the Wiley Classics Library.

Texts and References (Continued)

MURRAY · X-STAT 2.0 Statistical Experimentation, Design Data Analysis, and Nonlinear Optimization

PURI, VILAPLANA, and WERTZ · New Perspectives in Theoretical and Applied Statistics

RENCHER · Methods of Multivariate Analysis

RENCHER · Multivariate Statistical Inference with Applications

ROSS · Introduction to Probability and Statistics for Engineers and Scientists

ROHATGI · An Introduction to Probability Theory and Mathematical Statistics

RYAN · Modern Regression Methods

SCHOTT · Matrix Analysis for Statistics

SEARLE · Matrix Algebra Useful for Statistics

STYAN · The Collected Papers of T. W. Anderson: 1943–1985

TIERNEY · LISP-STAT: An Object-Oriented Environment for Statistical Computing and Dynamic Graphics

WONNACOTT and WONNACOTT · Econometrics, *Second Edition*

WILEY SERIES IN PROBABILITY AND STATISTICS

ESTABLISHED BY WALTER A. SHEWHART AND SAMUEL S. WILKS

Editors
Robert M. Groves, Graham Kalton, J. N. K. Rao, Norbert Schwarz, Christopher Skinner

Survey Methodology Section

BIEMER, GROVES, LYBERG, MATHIOWETZ, and SUDMAN · Measurement Errors in Surveys

COCHRAN · Sampling Techniques, *Third Edition*

COUPER, BAKER, BETHLEHEM, CLARK, MARTIN, NICHOLLS, and O'REILLY (editors) · Computer Assisted Survey Information Collection

COX, BINDER, CHINNAPPA, CHRISTIANSON, COLLEDGE, and KOTT (editors) · Business Survey Methods

*DEMING · Sample Design in Business Research

DILLMAN · Mail and Telephone Surveys: The Total Design Method

GROVES and COUPER · Nonresponse in Household Interview Surveys

GROVES · Survey Errors and Survey Costs

GROVES, BIEMER, LYBERG, MASSEY, NICHOLLS, and WAKSBERG · Telephone Survey Methodology

*HANSEN, HURWITZ, and MADOW · Sample Survey Methods and Theory, Volume 1: Methods and Applications

*HANSEN, HURWITZ, and MADOW · Sample Survey Methods and Theory, Volume II: Theory

KISH · Statistical Design for Research

*KISH · Survey Sampling

LESSLER and KALSBEEK · Nonsampling Error in Surveys

LEVY and LEMESHOW · Sampling of Populations: Methods and Applications, *Third Edition*

LYBERG, BIEMER, COLLINS, de LEEUW, DIPPO, SCHWARZ, TREWIN (editors) · Survey Measurement and Process Quality

SKINNER, HOLT, and SMITH · Analysis of Complex Surveys

*Now available in a lower priced paperback edition in the Wiley Classics Library.